中文翻译版

免疫治疗

Immunotherapy

原书第 2 版

主　编　Aung Naing　Joud Hajjar
主　译　苏春霞

科学出版社
北京

图字：01-2019-6725 号

内 容 简 介

本书主要介绍了免疫治疗在黑色素瘤、肺癌和急性髓系白血病和骨髓增生异常综合征中的临床进展，并重点关注了免疫检查点抑制剂治疗的不良事件，包括皮肤毒性、肺炎、结肠炎和肝炎。此外，由于免疫治疗药物与化疗药物在反应模式和毒性方面存在显著差异，在临床试验中评估其安全性和有效性仍然具有挑战性，因此，本书讨论了使用各种免疫治疗评估标准的临床意义和不足之处。本书是国外肿瘤免疫领域著作 Immunotherapy 第 2 版的首次中文翻译版，旨在为国内同行提供新的、有价值的知识参考。

本书适合于肿瘤及相关临床医学专业医生使用，也可作为国内高校临床医学专业学生的参考用书。

图书在版编目（CIP）数据

免疫治疗：原书第 2 版 /（美）昂奈（Aung Naing），（美）乔德·哈贾尔（Joud Hajjar）主编；苏春霞主译. —北京：科学出版社，2019.11

书名原文：Immunotherapy（Second Edition）

ISBN 978-7-03-063248-7

Ⅰ. ①免⋯　Ⅱ. ①昂⋯　②乔⋯　③苏⋯　Ⅲ. ①肿瘤免疫疗法–研究　Ⅳ. ①R730.51

中国版本图书馆 CIP 数据核字（2019）第 248765 号

责任编辑：陈若菲　戚东桂／责任校对：张小霞
责任印制：赵　博／封面设计：龙　岩

First published in English under the title
Immunotherapy（2nd Ed.）
edited by Aung Naing and Joud Hajjar
Copyright © SPRINGER NATURE Switzerland AG, 2018
This edition has been translated and published under licence from
Springer Nature Switzerland AG.

科学出版社 出版
北京东黄城根北街 16 号
邮政编码：100717
http://www.sciencep.com

北京画中画印刷有限公司 印刷
科学出版社发行　各地新华书店经销

*

2019 年 11 月第 一 版　开本：720×1000　1/16
2019 年 11 月第一次印刷　印张：10 3/4
字数：205 000
定价：108.00 元
（如有印装质量问题，我社负责调换）

《免疫治疗》（原书第2版）翻译人员

主　译　苏春霞

副主译　蔡修宇　李雪飞　赵　静

审　校　周彩存

译　者　（按姓氏汉语拼音排序）

蔡修宇	中山大学附属肿瘤医院
陈　健	上海市第一人民医院
程　超	海军军医大学附属长海医院
储香玲	同济大学附属上海市肺科医院
宫晓梅	同济大学附属上海市肺科医院
李雪飞	同济大学附属上海市肺科医院
乔　梦	同济大学附属上海市肺科医院
石　琴	福州肺科医院
苏春霞	同济大学附属上海市肺科医院
王　琪	同济大学附属上海市肺科医院
赵　超	同济大学附属上海市肺科医院
赵　静	同济大学附属上海市肺科医院
赵　沙	同济大学附属上海市肺科医院
周　娟	同济大学附属上海市肺科医院
周彩存	同济大学附属上海市肺科医院

Contributors

Hamzah Abu-Sbeih Department of Gastroenterology, Hepatology and Nutrition, Division of Internal Medicine, The University of Texas MD Anderson Cancer Center, Houston, TX, USA

Rana Alqusairi Baltimore, MD, USA

Christian Caglevic Medical Oncology Department, Clínica Alemana Santiago, Santiago, Chile

Luis Corrales Medical Oncology Department, CIMCA / Hospital San Juan de Dios-CCSS, San José, Costa Rica

Naval Daver Department of Leukemia, MD Anderson Cancer Center, Houston, TX, USA

Guillermo Garcia-Manero Department of Leukemia, MD Anderson Cancer Center, Houston, TX, USA

Isabella C. Glitza Oliva The University of Texas MD Anderson Cancer Center, Houston, TX, USA

Joud Hajjar Baylor College of Medicine and Texas Children's Hospital, Houston, TX, USA

Akash Jain Department of Pulmonary Medicine, The University of Texas MD Anderson Cancer Center, Houston, TX, USA

Hagop Kantarjian Department of Leukemia, MD Anderson Cancer Center, Houston, TX, USA

Lucia Masarova Department of Leukemia, MD Anderson Cancer Center, Houston, TX, USA

Tito R. Mendoza Department of Symptom Research, The University of Texas MD Anderson Cancer Center, Houston, TX, USA

Ken Miller Thoracic Oncology Program, University of Maryland Greenebaum Comprehensive Cancer Center, Baltimore, MD, USA

Julio Oliveira Medical Oncology Department, Portuguese Institute of Oncology of Porto, Porto, Portugal

Omar Pacha Department of Dermatology, The University of Texas MD Anderson Cancer Center, Houston, TX, USA

Anisha B. Patel Department of Dermatology, The University of Texas MD Anderson Cancer Center, Houston, TX, USA

Farhad Ravandi Department of Leukemia, MD Anderson Cancer Center, Houston, TX, USA

Christian Rolfo Thoracic Oncology Program, University of Maryland Greenebaum Comprehensive Cancer Center, Baltimore, MD, USA

Marlene and Stewart Greenebaum Comprehensive Cancer Center, University of Maryland School of Medicine, Baltimore, MD, USA

Katherine Scilla Thoracic Oncology Program, University of Maryland Greenebaum Comprehensive Cancer Center, Baltimore, MD, USA

Vickie R. Shannon Department of Pulmonary Medicine, The University of Texas MD Anderson Cancer Center, Houston, TX, USA

Padmanee Sharma Department of Immunotherapy Platform, MD Anderson Cancer Center, Houston, TX, USA

Ajay Sheshadri Department of Pulmonary Medicine, The University of Texas MD Anderson Cancer Center, Houston, TX, USA

Bettzy Stephen The University of Texas MD Anderson Cancer Center, Houston, TX, USA

Yun Tian Department of Oncology, Shanghai Dermatology Hospital, Tongji University, Shanghai, China

Tongji University Cancer Center, The Shanghai Tenth People's Hospital, Tongji University, Shanghai, China

Yinghong Wang Department of Gastroenterology, Hepatology and Nutrition, Division of Internal Medicine, The University of Texas MD Anderson Cancer Center, Houston, TX, USA

译者前言

目前，恶性肿瘤的治疗新增了靶向治疗和免疫治疗等新方法、让部分肿瘤患者有了治愈的可能性。但新的治疗方法和不同的联合治疗模式的复杂性，也给医生和患者带来了巨大的挑战，针对不同患者的疾病特征选择个体化的精准治疗模式是当前抗肿瘤诊疗中面临的新问题。因此，专业的抗恶性肿瘤相关治疗知识，尤其是免疫治疗的内容介绍非常有必要。这不仅可以帮助基层医生更深入地了解抗肿瘤治疗进展，使患者及家属能够及时、准确地接受专业的建议，也可以帮助恶性肿瘤患者及家属能更好地与医生沟通并做出正确的治疗选择，有效改善我国抗肿瘤治疗的现状。

本书邀请国内肿瘤诊疗领域多名青年专家共同翻译完成，旨在从专业的角度出发，带动基层医院医生肿瘤诊疗水平的提升，促进我国肿瘤诊疗规范化的普遍实施和治疗理念的实时更新，以使更多的患者真正受益于医疗水平的发展，提高我国恶性肿瘤患者的总体诊疗水平。

由于时间仓促，加之水平有限，翻译不妥之处敬请同道指正。

苏春霞
2019 年 11 月

目 录

第1章 基础免疫学概况及相关转化医学概念 ………………………………… 1

第2章 黑色素瘤的免疫治疗 ………………………………………………… 39

第3章 肺癌的免疫治疗：肿瘤治疗的新时代 ………………………………… 60

第4章 急性髓系白血病和骨髓增生异常综合征免疫治疗的更新：单克隆抗体和检查点抑制剂即将进入临床实践 ……………………………………… 88

第5章 免疫检查点抑制剂的皮肤不良事件 ………………………………… 106

第6章 免疫相关不良事件之肺炎 …………………………………………… 119

第7章 免疫检查点抑制剂诱发的结肠炎 …………………………………… 135

第8章 免疫检查点抑制剂诱发的肝炎 ……………………………………… 141

第9章 患者报告的症状结局 ………………………………………………… 147

第 1 章
基础免疫学概况及相关转化医学概念

Bettzy Stephen, Joud Hajjar

译者：赵 超 李雪飞

摘要 肿瘤存在于极其复杂的结构网络中，并在其发生和发展过程中不断进化而逃避宿主的免疫监视。肿瘤免疫微环境包含多种成分，如巨噬细胞、树突状细胞、自然杀伤细胞、中性粒细胞、肥大细胞等，这些成分可聚集在肿瘤组织中央、肿瘤边缘、相邻的基质、肿瘤淋巴管等多个部位。肿瘤组织中免疫细胞浸润的异质性广泛存在，同一例患者的不同肿瘤部位或者具有相同组织学类型肿瘤的不同患者之间，浸润都是不同的。肿瘤微环境中免疫细胞的浸润部位、密度、功能，以及和其他成分之间的相互作用都会影响患者的抗肿瘤免疫应答、预后和生存。因此，全面了解肿瘤微环境中免疫成分的特性及其在免疫监视中的作用，对正确选择免疫治疗靶点和制订抗肿瘤免疫治疗策略都是至关重要的。在本章，我们将对人体个性化的免疫系统，以及具有临床转化意义的预测生物标志物进行概述。

关键词 自适应 生物标志物 CTLA-4 免疫检查点 免疫 免疫治疗 自然免疫 PD-1 PD-L1 抵抗 反应 T淋巴细胞 转化

人体免疫系统是由不同细胞构成的复杂、动态的网络系统，在这些细胞共同作用下，该系统保护人体避免受到包括恶性细胞在内的外源性物质的攻击。人体内存在两种水平的免疫：固有免疫和适应性免疫。固有免疫是抵抗病原体的第一

B. Stephen
The University of Texas MD Anderson Cancer Center, Houston, TX, USA
e-mail: BAStephen@mdanderson.org

J. Hajjar (✉)
Baylor College of Medicine and Texas Children's Hospital, Houston, TX, USA
e-mail: joud.hajjar@bcm.edu

© Springer Nature Switzerland AG 2018
A. Naing, J. Hajjar (eds.), *Immunotherapy*, Advances in Experimental Medicine and Biology 995, https://doi.org/10.1007/978-3-030-02505-2_1

道防线，包括解剖学屏障和生理学屏障，具有吞噬功能的白细胞、树突状细胞（DC）、自然杀伤（NK）细胞，以及循环中的血浆蛋白[1]。其中，白细胞募集和吞噬微生物的概念首次被著名病理学家、自然免疫之父——Elie Metchnikoff 描述。适应性免疫系统以 B 淋巴细胞和 T 淋巴细胞为主，是功能更强大的免疫系统，这是基于另一位科学家 Paul Ehrlich 对抗体形成的侧链理论的阐述[3]。固有免疫和适应性免疫不同，但它们可以相互作用共同抵抗外源蛋白[4]。在本章，将会阐述免疫系统的基本成分及其发展，固有免疫和适应性免疫如何相互作用清除肿瘤细胞，以及抗肿瘤免疫治疗策略的发展。

固有免疫系统

长期以来人们对炎症和肿瘤形成之间的关系一直有所描述，但这种关系的确立是在 20 世纪初[5]。人体每天持续暴露在存有大量不同外源性病原体的环境中，这些病原体会迅速地被健康机体的固有免疫系统清除。反应快速是固有免疫的基本特性，然而，固有免疫是非特异性的，且持续时间短、缺乏免疫记忆[6]。传统上认为，固有免疫系统的细胞组分包括巨噬细胞、中性粒细胞、嗜酸性粒细胞、嗜碱性粒细胞、肥大细胞、NK 细胞、DC，它们与微生物菌剂的清除及固有免疫失败后更有效且具有抗原特异性的适应性免疫的激活相关[4,6]。固有免疫系统的体液成分包括补体蛋白和 C 反应蛋白，它们被认为是炎症过程中的调节因子[4]。越来越多的证据显示，固有免疫和适应性免疫可以被肿瘤抗原激发，并且在对恶性肿瘤细胞的识别和清除方面也发挥着重要的作用[7]。在此过程中，一些有害的化学物质、细胞因子和化学因子释放，将进一步损伤健康组织[8]。炎性的微环境同样也会诱发基因组的不稳定性和增加分子变异的概率[9]。慢性炎症导致的反复的细胞更新和增殖为细胞恶性转化提供了适宜的环境[10]。基于以上原因，肿瘤有时被描述为"无法痊愈的伤口"[11]。

固有免疫的细胞成分

免疫系统内的所有细胞都起源于骨髓中的多能造血干细胞（HSC）。HSC 可分化成共同淋巴祖细胞（CLP）和共同髓样祖细胞（CMP）。CLP 进一步分化为 T 淋巴细胞和 B 淋巴细胞，参与适应性免疫。而 CMP 进一步分化为各种白细胞（包括中性粒细胞、单核细胞、嗜酸性粒细胞和嗜碱性粒细胞）、肥大细胞、DC、红细胞和巨核细胞等。

白细胞

白细胞的首要功能是保护机体免受微生物病原体的侵袭。然而，炎症部位的微环境因素导致个体细胞表型和功能状态发生实质性变化，这将会有利于肿瘤的发生和发展[12,13]。

中性粒细胞

中性粒细胞在循环白细胞中占 50%~70%[14]，是构成抵御病原体侵袭第一道防线不可或缺的成分。中性粒细胞起源于骨髓中的 CMP，是在粒细胞集落刺激因子（G-CSF）、粒细胞巨噬细胞集落刺激因子（GM-CSF）等细胞因子刺激后分化而来的[14,15]。它们在血液循环中处于功能休眠状态，而在特异性的化学因子、细胞因子和细胞黏附分子刺激下可被募集到受感染的部位[16]。病菌随后会被吞噬，并且被高浓度的杀菌颗粒，或者被与包含病原体的液泡里高毒性活性氧产生相关的呼吸爆发而消灭[14]。此外，活化的中性粒细胞会上调对其他中性粒细胞、巨噬细胞、T 淋巴细胞的趋化和募集起关键作用的细胞因子[包括肿瘤坏死因子-α（TNF-α）、白细胞介素（IL）-1β、IL-1Rα、IL-12 和血管内皮生长因子]和化学因子（包括 IL-8）[17,18]。

除了其经典的吞噬作用，中性粒细胞在肿瘤生物学行为中也发挥着重要作用[1,19]。中性粒细胞可通过局部化学因子，如 IL-8、巨噬细胞炎症蛋白-1α（MIP-1α/CCL3）和人粒细胞趋化蛋白-2（huGCP-2/CXCL6）[20]募集到肿瘤微环境中（TME）。肿瘤相关中性粒细胞（TAN）和原始中性粒细胞显著不同，TAN 在不同分子水平显示出截然相反的作用[20]，可表现为抗肿瘤的 N1 型，以及促肿瘤发生的 N2 型[14,21]。在未经治疗的肿瘤中，肿瘤细胞中的转化生长因子-β（TGF-β）驱动 TAN 向 N2 型转化[13]。这些中性粒细胞在局部可以释放弹性蛋白酶（ELA2）[22]、抑瘤素 M[23]和 S100A8/9[24]，进一步促进肿瘤细胞的增殖、存活、转移和对化疗药物的耐药。另外，N2 型的 TAN 可以通过释放生长刺激信号、血管形成因子，以及基质降解酶而进一步引起抗肿瘤免疫抑制，促进肿瘤发展[13,20,25]。总之，中性粒细胞在肿瘤细胞的发生与发展过程中发挥了多重作用[26]。然而，在一些特殊条件下，如阻断 TGF-β，TAN 会分化为能表达更多促进免疫的细胞因子和化学因子、更少精氨酸酶的具有更强杀伤能力的 N1 型[13]。N1 型的 TAN 也可以和 DC 相互作用来激发适应性免疫应答[27]，另外，还能通过释放化学因子（如 CCL3、CXCL9 和 CXCL10）和促炎细胞因子（如 IL-12、TNF-α、GM-CSF 和 VEGF）[28]来促进肿瘤内 CD8$^+$T 淋巴细胞浸润。这种亚型的 TAN 具有抑制肿瘤发展的潜能，这提示其通过抑制 TGF-β 来刺激抗肿瘤免疫的可能[13]。

单核细胞和巨噬细胞

单核细胞从 CMP 分化而来。它们是一些体积大的单核细胞，占循环白细胞的 5%～7%。这些单核细胞迁移到不同组织，根据定植的组织类型进而迅速分化成熟为不同类型的巨噬细胞，如在表皮可分化为朗格汉斯细胞，在肝脏内可分化成库普弗细胞，在中枢神经系统可分化为小胶质细胞[29]。巨噬细胞可发挥多重功能，它们同时可以释放细胞因子和化学因子来募集免疫系统其他细胞至炎症部位。巨噬细胞也可以诱导抗原提呈细胞（APC）上共刺激分子的表达来启动适应性免疫，同时可以帮助处理被适应性免疫应答杀死的病原体[2]。

与 TAN 类似，单核细胞也会被肿瘤来源的化学因子（如 CCL2、CCL5、CCL7、CCL8）或细胞因子（如 VEGF、PDGF、TGF-β、GM-CSF、M-CSF）[30-33]募集到肿瘤微环境[34]，进而分化为具有组织特异性的巨噬细胞。肿瘤相关巨噬细胞（TAM）包括抗肿瘤的 M_1 型（经典活化型）和促肿瘤的 M_2 型（条件活化型），这反映了该类细胞的功能可塑性[35]。肿瘤微环境内的细胞因子谱对巨噬细胞向不同类型分化起了关键作用[36]。通常情况下，肿瘤微环境内主要的细胞因子，如 M-CSF、TGF-β、IL-10 等可以显著抑制 TAM 内 IL-12 的产生和 NF-κB 的活化[37]，这会导致单核细胞向 M_2 型的巨噬细胞分化，表现为 IL-12 高表达、IL-10 低表达的巨噬细胞[30,38]。这种类型巨噬细胞可以迁移至肿瘤组织内缺氧部位，通过分泌 VEGF、血管生成素、促血管因子、IL-1 等诱导血管形成，释放一系列基质金属蛋白酶，如 MMP1 和 MMP9，以重塑肿瘤基质，以及通过释放前列腺素、IL-4、IL-6、IL-10、TGF-β、IDO 和调节性 T 细胞 Treg 来抑制适应性免疫[33,38]，最终促进肿瘤的发展。这使得肿瘤细胞逃逸到外周基质，并且有利于转移到远处器官。然而，在特定条件下，会发生经典的巨噬细胞活化。例如，在 GM-CSF、微生物、脂多糖、IFN-γ 等存在的条件下，TAM 会具有更强的杀伤能力与抗原提呈功能，表现为 IL-12 高表达、IL-10 低表达的 M_1 型[33]。它们通过分泌丰富的促炎细胞因子，如 IL-12、IL-23、一氧化氮、活化氧介质和 TNF[30,33]来杀伤微生物和肿瘤细胞。这些细胞因子也可以启动 1 型辅助 T 淋巴细胞（Th1）适应性免疫。尽管巨噬细胞数目升高与乳腺癌[39,40]、膀胱癌[41]、子宫内膜癌[42]和宫颈癌[43]等患者更差的预后相关，但在前列腺癌[44]和结直肠癌[45]中，肿瘤组织内存在高 TAM 的患者更具有生存优势。通过药物作用，肿瘤组织内巨噬细胞由 M_2 型向 M_1 型分化，可能为癌症患者提供可获益的治疗手段。

嗜酸性粒细胞

嗜酸性粒细胞来源于 CMP，在循环白细胞中所占比例低于 5%[2,46]。通常，嗜酸性粒细胞与宿主抵御大的、多细胞的寄生虫或真菌的过敏反应相关[47]。嗜酸性粒细胞表面可表达多种受体，包括化学因子受体、细胞因子受体、免疫球蛋白受体、Toll 样识别受体和组胺受体[48]。这些受体的参与导致了高度细胞毒性蛋白质的释放，如主要的碱性蛋白质、嗜酸性细胞分泌的神经毒素或嗜酸性粒细胞过氧化物酶（EPO）、促炎细胞因子和生长因子（IL-2、IL-3、IL-4、IL-5、IL-6、IL-10、IL-12 和 IL-13、IFN-γ、TNF-α、GM-CSF、TGF-α/β）、趋化因子、[趋化因子配体 5（CCL5）、趋化因子-1（CCL11）、CXC 趋化因子配体 5（CXCL5）]，以及过敏反应部位的、大的、具有高度细胞毒性的胞质颗粒脂质分泌的介质（血小板活化因子和白三烯 C4）[48,49]。

另外，嗜酸性粒细胞可见于肿瘤浸润区[1]。肿瘤相关组织嗜酸性粒细胞增多与多种实体瘤 [包括结直肠癌[50]、口腔鳞状细胞癌（SCC）[51]、喉癌和膀胱癌[52]] 患者预后良好相关。尽管对嗜酸性粒细胞在癌症中发挥的功能仍然未能完全理解，但显而易见的是嗜酸性粒细胞表达主要组织相容性复合体（MHC）Ⅱ类和共刺激分子 [CD40、CD28/86、细胞毒性 T 淋巴细胞相关蛋白 4（CTLA-4）][53,54]，因此，它们可起到抗原提呈的作用，并进一步启动 T 淋巴细胞的抗原特异性免疫应答[55]。动力学方法研究表明，趋化因子如嗜酸细胞活化趋化因子（eotaxin）、损伤相关分子模式（DAMP）、坏死肿瘤细胞释放的高迁移率族蛋白 1（HMGB1），可优先诱导嗜酸性粒细胞早于 CD8$^+$T 淋巴细胞向肿瘤浸润[56-58]。活化的肿瘤相关的组织嗜酸性粒细胞可释放趋化因子，如 CCL5、CXCL9 和 CXCL10，募集 CD8$^+$T 淋巴细胞迁移到肿瘤组织[59]。在肿瘤特异性 CD8$^+$T 淋巴细胞存在的情况下，肿瘤相关组织嗜酸性粒细胞会引起肿瘤微环境（TME）内多种变化，如促使 TAM 向 M$_1$ 型极化和诱导肿瘤血管正常化，导致 T 淋巴细胞进一步增殖，增强抗肿瘤免疫反应，并最终改善患者的生存状况[58]。

嗜碱性粒细胞

嗜碱性粒细胞起源于骨髓中的 CMP，并作为成熟细胞释放到外周循环系统[2]。它们在循环白细胞中占比不到 1%，该类细胞一直被认为是肥大细胞的冗余，直到大约 15 年前这种认知才被改变[60]。嗜碱性粒细胞会响应过敏性和微生物侵袭的部位释放的细胞因子和趋化因子的趋化，从而进入到炎症部位[60]。IgE 介导的嗜碱性粒细胞活化可诱导多种炎性介质的增殖和释放，如组胺、白三烯 C4、前列腺素，以及大量 IL-4、IL-13[61]。在嗜酸性粒细胞活化后 1 小时内释放的 IL-4 和 IL-13，对其他免疫细胞可起到化学趋化作用，并诱导未成熟的 T 淋巴细胞向 Th2 型分化，通过 IgE 依赖性和 IgE 非依赖型模式诱导 Th2（过敏）型免疫应答[62,63]。此外，嗜碱性粒细胞表达的 CD40 配体可与 B 细胞上的 CD40 配体结合，诱导 B 细胞转化为浆细胞，并进一步促进 IgE 抗体的产生[63]。

尽管嗜碱性粒细胞在肿瘤发生中的作用尚未被完全诠释，但可以肯定的是，嗜碱性粒细胞可以促进肿瘤血管的生成[64]。嗜碱性粒细胞在细胞质空泡中可表达血管生成素-1和血管生成素-2的信使RNA（mRNA），并在细胞表面表达VEGFR-2和Tie-1受体。同时，被激活的嗜碱性粒细胞可通过嗜碱性粒细胞和肥大细胞之间的相互交流作用释放促血管生成因子VEGF-A和VEGF-B，以促进肿瘤血管形成。此外，胰腺导管腺癌患者的肿瘤引流淋巴结中的嗜碱性粒细胞与Th2细胞炎症反应具有相关性，以及嗜碱性粒细胞可作为术后不良生存预后的独立预测因子，这些均提示嗜碱性粒细胞在肿瘤发生、发展和复发中起重要作用[65]。

肥大细胞

肥大细胞是一类基于组织的造血起源的炎性细胞[66]。长期以来，肥大细胞的起源尚存争议。最近，Qi等确定了嗜碱性粒细胞前体和肥大细胞祖细胞（BMP前体）都属于粒细胞-巨噬细胞祖细胞群（GMP），分别具有分化为嗜碱性粒细胞和肥大细胞的能力，同时保留了部分分化成髓样细胞的能力[67]。BMP前体细胞（pre-BMP）在血液中循环并到达外周组织，在相互独立的转录因子CCAAT增强子结合蛋白α（C/EBPα）和小眼畸形相关转录因子（MITF）存在下，分别分化为嗜碱性粒细胞和肥大细胞[67]。嗜碱性粒细胞和肥大细胞具有许多共同特征，如IgE受体的表达、相同颗粒的存在及受刺激时产生相似的免疫应答介质和细胞因子等。这两类细胞都能产生保护性蛋白来抵御寄生虫的感染，并且都在Th2（过敏）型免疫应答中起到关键作用[68,69]。然而，根据肥大细胞表型和其所处细胞因子环境，不同肥大细胞在其组织化学、生物化学和功能特征等方面有着显著性差异，这种现象称为"肥大细胞异质性"[70]。肥大细胞表达多种表面受体，包括IgG受体和Toll样受体（TLR）[70]。肥大细胞的特征是在含有组胺和肝素的细胞质中存在致密异种颗粒，这些颗粒在与过敏原接触时会爆发性释放[71]。组织肥大细胞除在胃肠道和中枢神经系统中是最大的组胺库外，同时其内还储存了几种介质的前体，如肝素、5-羟色胺、类胰蛋白酶和糜蛋白酶，脂质介质，细胞因子如TNF-α/β、IFN-α/β、IL-1α/β、IL-5、IL-6、IL-13、IL-16和IL-18，趋化因子如IL-8（CXCL8）、I-309（CCL1）、MCP-1（CCL2）、MIP-1αS（CCL3）、MIP1β（CCL4）、MCP-3（CCL7）、RANTES（CCL5）、eotaxin（CCL11）和MCAF（MCP-1），生长因子如SCF、M-CSF、GM-CSF、bFGF、VEGF、NGF和PDGF[71]，它们在肥大细胞被IgE或IgG依赖性机制活化时，被迅速合成并释放。肥大细胞通常定植在黏膜和环境表面等关键位置（如靠近血管、神经、腺体和上皮表面下的界面）[68,70]，并且它们具有预先储存TNF-α的能力，使得它们成为构成抵御病原体的第一道防线[66]。不同来源的刺激会激活不同的免疫反应途径，导致肥大细胞释放不同的鸡尾酒式的反应分子，这会显著影响T淋巴细胞分化和随后的适应性免疫反应[66]。

肿瘤组织中肥大细胞数量的增加在肿瘤发展过程中可能起到双重作用。肿瘤内肥大细胞的浸润与某些癌症（如前列腺癌[72]、唇癌[73]和弥漫性大 B 细胞淋巴瘤[74]）的预后不良相关。这可能是因为肿瘤内肥大细胞（促血管生成因子和促肿瘤生长介质的丰富来源）可以刺激或调节肿瘤血管生成，同时，具有丰富类胰蛋白酶和糜蛋白酶来源的周围肥大细胞可以促进细胞外基质的降解和肿瘤细胞的侵入，这导致了肿瘤的进展[73,75,76]。相反，乳房中肥大细胞与乳腺癌[77]、卵巢癌[78]、肺癌[79]和结直肠癌[80]的预后良好相关。这是由于基质肥大细胞可释放一些抗肿瘤因子，包括细胞毒性内源性过氧化物酶，细胞因子如 IL-1、IL-4、IL-6 和 TNF-α，来诱导内皮细胞凋亡和抑制血管生成的胃促胰酶分泌，并分泌类胰蛋白酶导致肿瘤性纤维化[78,81,82]。由于肥大细胞参与免疫调节，因此，肿瘤样本中肥大细胞的密度和位置，以及肥大细胞和基质细胞之间的串扰能够更好地预测患者的生存期[1]。

树突状细胞

DC 是专职的抗原提呈细胞，它们存在于体内大部分组织中，并集中在次级淋巴组织[83]。在稳定状态下，它们起源于来自骨髓 CMP 的单核细胞和树突状细胞祖细胞（MDP）[84]。MDP 在骨髓中可以产生单核细胞和普通 DC 祖细胞（CDP）[85]。CDP 产生 DC 前体，前体细胞从骨髓通过血液循环迁移到淋巴组织和非淋巴组织，它们在组织中可分化产生常规 DC（cDC）。DC 前体缺乏成熟 DC 的形式和功能，但是在微生物或炎症刺激下可发展为成熟 DC[86]。浆细胞样 DC 是在血液、胸腺、骨髓和次级淋巴组织中发现的 DC 前体的一种，其暴露于病毒时可产生Ⅰ型 IFN-α。cDC 大致分为迁移性 DC 和淋巴组织驻留型 DC。迁移性 DC（朗格汉斯细胞和皮肤 DC）是外周组织中存在的未成熟 DC，对捕获抗原非常有效。该类细胞使用几种感受器对环境进行取样，包括 TLR 和 NOD 样受体（NLR）在内的多种受体。在遇到病原体时，细胞内吞作用会短暂增强，以促进外周组织中未成熟 DC 的吞噬细胞和巨噬细胞的大量积聚[3]。由于抗原肽的形成减少[3]，溶酶体中 MHCⅡ类分子的泛素化和共刺激配体（CD80、CD86）的不良表达，未成熟的 DC 在细胞表面呈递肽-MHC 复合物时相对不够有效[3,87]。但随后，功能成熟的 DC 很快会触发抗原提呈机制，这也是固有免疫和适应性免疫之间的关键联系[88]。MHCⅡ类分子泛素化的停止可能会导致 DC 内吞作用的降低，以及 MHCⅠ、MHCⅡ和共刺激分子表达的上调[87]。最终，成熟的 DC 会降解病原体，并将 MHCⅠ类或 MHCⅡ类分子上的抗原肽提呈给原始 T 淋巴细胞，同时表达共刺激配体（CD80、CD86），并迁移至淋巴组织的 T 淋巴细胞区域[3]。配体与 T 淋巴细胞上共刺激分子的结合会导致 T 淋巴细胞的活化[87]。根据接收到的病原体类型和其他成熟的信号，活化的 T 淋巴细胞会进一步增殖、分化为有效的效应细胞毒性 T 淋巴细胞或辅助性 T 淋巴细胞[3]。DC 也可以直接提呈完整抗原以激活具有抗原特异性的 B 淋巴细胞[3]。淋巴组织驻留的 DC（CD8$^+$和 CD8$^-$、脾脏 cDC 和胸腺 cDC）是未成熟的 DC，特异性地位于原始 T 淋巴细胞被激活的区域[87]。cDC 可将淋巴器官中的抗原提呈给 T 淋巴细胞[86]。它们可能参与维持稳定状态下的外周免疫耐受。而在炎症条件下，部分 DC 可能来自于 CLP 细胞和单核细胞[2]，并可产生肿瘤坏死因子和诱导型一氧化氮合酶 DC（TipDC），是炎症性 DC 的一个很好的例子[86]。

在正常情况下，DC 负责维持对宿主细胞的免疫耐受[3]。DC 在稳定状态下通常在表型和功能上并不成熟，其未成熟状态的特征是 MHC Ⅱ 类分子的泛素化和细胞内堆积低水平的共刺激分子[83]。在没有感染的情况下，虽然 DC 可以持续地将自身抗原和非致病性环境抗原提呈给 T 淋巴细胞，但是这仅诱导 Treg 的产生而不是效应 T 淋巴细胞的产生。在癌症的发展中，肿瘤细胞与机体正常细胞相似，因此，DC 会在这种缺乏炎症的情况下表现为诱导外周耐受。此外，其他免疫抑制机制如 PD-L1 和 PD-L2，TGF-β 和 IDO 的表达，也可以抑制 DC 和 T 淋巴细胞功能，促进肿瘤细胞逃避免疫系统识别。这也就可以解释为什么疫苗不能成功作为癌症患者的有效治疗方式[3]。由于 DC 能够监控微环境，发现环境中的病原体并指导免疫细胞在免疫耐受和免疫抵抗之间做出快速适当的反应[83]，因此 DC 通常被比喻为免疫系统的守门人。

自然杀伤细胞

NK 细胞是固有免疫系统中功能最强大的淋巴细胞，具有强大的细胞毒活性。它们起源于骨髓中的 CLP，占所有循环淋巴细胞的 15%[1]，此外，它们还存在于许多外周组织中。尽管 NK 细胞不表达如 B 淋巴细胞的典型膜结合 Ig 或 T 淋巴细胞的 T 淋巴细胞受体（TCR）的抗原特异性表面受体，它们可表达广泛的活化和抑制性细胞表面受体。由于 NK 细胞的主要功能是识别和消除不能产生自我 MHC Ⅰ 类分子的细胞，成熟的 NK 细胞会通过表达几种细胞表面抑制因子来识别"缺失的自我"受体，如杀伤细胞抑制性受体 L（KIR-L）可以特异性结合 MHC Ⅰ 类配体[89]。NK 通过 MHC Ⅰ 配体与正常细胞上同源的受体相整合，转导抑制性信号，确保了机体在稳态条件下的免疫耐受[90]。而在肿瘤细胞和被感染的细胞（如被病毒感染后被 NK 细胞识别破坏的细胞）上并不存在这些 MHC Ⅰ 类配体[89]。

细胞表面活化受体[包括有效的 NKG2D 受体、杀伤细胞 Ig 样受体（KIR-S）、TLR 和 NLR]可参与激发 NK 细胞的效应功能，这些细胞表面活化受体通过识别病原相关分子模式（PAMP）来决定受应激的细胞是非自我感染细胞还是自我感染细胞[91]。然而，NK 细胞的活化依赖于与辅助细胞，如 DC、中性粒细胞、巨噬细胞、肥大细胞和（或）包含 IL-2、IFN-α/β、IL-12、IL-15、IL-18 或 IL-21 等细胞因子的微环境中的细胞之间相互交流作用[92,93]。DC 位于 NK 细胞附近，是和 NK 细胞相互作用的关键细胞，可以通过直接接触或分泌细胞因子如 IFN-α、IL-2、

IL-12、IL-15 或 IL-18 等来启动 NK 细胞活化[94]。被激活的 NK 细胞诱导细胞毒性和（或）促进细胞因子的产生[94]。NK 细胞可通过释放穿孔素和颗粒酶等细胞质颗粒，或通过表达 Fas 配体（CD95）或 TNF-α 相关的凋亡诱导配体（TRAIL）来与肿瘤细胞表面死亡受体结合，诱导肿瘤细胞凋亡[95]。然而，肿瘤细胞会进化并逃避 NK 细胞的破坏[95]。肿瘤细胞常见的逃避 NK 细胞杀伤的机制是使细胞表面 NKG2D 配体水解并脱落[96]。此外，通过肿瘤相关的 TGF-β 和 NKG2D 配体（包括 MHC I 类同系物 MICA 和 MICB）对肿瘤细胞表面的 NKG2D 通路慢性刺激，可以诱导 NK 细胞上的 NKG2D 受体的内吞和破坏，最终导致 NKG2D 途径功能的损害[97,98]。这导致 NK 细胞上 NKG2D 表达水平的显著降低，并导致 T 淋巴细胞沉默，促进肿瘤细胞逃避免疫监视。然而，NK 细胞还可以通过其他机制来攻击肿瘤细胞，如抗体依赖性细胞毒性作用[99]。NK 细胞可表达其他激活受体，如 CD16、Fc-γ 受体Ⅲa（FCGR3A），来结合 Ig 的 Fc 区[100]。这使得 NK 细胞能够识别抗体包被的肿瘤细胞并通过释放穿孔素将其破坏。

基于 CD56 和 CD16 的表达，NK 细胞至少有两种功能已被详细阐述[101]。$CD56^{dim}CD16^{+}$ NK 细胞占循环 NK 细胞的 90%。这些细胞可被趋化因子募集到外周组织，它们可表达穿孔素、天然细胞毒性受体（NCR）和杀伤细胞抑制性受体（KIR）。在活化时，一方面，$CD56^{dim}CD16^{+}$ NK 细胞更具细胞毒性并分泌低水平的细胞因子。另一方面，$CD56^{bright}CD16^{-}$ NK 细胞主要位于次级淋巴组织中，在循环 NK 细胞中所占比例不到 10%，该类 NK 缺乏穿孔素、NCR 和 KIR 的表达。在被 IL-2 活化时，$CD56^{bright}CD16^{-}$ NK 细胞可产生细胞因子，主要包括 IFN-γ、GM-CSF 和 TNF-α。然而，在 IL-2 长时间刺激下，$CD56^{bright}CD16^{-}$ NK 细胞可表达穿孔素、NCR 和 KIR，并获得细胞毒性功能。

虽然 NK 细胞传统上被定性为固有免疫细胞，但其也表现出 T 淋巴细胞特征，并且能够在二次暴露时产生快速而强大的免疫反应[102]。NK 细胞的免疫记忆功能在初次暴露后可持续数月，并且是抗原特异性的，可转移到其他未接触过病原暴露的动物体内[102]。尽管 NK 细胞是具有记忆功能的强效免疫杀手，但由于它们对肿瘤细胞的杀伤能力有限，NK 细胞在临床上的治疗作用并未取得很大成功[103]。

适应性免疫系统

适应性免疫由 T 淋巴细胞和 B 淋巴细胞介导，其标志是特异性抗原刺激的免疫应答。适应性免疫的另一个独特特征是其具有持续免疫记忆的能力，从而在暴露于相同的抗原后可以做出更快速和更强的免疫应答[2]。与固有免疫反应（存在生殖细胞系编码的细胞表面受体，可立即发生）相反，适应性免疫反应是较慢的过程,因为活化的淋巴细胞产生免疫效应之前先克隆扩增至足够的数量[29]。适应性免疫应答包括两种类型:体液免疫和细胞免疫。体液免疫应答由 B 淋巴细胞介导,用以抵抗血液和组织内的细胞外抗原。细胞免疫应答由 T 淋巴细胞介导,主要用于抵抗可在 MHC 分子上呈现小抗原决定簇的细胞内病原体。

适应性免疫系统的细胞成分

T 淋巴细胞和 B 淋巴细胞起源于 CLP,这是一类来源于多能干细胞的特殊类型的干细胞[2]。

T 淋巴细胞

CLP 从骨髓迁移到胸腺,在胸腺内经历 4 个分化和增殖阶段,包括产生确保细胞不识别抗原-MHC 复合物或可区分不成熟的自身抗原的检查点分子[104]。CLP 在通过皮层的迁移过程中,会接受与胸腺上皮细胞(TEC)的不断相互作用而得到不断发育进化[105]。CLP 不表达 TCR 或 CD4 或 CD8 共同受体,因此称为 CD4/CD8 双重阴性(DN)淋巴细胞(DN1)[106]。当 CLP 从皮质髓质交界处通过皮层迁移到被膜时,它们会丧失形成 B 淋巴细胞或 NK 细胞的能力,并成为定向 T 淋巴细胞前体(DN2)[107]。在确认向 T 淋巴细胞系分化和重组激活基因 1(RAG1)的表达后,细胞内 TCRβ 链会被重排并与前 Tα 链配对,导致 TCR 前体(DN3)的表达[104]。随后,DN3 大量的增殖可导致多种胸腺细胞(DN4)的产生,通过相应的细胞因子刺激,DN4 首先表达 CD8 辅助受体,然后表达 CD4 辅助受体,最后变成双阳性(DP)胸腺细胞。这伴随着 TCRα 链重排,完整的 αβTCR 随之产生。然后,DP 胸腺细胞与 TEC 相互作用,同时基于它们与 MHC I 类或与自身肽相关的 MHC II 类分子结合能力的强弱来进一步发育成原始的 T 淋巴细胞[104,108]。大约 90% 的 DP 胸腺细胞会表达不能与 MHC 分子结合的 TCR,这将导致这类细胞的延迟凋亡(非选择的死亡)。基于 DP 胸腺细胞与 MHC 分子的相互作用,并可通过沉默共受体基因座的转录而进一步分化为单一阳性的 T 淋巴细胞[105,109]。

在髓质中,根据包括 T 淋巴细胞对胸腺髓质上皮细胞表达的自身肽在内的各种组织特异性蛋白质的反应性,T 淋巴细胞将进一步被筛选[29]。表达 TCR 的 T 淋巴细胞对自身肽具有高度亲和力,在髓质内会经历快速凋亡并且随后被胸腺巨噬细胞清除(阴性选择)。表达中等水平 TCR 信号的 T 淋巴细胞则通过正选择过程进入成熟阶段。表达与 MHC I 类分子结合的 TCR 的 T 淋巴细胞可分化成熟为单个 CD8[+] 成熟 T 淋巴细胞,而表达与 MHC II 类分子结合的 TCR 的 T 淋巴细胞分化成熟为单个 CD4[+] 成熟 T 淋巴细胞。原始的 T 淋巴细胞在髓质可识别被 DC 提呈的抗原。在暴露于由 APC 提呈的抗原决定簇时，T 淋巴细胞在 CD28 的共刺激下被 APC 上的 B7 分蛋白（CD80 和 CD86）激活以形成效应 T 淋巴细胞，效应 T 淋巴细胞可破坏病原体或募集其他免疫细胞。在髓质中不存在抗原刺激时，原始 T 淋巴细胞会经血液循环到达周围淋巴组织并进入淋巴结的副皮质区域。在肿瘤引流的淋巴结中，原始 T 淋巴细胞可被表达 MHC 分子的肿瘤抗原，以及通过 APC 上的 B7 蛋白（CD80 或 CD86）与 T 淋巴细胞表面上的共刺激分子 CD28 结合而激活[110]。这导致淋巴结中原始 T 淋巴细胞克隆扩增和分化成辅助性 T 淋巴细胞（CD4$^+$T 淋巴细胞）或细胞毒性效应 T 淋巴细胞（CD8$^+$T 淋巴细胞），然后它们迁移回肿瘤并杀伤肿瘤细胞。根据肿瘤微环境中的细胞因子类型和转录因子类型，CD4$^+$T 淋巴细胞可分化成多种亚型，包括辅助性 T 淋巴细胞 Th1[111]、Th2[112]、Th17[113]、诱导 Treg（iTreg）[114]、滤泡辅助性 T 细胞（Tfh）[115]和 Th9[116]。Th 细胞可分泌调节免疫应答的细胞因子和趋化因子。Th1 细胞通过激活 CD8$^+$T 淋巴细胞促进抗细胞内病原体的免疫应答而促进细胞免疫，而 Th2 细胞通过激活 B 淋巴细胞抗细胞外寄生虫来促进体液免疫。另外，通过 MHC I 类分子上的抗原提呈或通过 CD4 辅助 T 淋巴细胞活化的 CD8$^+$T 淋巴细胞直接具有细胞毒性。此外，一些活化的 T 淋巴细胞和 B 淋巴细胞分化成负责长效免疫记忆的记忆细胞[117]，当再次暴露于相同的抗原时可介导更快更强的免疫应答。

免疫检查点的共刺激信号和抑制信号之间的平衡调节 T 淋巴细胞的免疫应答。共刺激受体包括 CD28、诱导 T 淋巴细胞联合刺激器（ICOS）、4-1BB（CD-137）、OX40（CD-134）和糖皮质激素诱导蛋白（GITR），而 CTLA-4、程序细胞死亡 1（PD-1）、淋巴细胞活化因子 3（Lag-3）、T 淋巴细胞免疫球蛋白 3（Tim-3）、T 淋巴细胞免疫受体与 T 淋巴细胞免疫球蛋白 ITIM 结构域（TIGIT）具有共抑制作用[118]。CD28 是原始 T 淋巴细胞表面组成性表达的主要共刺激分子，在相应配体与 APC 上的 B7-1 和 B7-2 结合后，它们为 T 淋巴细胞的活化和下游信号传导提供了重要的共刺激信号[119]。除 CD28 外，还存在其他 TNF 受体超家族（4-1BB[120]、OX40[121]、GITR[122]）的共信号受体，与 TCR 信号协同促进细胞因子产生和 T 淋巴细胞存活。为了维持免疫平衡，T 淋巴细胞的刺激作用被抑制机制抵消。活化的 T 淋巴细胞在其表面上同时表达 CTLA-4 和 PD-1 作为免疫检查点[123-125]。CTLA-4 是具有较高亲和力的 CD28 同源物，可与 B7 分子结合。CTLA-4 是一种与 B7 分子具有较高亲和力的 CD28 同系物，是一种在启动阶段调节 T 淋巴细胞活性的早期共抑制信号。当与 B7 结合时，CTLA-4 阻断 CD28 共刺激，并抑制 T 淋巴细胞活性和细胞因子产生。另外，作为 CD28 家族成员的 PD-1 是一种晚期共抑制信号，在外周组织的效应阶段调节 T 淋巴细胞活性。PD-1 与两种配体 PD-L1 和 PD-L2 相互作用。PD-L1 在包括肿瘤细胞在内的许多细胞上表达，包括肿瘤细胞、受活化的 T 淋巴细胞分泌的 IFN-γ 激活的 B 淋巴细胞和 T 淋巴细胞；而 PD-L2 可表达于巨噬细胞和DC[126]。与CTLA-4不同，PD-1与其配体PD-L1的结合不干扰共刺激信号，但可以通过干扰TCR和BCR下游信号通路下调B淋巴细胞和T淋巴细胞的增殖和相应细胞因子的产生[127]。除CTLA-4和PD-1外，还有其他新一代共抑制受体，如Lag-3、Tim-3和TIGIT，在不同的淋巴细胞亚群上表达，这些亚群负责差异性抑制免疫反应[128]。例如，Tim-3途径可以调节肠道的免疫反应，而TIGIT则可以调节肺部和胰腺的Lag-3。同样地，TIGIT可以选择性地抑制Th1细胞和Th17细胞的促炎反应，同时促进Th2细胞的反应[129]。除了免疫检查点，对免疫抑制效应贡献最大的是调节性T淋巴细胞（Treg），Treg是抑制其他T淋巴细胞细胞毒性的特殊T淋巴细胞[130]。它们被分为胸腺分化的天然Treg（nTreg）和外周诱导的Treg（iTreg）。nTreg特征是细胞表面表达CD4抗原和CD25抗原，细胞核表达Foxp3，是高表达自身抗原MHCⅡ类分子的正选择胸腺细胞。相反，iTreg从表达TGF-β的幼稚$CD4^+T$淋巴细胞分化而来，它们通过表达免疫抑制细胞因子（如IL-10和TGF-β）发挥免疫抑制作用[114]。降低Treg活性可增强固有免疫反应和适应性免疫反应，可用于治疗癌症[131]。因此，在正常情况下，调节好免疫激活和免疫抑制通路在维持外周耐受和调节T淋巴细胞反应程度和持续时间中起着重要作用[132]。

B淋巴细胞

B淋巴细胞从胎儿时期肝脏中的造血干细胞发育而来，并在成年后继续存在于骨髓中[2]。前原B淋巴细胞、早期前B淋巴细胞、后期前B淋巴细胞和前B淋巴细胞是B淋巴细胞的四种前体细胞，由CLP发育而来，表面不表达Ig[133]。在RAG1和RAG2存在下，这些细胞不断与骨髓基质细胞相互作用，为B淋巴细胞发育提供关键的生长因子、趋化因子和细胞因子。B淋巴细胞前体经历了编码重链（H）的基因顺序重排[134]。早期DJ重排发生在早期前B淋巴细胞中，随后在晚期前B淋巴细胞中发生VDJ重排，导致在细胞质中形成一个完整Igμ重链的大型前B淋巴细胞[2]。μ重链与替代轻链（L）和两条不变辅助链Igα和Igβ结合以形成前B淋巴细胞受体（BCR），其在前B淋巴细胞表面上瞬时表达，促进细胞进一步发展。此过程同时启动了负反馈循环，通过该循环可关闭RAG表达，阻止前B淋巴细胞中的H基因重排，阻止第二H基因（等位基因排斥）的重排，并且发出信号介导前B淋巴细胞的增殖。RAG基因被重新表达，在正选择的前B细胞中可诱导编码L的基因重排，导致在细胞表面上形成完整的IgM BCR，进而形成不成熟的B淋巴细胞，这也触发了L基因重排的停止。由于能够识别包括自身抗原的大量多样的BCR表达，因此在离开骨髓之前，未成熟的B淋巴细胞会被测试对自身抗原的反应性。当未成熟的B淋巴细胞表达具有最佳下游信号传导的非自身反应性BCR时，则RAG表达下调，这使得该类细胞经过阳性选择，并作为过渡 B 淋巴细胞进入脾脏。然而，当未成熟 B 淋巴细胞表达具有低基础 BCR 信号传导的非自身反应 BCR 时，则不足以下调 RAG 表达和表现强烈的自反应能力，因而会被消极选择，最终通过细胞凋亡（克隆缺失）而被消除。而有时，这些细胞可能失活（无反应性）或可能进行受体编辑，经历 L 基因的二次重排，导致形成非自反应的新 BCR，这使得该类未成熟 B 淋巴细胞随后被正向选择而进一步发育[135]。

未成熟的 B 淋巴细胞作为移行细胞进入脾脏。由于外周组织表达的自身抗原具有强反应性，大部分 T1 淋巴细胞会经历克隆缺失或无反应性，因此极少数细胞从 T1 阶段向 T2 阶段发展[136]。而且，从 T1 淋巴细胞到 T2 淋巴细胞的转变依赖于基础的 BCR 信号，T2 淋巴细胞通过 B 淋巴细胞活化因子（BAFF）-R 接受促生存信号并分化为表达 IgM 和 IgG 表面受体的原始 B 细胞。根据 BCR 信号强弱程度，原始 B 淋巴细胞分化成表达中等程度 BCR 信号和酪氨酸激酶（BTK）的卵泡（FO）B 淋巴细胞，以及表达弱 BCR 信号和 NOTCH2 的边缘区（MZ）B 淋巴细胞[136,137]。位于脾白髓中的 MZ B 淋巴细胞是静止的、不参与循环的成熟 B 淋巴细胞。它们具有有限的抗原特异性，并且可被非蛋白抗原激活，如独立于 T 淋巴细胞的常见血源性病原体。在被激活时，它们迅速发展成可分泌低亲和力 IgM 抗体的短寿命浆细胞，且不具备记忆功能。在血液和脾脏之间循环的 FO B 淋巴细胞位于次级淋巴器官的 T 淋巴细胞富含区域附近，并且可被外源蛋白以 T 淋巴细胞依赖的方式激活[138]。与膜结合 Ig 结合的抗原被 FO B 淋巴细胞摄取，并提呈给表达 MHC Ⅱ 类分子的 CD4$^+$ T 淋巴细胞。活化的 T 淋巴细胞可表达共刺激分子 CD40L 和 B 淋巴细胞活化所需的其他细胞因子[2]。激活的 B 淋巴细胞进行克隆扩增以分化成可产生大量高亲和性分泌抗体的浆细胞。一些活化的 B 淋巴细胞迁移到淋巴滤泡形成生发中心，在那里经历广泛增殖、Ig 类转换和体细胞超突变，从而形成长寿命浆细胞或记忆 B 淋巴细胞。这些浆细胞离开生发中心并迁移至骨髓中，即使在消除抗原后仍可继续产生抗体。在二次感染时，这些循环抗体可提供即时保护并激活位于外周淋巴组织中的记忆细胞。

免疫球蛋白

免疫球蛋白是由两条相同的 L 链和两条相同的 H 链组成的 Y 形异二聚体[139]。两条 H 链通过多个二硫键相互连接，并且每条 L 链通过二硫键连接到 H 链。每个 L 链和 H 链分为一个可变区和恒定区域。每条 L 链和 H 链中的变异区有三个互补决定区（CDR）。一个 L 链中的三个 CDR 与 Y 的每个臂中 H 链中的三个 CDR 配对以形成抗原结合位点。每个互补位特异性针对抗原的表位决定了 Ig 的特异性。H 链的恒定区域对于同一类别的所有 Ig 是相同的，但类别不同。所以，一个类别中的所有 Ig 都有 λ 链或 κL 链。用木瓜蛋白酶进行蛋白水解消化，可将 Ig 分成三个功能单位，即两个抗原结合片段（Fab）和可结晶片段（Fc）。每个 Fab 片段含有完整的 L 链和 H 链的一个可变结构域与一个恒定结构域,其包含抗原结合位点。Fc 片段含有 H 链的两个恒定结构域,这是活化的 NK 细胞、经典补体途径和吞噬作用的 Ig 效应结构域[140]。

根据 H 链恒定区中的氨基酸序列,人类抗体被分为 IgM、IgD、IgG、IgE 和 IgA[139],因此它们具有不同的生物功能。IgM 是在 B 淋巴细胞发育过程中细胞表面表达的最早的抗体,并且它是在首次暴露于抗原时分泌的主要 Ig 类别。IgG 是血液中的主要抗体,在二次免疫反应期间大量产生,并负责清除经处理后的病原体,中和毒素和病毒。IgA 是人体分泌物中的主要抗体,约占初乳蛋白质含量的 50%,并可保护黏膜表面免受毒素、病毒和细菌的侵害。当未成熟的 B 淋巴细胞离开骨髓时,膜结合的 IgD 少量地表达,并且参与调节细胞的活化。在血液中 IgE 极少量地存在,但它在超敏反应或过敏反应和寄生虫感染过程中至关重要。

体内的每个 B 淋巴细胞只能产生一种抗体[140]。原始 B 淋巴细胞被激活时,可增殖并分化成浆细胞,分泌大量与 BCR 具有相同抗原结合位点的抗体,且每个抗体只针对一个抗原表位,因此这类抗体被称为单克隆抗体(mAb)。多克隆抗体是由与相同抗原上的不同表位结合的不同 B 淋巴细胞克隆增殖并分泌而来。

单克隆抗体已经彻底改变了 Ig 作为治疗药物的应用。但是,工程化的单克隆抗体还存在多种挑战。首个为人类设计并使用的 mAb 是鼠抗体[141]。它们具有高度免疫原性、有限的生物有效性且半衰期很短。通过基因工程改造,将鼠可变区与人恒定区融合,产生 70%的人类嵌合单克隆抗体,可以克服鼠抗体的局限性[142]。后来,开发出的人类 mAb 已达到 85%~90%的人源化,其中只有 CDR 是鼠源性[143]。目前,通过噬菌体重组技术产生的完全人类单克隆抗体也已被应用[144]。人源化的生产过程使得这类 mAb 的免疫原性远低于鼠单克隆抗体。因此,几种靶向生长因子受体[如表皮生长因子(西妥昔单抗),人表皮生长因子受体 2(曲妥珠单抗)]、TME 和肿瘤抗原的 mAb 已被批准用于治疗结直肠癌、乳腺癌和肺癌[145]。单克隆抗体命名可体现抗体的人源性与否。例如,-xi-表示嵌合 mAb(利妥昔单抗),"-zu-"表示人源化(贝伐珠单抗),"-u-"表示完全人类 mAb(易普利姆玛)。

免疫系统在行动!

抗肿瘤免疫应答的概述

在抗癌方面,更深入地了解肿瘤微环境(TME)内的免疫调节过程,对免疫治疗的发展至关重要。TME 是复杂的,存在于 TME 中的免疫细胞包括巨噬细胞、DC、NK 细胞、肥大细胞、初始淋巴细胞、B 淋巴细胞、细胞毒性 T 淋巴细胞、辅助性T淋巴细胞、记忆细胞、Treg、骨髓源性抑制细胞（MDSC）和基质细胞等[146]。尽管TME中的这些因素与肿瘤之间存在动态相互作用，但癌细胞仍会改变其细胞内的流程，抵抗免疫攻击并变得适应这种微环境。因此，全面了解肿瘤和TME中各种因素之间的相互作用，将有助于识别新的靶点并形成新的治疗策略。

人体免疫系统在癌症中通常表现出双重作用。尽管免疫系统的主要功能是抑制肿瘤的生长，但它也可以通过一种称为癌症免疫编辑的动态过程来重塑免疫原性并促进肿瘤发展[147]。此过程包括三个不同阶段：消除、平衡和逃避。在消除阶段（肿瘤免疫监视），免疫系统对自身正常细胞与恶性细胞的识别存在挑战[148]。肿瘤细胞表达多种危险信号，如NKG2D配体和表面钙网蛋白，并可降解周围组织，介导如IFN-γ、IFN-α/β、TNF和IL-12的炎症信号释放，招募NK细胞、DC和巨噬细胞至肿瘤部位，这些将导致肿瘤细胞凋亡和死亡。死亡后的肿瘤细胞可释放肿瘤抗原，通过APC上MHC分子提呈给T淋巴细胞。这会启动肿瘤特异性适应性免疫应答。细胞毒性T淋巴细胞可与肿瘤细胞上的Fas和TRAIL受体直接相互作用，或通过分泌颗粒酶和穿孔素以诱导肿瘤细胞凋亡。固有免疫细胞和适应性免疫细胞具有完全消除肿瘤细胞并阻断肿瘤细胞免疫编辑过程的能力。

而在平衡期间，免疫细胞和逃避了消除阶段的肿瘤细胞之间继续相互作用，这可防止肿瘤细胞的扩增。然而，这种持续的免疫压力会选择或促进肿瘤细胞新型变体的形成，导致肿瘤细胞免疫原性降低，从而使其逃避免疫系统的识别[148]。该阶段是免疫编辑过程中最长的阶段，在肿瘤细胞新变异体最终逃逸之前，以隐匿形式存在[149]。

在逃避阶段，肿瘤细胞可通过多种机制逃避免疫系统监视[150]。肿瘤细胞可下调肿瘤抗原或MHCⅠ类分子的表达，以减少肿瘤特异性T淋巴细胞的免疫识别和抗原提呈，并组织T淋巴细胞的活化。肿瘤细胞也可能上调促生长因子的表达，如上调EGFR和HER2表达。此外，肿瘤细胞通常还可以发展出一系列免疫抑制机制，通过免疫耐受过程逃避免疫监视[7]。例如，肿瘤细胞可以表达与活化T淋巴细胞上的PD-1受体结合导致T淋巴细胞耗竭的抑制性表面配体PD-L1或PD-L2，或释放免疫抑制分子IDO等[151]。在低氧条件下，TME还可以释放VEGF，通过VEGF抑制T淋巴细胞与肿瘤内内皮细胞的黏附，来阻止T淋巴细胞进入肿瘤组织。类似地，在TME中存在大量IL-4、IL-10和TGF-β的情况下，TAM极化呈现M2型并表达高水平的IL-10和低水平的IL-12。这类巨噬细胞可抑制T淋巴细胞活性，并促进血管生成和肿瘤生长[152]。此外，TME中未成熟的、来源于固有免疫细胞的骨髓来源抑制细胞（MDSC）还可通过各种机制促进肿瘤的发展，如高表达IL-10、TGF-β和促进Treg表达等[153,154]。总之，发生免疫逃逸的肿瘤细胞具有更强的抵抗免疫系统攻击的能力，可导致具有明显临床症状的恶性肿瘤的不可控生长。因此，克服肿瘤对免疫系统的逃逸，开发能产生显著临床疗效的治疗方案至关重要。

肿瘤免疫学

免疫治疗在晚期肿瘤患者中产生持续应答的能力彻底改变了肿瘤治疗。尽管很多免疫药物如 IL-2、IFN-α 和 Sipuleucel-T 疫苗处于研究中，但只观察到很小的疗效提高。很多单克隆抗体[155]通过抑制配体结合和下游信号通路（cetuximab）、靶向肿瘤微环境（bevacizumab）及靶向免疫抑制细胞因子（GC-1008 和抗 TGF-β 抗体）[156]的作用被用于肿瘤治疗。

然而，免疫检查点 CTLA-4 的发现和对免疫调节途径的深入理解使得癌症免疫治疗有了重大突破[157]。在发现活化的 T 淋巴细胞表达 CTLA-4（与 APC 上的 B7 分子相结合，阻断 T 淋巴细胞的共刺激，导致免疫抑制）之后，科学家们进行了一系列的试验，试图通过释放 T 淋巴细胞的免疫调控能力来抗击癌症。这一切的发展形成了"免疫检查点阻断"的概念并由此研发出了伊匹木单抗（一种 CTLA-4 抑制剂），伊匹木单抗在约 20% 的转移性黑色素瘤患者中产生持久应答并且可使得总生存期（OS）得到显著延长，因此在 2011 年获得美国食品药品监督管理局（FDA）批准上市[158]。伊匹木单抗引人注目的反应奠定了探索其他 T 淋巴细胞抑制通路的基础。PD-1 是另一个免疫检查点，它与 PD-L1/PD-L2 结合产生免疫抑制。在应对免疫攻击时，肿瘤细胞过表达 PD-L1 和 PD-L2 而导致免疫抑制，这有利于免疫逃避和肿瘤进展。基于切实的临床前证据，用单克隆抗体阻断 PD-1/PD-L1 通路在多个肿瘤类型中产生了持久反应[159-163]。鉴于几种肿瘤类型的持久反应和生存益处，FDA 加速批准了几种免疫检查点抑制剂 ICPi[164]。这提供了一个有意义的概念，即检查点抑制药物可以在一系列敏感肿瘤患者中提供持久和有意义的反应（表 1.1）。

除了 CTLA-4 和 PD-1/PD-L1 信号通路外，其他免疫调节通路也被作为潜在的治疗靶点。IDO 是肿瘤细胞用来逃避免疫监视的免疫抑制途径之一[165]。一些 IDO 抑制剂正在临床开发中，包括 INCB024360[166,167]、indoximod[168]、IDO 多肽疫苗[169]、BMS-986205[170]和 NLG919[171]。一个强大的治疗性免疫反应不仅释放 T 淋巴细胞上的"刹车"，而且踩下"油门"。T 淋巴细胞通过共刺激受体（如 OX40 或 4-1BB）提供一个有效的"走"信号，积极促进最佳的"杀手"CD8$^+$T 淋巴细胞反应[172]。一些在进行中的临床试验正在研究免疫检查点激动剂，单一药物或与其他免疫疗法、化学治疗、靶向治疗或放射治疗相结合。

尽管 ICPi（CTLA-4，PD-1/PD-L1 抑制剂）在多种肿瘤中取得了成功，但很多患者在开始反应后不久就产生原发耐药或继发耐药[173]。在临床中正在研究的克服 ICPi 原发耐药和继发耐药的几种机制中,越来越多的证据表明,联合治疗可能具有协同作用,并且比单药治疗克服耐药更有效,因为肿瘤使用多种途径逃避免疫清除[174]。此外,由于这些共抑制受体具有非冗余的信号通路,对这些机制上不同通路的联合阻断可能在恢复 T 淋巴细胞介导的免疫反应中起协同作用[128]。最近,FDA 批准纳武单抗联合伊匹木单抗用于治疗 BRAFV600 野生型不可切除或转移性黑色素瘤患者[164]。目前有大量的研究以确定最佳组合,提高反应率和持续时间。众所周知,靶向治疗能使肿瘤迅速消退[175]。然而,这种反应是短暂的。相反,免疫疗法产生更持久的反应,但是,启动肿瘤消退需要更长的时间。由于其相互补充,靶向治疗和免疫治疗的组合正在几个临床试验中进行研究,新的数据表明,这种组合可能具有协同作用[176]。同样,放疗诱导的免疫调节变化可以使局部得到控制和延长生存期,但不足以改变免疫抑制性的 TME 获得抗肿瘤的效果[177]。为了克服这一局限性,目前正在进行临床研究,评估放疗和 ICPi 的结合疗法[178,179]。

新的数据表明,固有免疫系统的激活可以破坏 TME 的免疫抑制状态,从而引起有效的抗肿瘤免疫反应。重要的是,这个过程通过增强 T 淋巴细胞活化过程来启动适应性免疫反应。TLR 是固有免疫中最重要的受体,在癌症中具有双重作用[180]。虽然一些肿瘤细胞的 TLR 有利于肿瘤的进展[181,182]和增强对化疗的抵抗,但大多数免疫细胞的 TLR 起着传感器的作用[180]。外来抗原激活这些 TLR,引发一系列促炎反应,最终引发适应性免疫反应。因此,TLR 已被确定为潜在的靶点,正在研究几种 TLR 激动剂(TLR3、TLR4、TLR5 和 TLR7 激动剂)以供临床应用[183,184]。同样,在 APC 中高度表达的内质网膜蛋白 STING(干扰素基因刺激因子)通过诱导固有免疫和启动适应性免疫来介导有效的抗肿瘤活性[184]。通常,自身 DNA 位于细胞核或线粒体中,而微生物/肿瘤衍生的 DNA 位于细胞质中。根据它们的位置和肿瘤衍生的 DNA 可以被多个细胞溶质 DNA 传感器识别,从而触发 APC 中 STING 信号的激活[185]。通过 STING 途径产生的下游信号导致干扰素调节因子 3(IRF3)和核因子-κB 磷酸化,随后诱导促炎分子、IFNβ 和细胞因子,如 TNF、IL-1β 和 IL-6。在此过程中,IFN 还促进 DC 对 T 淋巴细胞的交叉启动,从而引发适应性免疫反应[186]。由于 STING 通路的激活促进 T 淋巴细胞启动和适应性免疫机制的诱导,一些 STING 激动剂作为疫苗佐剂及与其他免疫调节剂的合用正在研究中[187-189]。因此,连接固有免疫和适应性免疫反应的策略可能具有治疗效果。

表 1.1　FDA 批准的 ICPi 和适应证 [a]

药物	免疫检查点	FDA 批准的肿瘤类型 [b]
伊匹木单抗(ipilimumab)	CTLA-4	不可切除或转移性黑色素瘤

续表

药物	免疫检查点	FDA 批准的肿瘤类型 [b]
纳武利尤单抗（nivolumab）	PD-1	不可切除或转移性黑色素瘤
		转移性非小细胞肺癌
		晚期肾细胞癌
		经典霍奇金淋巴瘤
		复发性或转移性头部和颈部鳞状细胞癌
		局部晚期或转移性尿路上皮癌
		失配修复缺陷和微卫星不稳定的转移性结直肠癌
		肝细胞癌
帕博利珠单抗（pembrolizumab）	PD-1	不可切除或转移性黑色素瘤
		PD-L1 阳性的非小细胞肺癌
		复发性或转移性头部和颈部鳞状细胞癌
		经典霍奇金淋巴瘤
		局部晚期或转移性尿路上皮癌
		不可切除或转移性的失配修复缺陷和微卫星不稳定实体瘤
		复发性局部晚期或转移性 PD-L1 阳性胃或胃食管交界处腺癌
阿特珠单抗（atezolizumab）	PD-L1	转移性尿路上皮癌
		转移性非小细胞肺癌
度伐鲁单抗（durvalumab）	PD-L1	局部晚期或转移性尿路上皮癌
		不可切除的Ⅲ期非小细胞肺癌
阿维鲁单抗（avelumab）	PD-L1	转移性默克尔细胞癌
		局部晚期或转移性尿路上皮癌
纳武利尤联合伊匹单抗	PD-1 和 CTLA-4	不可切除或转移性黑色素瘤
		晚期肾癌

a 截至 2018 年 5 月 15 日，FDA 批准的 ICPi 列表，信息来源于 https://www.fda.gov/Drugs/InformationOnDrugs/ApprovedDrugs/ucm279174.htm。

b 肿瘤类型必须符合上述网站列出的标准。

转化相关性

免疫治疗药物彻底改变了晚期肿瘤患者的治疗模式。然而仅在少部分患者中观察到显著的生存获益。因此，生物标志物驱动的药物开发至关重要，它可以帮助医生预先选择最有可能从中获益的患者，并使这些患者免于可避免的免疫相关的毒性和费用治疗[190]。这些生物标志物适用于多种对治疗有反应的肿瘤类型。其中一些重要的预测标志物包括下述几项。

PD-L1 表达

早期 I 期试验表明，治疗前组织样本肿瘤细胞表面的 PD-L1 表达可作为抗 PD-1/PD-L1 治疗反应的生物标志物。在抗 PD-1 抑制剂 MDX-1106 的 I 期研究中，39 例晚期肿瘤患者，其中 9 例患者的肿瘤活体组织检查（活检）标本用于免疫组化（IHC）分析 PD-L1 的表达[159]。在 4 例 PD-L1 阳性患者中有 3 例观察到客观缓解（75%），而 5 例 PD-L1 阴性的患者没有反应。在其他抗 PD-1 药物 BMS-936558（纳武单抗）的 I 期研究中观察到相似的结果，42 例晚期肿瘤患者的治疗前组织标本用 IHC 进行 PD-L1 表达分析[191]。25 例 PD-L1 阳性患者中有 9 例（36%）客观缓解，而 17 位 PD-L1 阴性患者没有反应，提示在治疗前组织标本中 PD-L1 的表达与客观缓解具有某种关系。最近，FDA 批准 IHC 使用 22C3 抗体检测 PD-L1 的表达用于选择使用帕博利珠单抗（pembrolizumab）的 NSCLC 患者[192]。然而，将治疗前肿瘤标本中的 PD-L1 的表达作为绝对的生物标志物预测 PD-1/PD-L1 通路抑制剂的疗效由于多种原因而受到质疑。在一项评估抗 PD-L1 抗体 MPDL3280A 的安全性和有效性的 I 期研究中，整体客观缓解率（ORR）在治疗前肿瘤组织 PD-L1 高表达的患者中为 46%，在 PD-L1 中等表达的患者中为 17%，在 PD-L1 最小表达的患者中为 21%，在 PD-L1 无表达的患者中为 13%[193]。令人吃惊的是在 PD-L1 无表达的患者中也有治疗反应。另外，PD-L1 表达与治疗反应在肿瘤细胞和肿瘤免疫细胞之间是不一致的。肿瘤浸润免疫细胞上的 PD-L1 表达与对 MPDL3280A 的反应呈显著性相关（$P=0.007$），而 PD-L1 在肿瘤细胞上的表达与对 MPDL3280A 的反应无相关性（$P=0.079$）。此外，在一项 III 期研究中，无论肿瘤或免疫细胞中 PD-L1 的表达如何，与多西紫杉醇相比，阿特珠单抗治疗的非小细胞肺癌患者的生存率有所提高[194]。在同一个体的原发灶和转移灶样本中，PD-L1 表达也存在明显的异质性[195]。此外，免疫检测使用不同的 PD-L1 抗体进行 IHC 染色，并采用不同的染色步骤和评分模式[196]。因此，缺乏经过定义的标准来确定 PD-L1 阳性肿瘤。上述发现表明，虽然肿瘤组织中的 PD-L1 表达表明对 PD-1/PD-L1 抑制剂有治疗反应的可能性增加，但它可能不将 PD-L1 阴性患者排除在治疗之外[193,197]。

肿瘤内 T 淋巴细胞浸润

有大量证据表明，T 淋巴细胞浸润肿瘤组织，特别是侵袭性肿瘤边缘的 $CD8^+$ T 淋巴细胞密度与黑色素瘤、乳腺癌、卵巢癌、肺癌、肾细胞癌、结直肠癌、膀胱癌及其他实体瘤患者的生存期提高有关[198-200]。与之相反，Treg 对肿瘤组织的浸润与卵巢癌、乳腺癌和肝细胞癌患者的生存率有关[201-203]。然而错配修复基因缺陷的结直肠癌患者中，$CD8^+$T 淋巴细胞和 Th1 淋巴细胞的强烈肿瘤内浸润不利于肿瘤免疫[204]。尽管在不利的 TME 中，肿瘤仍然能存活，是因为在侵袭边缘、间质及 TIL 中，几个免疫检查点如 PD-1、PD-L1、CTLA-4、Lag-3 和 IDO 有强烈共表达。一旦有这样的情况，表明肿瘤可能对检查点抑制剂有反应。因此，错配修复（MMR）状态可以预测 ICPi 的反应。

此外，肿瘤内免疫细胞的类型、密度和位置（统称为免疫结构）具有预后价值。用免疫组化对 415 例结直肠癌患者的肿瘤中心及侵袭边缘中的 T 淋巴细胞总数（CD3）、T 淋巴细胞效应物（CD8）、相关细胞毒性分子（GZMB）、记忆 T 淋巴细胞（CD45RO）、肿瘤中心（CT）和侵袭边缘（IM）等多个免疫标志物进行定量分析[205]。无复发患者的每个肿瘤区域的免疫细胞密度均高于复发患者，且可预测无病生存期（DFS）和 OS。这些结果与肿瘤分期无关，表明适应性免疫应答在预防肿瘤复发中的作用。另外 Th1 极化、细胞毒性和记忆细胞标志物的存在预示着低复发率。

TIL 的基线表达可能并不总是提示对 ICPi 有反应。TIL 可能并不总是能预测对 ICPi 的反应。例如，在转移性黑色素瘤患者中，IM 处的 $CD8^+$T 淋巴细胞与帕博利珠单抗的应答呈正相关[206]，但在用伊匹木单抗治疗的不能切除的Ⅲ/Ⅳ期黑色素瘤患者中，则与之无关[207]。然而，在一些研究中，治疗时 CT 处和 IM 处肿瘤浸润性 T 淋巴细胞水平的增加是对 ICPi 治疗有反应的有效预测因子[206-208]。抗肿瘤活性在很大程度上依赖于预先存在的适应性免疫机制，如样本基线时存在更多的 CD8、PD-1 和 PD-L1 表达细胞[206]。

免疫评分

免疫评分是对原位免疫浸润进行定量的方法。TNM 肿瘤分期被免疫评分所取代用于评估肿瘤的进展程度，制订明智的治疗决策[205]。采用 TNM 分类法观察到同一疾病阶段患者临床结果的显著性差异，部分原因是在肿瘤的 TNM 分类中，TME 中的免疫细胞没有包括在内。肿瘤细胞与免疫细胞之间的相互作用在肿瘤的免疫逃逸和进展中起着重要作用，因此，上述的免疫结构比 TNM 分类更能预测肿瘤的预后[209]。因此，从免疫系统中衍生出一种新的评分系统，被称为"免疫评分",即 CT 处和 IM 处两个淋巴细胞群 CD3/CD45RO、CD3/CD8 或 CD8/CD45RO 密度的比值。由于染色方法的困难,国际免疫评分共识已将 CT 和 IM 中的两个标志物（$CD3^+$ 和 $CD8^+$）组合用于开发和验证不同患者群体的免疫评分作为预后标志物。评分范围为免疫评分 0（I0,当两个区域的淋巴细胞密度均较低时）至免疫评分 4（I4,当两个区域的淋巴细胞密度均较高时）。该评分是局部性和转移性肿瘤患者的最有力的 DFS 和 OS 预后指标[210]。最近,这一免疫评分共识在一项由国际中心联盟的 13 个国家共同进行的临床研究中得到了证实[211]。在一项 2681 例结直肠癌患者的组织样本的研究中,免疫评分高的患者 5 年内复发风险最低,DFS 和 OS 延长,这一发现已在多个内部和外部验证中得到证实。这个评分系统将有助于根据复发风险对患者进行分层。目前必须推广免疫评分在肿瘤分型中的普遍应用。

T 淋巴细胞受体多样性

T 淋巴细胞在肿瘤细胞的识别和根除中起着重要作用。不同的 TCR 序列可以检测各种外来抗原。TCR 激活后,进行克隆扩增。因此,通过高通量测序（NGS）对 CDR3 序列中 TCR 基因测序,进行多样性的鉴定和评估,可以为深入了解 ICPi 的抗肿瘤活性提供依据。有一例伴脑转移的黑色素瘤患者使用伊匹木单抗后仍然进展,使用连续的全脑放疗和帕博利珠单抗获得持久的临床完全缓解（CR）[212]。对治疗前脑转移瘤内 T 淋巴细胞和治疗过程中的循环外周 T 淋巴细胞进行 CDR3 高通量测序。结果表明,在帕博利珠单抗治疗后,脑转移瘤（治疗前）中的主要 $CD8^+$T 淋巴细胞克隆性扩增,同时在外周血中也是最常见的克隆。这表明预先就有但不充分的适应性免疫反应通过使用帕博利珠单抗治疗得到了加强。同样,在治疗过程中,在治疗前转移部位存在的 $CD8^+$T 淋巴细胞的克隆扩增也见于一例非小细胞肺癌患者,该患者获得了纳武利尤单抗的病理上 CR[213]。在纳武利尤单抗治疗的 10 例转移性黑色素瘤患者中[214],有治疗效果的患者的治疗后,在肿瘤组织中观察到某些 TCR-β 寡克隆扩增。25 例接受帕博利珠单抗治疗的转移性黑色素瘤患者中也观察到类似的结果[206]。治疗前和治疗后样本的 TCR 序列分析显示,有效者体内扩增的克隆数是无反应者的 10 倍。此外,在给药前样本中,临床效果与更严格的 TCR-β 链序列相关。因此,在基线和治疗过程中肿瘤抗原特异性克隆扩增时,不同的 TCR 序列可预测 ICPi 治疗的反应。

突变负荷与分子改变

有高突变负荷的肿瘤如黑色素瘤、NSCLC 和头颈部鳞状细胞癌（HNSCC）

可能有体细胞基因突变带来的新抗原，更可能对检测点抑制剂产生反应，并引发快速的免疫反应[215]。在一些临床试验中，ICPi 治疗的高突变患者的临床受益率更高，无进展生存期（PFS）更长[215-217]。同样的原因是，在实体瘤患者，尤其是结直肠癌患者，MMR 机制缺陷的患者，ICPi 的治疗效果有所改善[218,219]。然而 Snyder 等却认为在黑色素瘤患者中，高突变负荷与阻断 CTLA-4 的持续应答相关，但并不是所有有高突变负荷肿瘤的患者都对这种治疗有反应[216]，不过这些患者的新抗原标签肽与 OS 强烈相关。相反，低突变负荷肿瘤，比如胰腺癌和前列腺癌等对检测点抑制治疗可能没有反应。而且 PI3K 通路中的分子改变可能通过 PD-L1 组成性的表达促进肿瘤的免疫逃逸[220]。在这些情况下，对 PD-L1 表达水平的评估能够预测对 PD-1/PD-L1 抑制剂治疗的反应。同样，VEGF 的表达水平可增加促进血管生成，并与预后不良有关[199]。

免疫基因信号

基因的差异表达可能有助于识别对 ICPi 治疗反应的表型。例如，在从接受抗 PD-1 药物治疗的患者取样的黑色素瘤的瘤组织中发现了具有特定突变特征的丧失功能的 *BRCA2* 基因突变[217]。同样，在接受帕博利珠单抗治疗的黑色素瘤患者中，治疗前组织中的 IFN-γ10 基因和过表达的免疫 28 基因特征与 ORR 和 PFS 呈显著性相关[221]。在进一步的评估中，我们发现更精细的免疫信号在 HNSCC 和胃癌患者中产生类似的结果[222]。治疗前高水平的 IFN-γmRNA 和 PD-L1 蛋白表达与度伐鲁单抗治疗的非小细胞肺癌患者 ORR 和 OS 增加相关[223]。阿特殊单抗治疗的非小细胞肺癌患者肿瘤组织中相关效应 T 淋巴细胞、IFN-γ 和 PD-L1 基因的高表达与 OS 改善之间也存在类似的关联[224]。T 淋巴细胞相关效应和 IFN-γ 相关基因的表达与免疫细胞而非肿瘤细胞的 PD-L1 表达相关，提示了本已经存在的适应性免疫反应的作用。相反，在抗 PD-1 治疗前的黑色素瘤中，发现了一组 26 个先天性抗 PD-1 抵抗（IPRE）信号，其特征是高表达的间质转换、血管生成、缺氧和伤口愈合基因[217]。在肺腺癌、结肠腺癌、胰腺癌和肾透明细胞癌等实体瘤患者的治疗前肿瘤样本中也发现了 IPRE 标记。因此，免疫相关基因表达特征可能与治疗结果相关。

肿瘤免疫雷达图

为了克服单个生物标志物不能真实反映免疫细胞与肿瘤的动态相互作用的局限性，建立了肿瘤免疫图模型。在假设 T 淋巴细胞是抗肿瘤活性的最终效应器的基础上，将 7 个参数纳入模型中，以了解肿瘤与患者 TME 中免疫细胞的相互作用[225]。7 个参数及其潜在的生物标志是：①肿瘤异物（突变负荷）；②一般免疫状态（淋巴细胞计数）；③免疫细胞浸润（肿瘤内 T 淋巴细胞）；④缺乏检查点（PD-L1）；⑤缺乏可溶性抑制剂[IL-6 和 C 反应蛋白（CRP）]；⑥缺乏抑制性肿瘤代谢[乳酸脱氢酶（LDH），葡萄糖利用]；⑦肿瘤对免疫效应物的敏感性（MHC 表达，IFN-γ 敏感性）。7 个参数中每个参数的数据点都绘制在雷达图中，连接各个数据点的线提供了反映 TME 中交互作用的个性化框架。雷达图中的空白表明了潜在的治疗策略，可能会在患者身上引起有效的免疫反应。

基于肿瘤免疫循环中的 7 个步骤，开发了一种用于非小细胞肺癌患者的改良免疫图[226]。免疫图评分（IGS）的 8 个轴是：IGS_1，肿瘤中存在 T 淋巴细胞免疫；IGS_2，肿瘤抗原性（存在新抗原和肿瘤种系抗原）；IGS_3，启动和激活（存在激活的树突状细胞）；IGS_4，运输和 T 淋巴细胞过滤；IGS_5，肿瘤抗原的识别；IGS_6，缺乏抑制性细胞（Treg 和 MDSC）；IGS_7，检查点表达缺失（PD-1、PD-L1 等）；IGS_8，抑制分子缺失（IDO1、精氨酸酶 1 等）。$IGS_{1\sim5}$ 得分高提示 T 淋巴细胞免疫有利环境。相反，$IGS_{6\sim8}$ 得分高提示 T 淋巴细胞免疫抑制环境。根据雷达图确定了三组患者：$IGS_{1\sim5}$ 高表达和 $IGS_{6\sim8}$ 低表达的 T 淋巴细胞表型患者其抗肿瘤活性受到免疫抑制性 TME 的抑制；IGS_1 和 $IGS_{3\sim5}$ 低表达的 T 淋巴细胞缺乏表型的患者在 T 淋巴细胞启动过程中存在缺陷；IGS_2，$IGS_{6\sim8}$ 的 T 淋巴细胞表型患者则处于中间。因此，免疫图有助于确定治疗的重点区域，以引发有效的抗肿瘤反应，癌症免疫图有望用于个性化免疫疗法。

血清生物标志物

一些常规可用的外周血参数被评估为 ICPi 治疗反应的生物标志物[208,227-234]。其中最常见的是绝对淋巴细胞计数（ALC）、绝对嗜酸性粒细胞计数（AEC）、LDH 和 CRP。在一项对伊匹木单抗治疗晚期难治性黑色素瘤患者的试验中，伊匹木单抗两次治疗后的 ALC≥1000/µl 与临床获益和 OS 呈显著性相关[230,231]。尽管基线时和一剂伊匹木单抗治疗后的 ALC 仅显示改善治疗结果的趋势，但它们可能有指导预后的意义，因为患者需要 ALC 的阈值达到每微升 1000 个细胞才能充分激活免疫系统，从而获得有意义的抗肿瘤效果。在用伊匹木单抗治疗的黑色素瘤患者的几个临床试验中也发现了类似的结果[230-234]，与稳定或降低水平的患者相比，从基线水平增加的 ALC 水平与改善的 OS 和疾病控制相关。同样，两个疗程的伊匹木单抗治疗后，AEC 水平的增加与 OS 相关[230]，而且是黑色素瘤患者反应的独立预测因子[235]。另外，基线时的 LDH 水平升高是生存率低的独立预测因子[230,236]。尽管这些外周血液参数与治疗结果之间存在关联，但没有有效的生物标志物可用于临床。

循环生物标志物

循环肿瘤细胞（CTC）和循环肿瘤 DNA（ctDNA）的连续评估是衡量肿瘤负荷的一个指标，可以预测检查点抑制剂治疗的反应。在三组接受 PD-1 抑制剂单药治疗或联合伊匹木单抗治疗的患者中，评估了 ctDNA 与治疗结果的相关性[237]。A 组为基线和治疗期间 ctDNA 检测不到的患者；B 组为基线时检测到 ctDNA，但在治疗期间早期检测不到的患者；C 组包括基线和治疗期间都能检测到 ctDNA 的患者。与基线 ctDNA 相比，持续治疗水平的 ctDNA 与 ORR 降低和生存率低相关。另一方面，接受 PD-1 抑制剂治疗的非小细胞肺癌患者的外周血循环中的免疫细胞、Ki-67$^+$T 淋巴细胞的增加与临床获益相关[238]。如果这些发现在大型前瞻性队列临床研究中得到验证，在肿瘤异质性的背景下，微创和容易获得的液体活检可能是一种更全面的生物标志物评估替代技术。

微生物组评估

新的数据表明，肠道微生物群可能与 PD-1 抑制剂治疗的反应有关。转移性黑色素瘤患者[完全缓解（CR）/部分缓解（PR）/稳定疾病（SD）≥6 个月]接受 PD-1 抑制剂治疗后，粪便样本中肠道微生物群的 α 多样性显著增高[239]。与低度或中度多样性患者相比，肠道微生物 α 多样性较高的患者的 PFS 更长。此外，肠道微生物群在有效患者中富集梭状芽孢杆菌，而在无应答患者中富集拟杆菌。与拟杆菌数量较多的患者相比，梭状芽孢杆菌中粪杆菌属数量较多的患者 PFS 明显较长。因此，良好的肠道微生物群可增强检查点抑制剂治疗患者的抗肿瘤反应。

由于免疫应答的动态特性，肿瘤免疫生物标志物的发展越来越具有挑战性。为此，免疫监测试验已发展到从基因组学、蛋白质组学及功能学等方面对免疫药物治疗前、后的肿瘤与血液配对样本进行研究[197]。预计这些生物标志物的变化与治疗效果之间的联系能使我们从信号通路的机制角度对免疫药物应答和耐药进行研究，引导对生物标志物驱动的协同的基于免疫治疗的联合治疗的发展。此外，需要根据免疫治疗药物的作用机制来选择生物标志物[159,191]。因此，单个免疫生物标志物的鉴别不足以预测免疫应答的状况[197]。这就需要我们制订一个多因素生物标志物模块，以确定肿瘤的免疫原性并预测肿瘤的免疫反应和耐药性，如当肿瘤内 CD8$^+$T 淋巴细胞存在，肿瘤细胞表达 PD-L1 及突变负荷增加时，通常会有更大的可能对 PD-1/PD-L1 检验点抑制剂起反应[240]。

结论

一些开创性的研究已经阐明了固有免疫系统与适应性免疫系统的不同组分。尽管它们是人体免疫系统中两个独立分支，却在时间和空间上相互交织并相互依赖。虽然通过单克隆抗体阻断免疫检查点释放 T 淋巴细胞抗肿瘤免疫应答的潜能已成为在晚期肿瘤治疗中强有力的新工具，但固有免疫系统的组分对适应性免疫的激活和发育也有所贡献。所以通过严格的分子图谱进一步理解 TME 中肿瘤细胞与免疫细胞的相互作用，对发展新的免疫治疗策略及找出有临床反应的潜在生物标志物具有指导意义。

参考文献

1. Benito-Martin A, Di Giannatale A, Ceder S, Peinado H. The new deal: a potential role for secreted vesicles in innate immunity and tumor progression. Front Immunol. 2015;6:66.
2. Murphy K, Weaver C. Janeway's immunobiology. 9th ed. New York: Garland Science, Taylor & Francis; 2016.
3. Mellman I. Dendritic cells: master regulators of the immune response. Cancer Immunol Res. 2013;1:145–9.
4. Turvey SE, Broide DH. Innate immunity. J Allergy Clin Immunol. 2010;125:S24–32.
5. Balkwill F, Mantovani A. Inflammation and cancer: back to Virchow? Lancet. 2001;357:539–45.
6. Janeway CA Jr, Medzhitov R. Innate immune recognition. Annu Rev Immunol. 2002;20:197–216.
7. Finn OJ. Immuno-oncology: understanding the function and dysfunction of the immune system in cancer. Ann Oncol. 2012;23(Suppl 8):viii6–9.
8. Lin WW, Karin M. A cytokine-mediated link between innate immunity, inflammation, and cancer. J Clin Invest. 2007;117:1175–83.
9. Grivennikov SI, Greten FR, Karin M. Immunity, inflammation, and cancer. Cell. 2010;140:883–99.
10. Fedeles BI, Freudenthal BD, Yau E, Singh V, Chang SC, Li DY, Delaney JC, Wilson SH, Essigmann JM. Intrinsic mutagenic properties of 5-chlorocytosine: a mechanistic connection between chronic inflammation and cancer. Proc Natl Acad Sci U S A. 2015;112:E4571–E80.
11. Dvorak HF, Flier J, Frank H. Tumors - wounds that do not heal - similarities between tumor stroma generation and wound-healing. N Engl J Med. 1986;315:1650–9.
12. Galli SJ, Borregaard N, Wynn TA. Phenotypic and functional plasticity of cells of innate immunity: macrophages, mast cells and neutrophils. Nat Immunol. 2011;12:1035–44.
13. Fridlender ZG, Sun J, Kim S, Kapoor V, Cheng G, Ling L, Worthen GS, Albelda SM. Polarization of tumor-associated neutrophil phenotype by TGF-beta: "N1" versus "N2" TAN. Cancer Cell. 2009;16:183–94.
14. Mayadas TN, Cullere X, Lowell CA. The multifaceted functions of neutrophils. Annu Rev Pathol. 2014;9:181–218.
15. Borregaard N. Neutrophils, from marrow to microbes. Immunity. 2010;33:657–70.

16. Kobayashi Y. Neutrophil infiltration and chemokines. Crit Rev Immunol. 2006;26:307–15.
17. Scapini P, Carletto A, Nardelli B, Calzetti F, Roschke V, Merigo F, Tamassia N, Pieropan S, Biasi D, Sbarbati A, Sozzani S, Bambara L, Cassatella MA. Proinflammatory mediators elicit secretion of the intracellular B-lymphocyte stimulator pool (BLyS) that is stored in activated neutrophils: implications for inflammatory diseases. Blood. 2005;105:830–7.
18. Theilgaard-Monch K, Knudsen S, Follin P, Borregaard N. The transcriptional activation program of human neutrophils in skin lesions supports their important role in wound healing. J Immunol. 2004;172:7684–93.
19. Fridlender ZG, Albelda SM. Tumor-associated neutrophils: friend or foe? Carcinogenesis. 2012;33:949–55.
20. Piccard H, Muschel RJ, Opdenakker G. On the dual roles and polarized phenotypes of neutrophils in tumor development and progression. Crit Rev Oncol Hematol. 2012;82:296–309.
21. Gregory AD, Houghton AM. Tumor-associated neutrophils: new targets for cancer therapy. Cancer Res. 2011;71:2411–6.
22. Houghton AM, Rzymkiewicz DM, Ji H, Gregory AD, Egea EE, Metz HE, Stolz DB, Land SR, Marconcini LA, Kliment CR, Jenkins KM, Beaulieu KA, Mouded M, Frank SJ, Wong KK, Shapiro SD. Neutrophil elastase-mediated degradation of IRS-1 accelerates lung tumor growth. Nat Med. 2010;16:219–23.
23. Queen MM, Ryan RE, Holzer RG, Keller-Peck CR, Jorcyk CL. Breast cancer cells stimulate neutrophils to produce oncostatin M: potential implications for tumor progression. Cancer Res. 2005;65:8896–904.
24. Acharyya S, Oskarsson T, Vanharanta S, Malladi S, Kim J, Morris PG, Manova-Todorova K, Leversha M, Hogg N, Seshan VE, Norton L, Brogi E, Massague J. A CXCL1 paracrine network links cancer chemoresistance and metastasis. Cell. 2012;150:165–78.
25. Shojaei F, Singh M, Thompson JD, Ferrara N. Role of Bv8 in neutrophil-dependent angiogenesis in a transgenic model of cancer progression. Proc Natl Acad Sci U S A. 2008;105:2640–5.
26. Liang W, Ferrara N. The complex role of neutrophils in tumor angiogenesis and metastasis. Cancer Immunol Res. 2016;4:83–91.
27. van Gisbergen KPJM, Geijtenbeek TBH, van Kooyk Y. Close encounters of neutrophils and DCs. Trends Immunol. 2005;26:626–31.
28. Scapini P, Lapinet-Vera JA, Gasperini S, Calzetti F, Bazzoni F, Cassatella MA. The neutrophil as a cellular source of chemokines. Immunol Rev. 2000;177:195–203.
29. Chaplin DD. Overview of the immune response. J Allergy Clin Immunol. 2010;125:S3–23.
30. Mantovani A, Schioppa T, Porta C, Allavena P, Sica A. Role of tumor-associated macrophages in tumor progression and invasion. Cancer Metastasis Rev. 2006;25:315–22.
31. Lin EY, Nguyen AV, Russell RG, Pollard JW. Colony-stimulating factor 1 promotes progression of mammary tumors to malignancy. J Exp Med. 2001;193:727–40.
32. Duyndam MC, Hilhorst MC, Schluper HM, Verheul HM, van Diest PJ, Kraal G, Pinedo HM, Boven E. Vascular endothelial growth factor-165 overexpression stimulates angiogenesis and induces cyst formation and macrophage infiltration in human ovarian cancer xenografts. Am J Pathol. 2002;160:537–48.
33. Sica A, Schioppa T, Mantovani A, Allavena P. Tumour-associated macrophages are a distinct M2 polarised population promoting tumour progression: potential targets of anti-cancer therapy. Eur J Cancer. 2006;42:717–27.
34. Sica A, Allavena P, Mantovani A. Cancer related inflammation: the macrophage connection. Cancer Lett. 2008;267:204–15.
35. Solinas G, Germano G, Mantovani A, Allavena P. Tumor-associated macrophages (TAM) as major players of the cancer-related inflammation. J Leukoc Biol. 2009;86:1065–73.
36. Pollard JW. Tumour-educated macrophages promote tumour progression and metastasis. Nat Rev Cancer. 2004;4:71–8.
37. Sica A, Saccani A, Bottazzi B, Polentarutti N, Vecchi A, van Damme J, Mantovani A. Autocrine production of IL-10 mediates defective IL-12 production and NF-kappa B activation in tumor-associated macrophages. J Immunol. 2000;164:762–7.
38. Mantovani A, Allavena P, Sica A. Tumour-associated macrophages as a prototypic type II polarised phagocyte population: role in tumour progression. Eur J Cancer. 2004;40:1660–7.

39. Tsutsui S, Yasuda K, Suzuki K, Tahara K, Higashi H, Era S. Macrophage infiltration and its prognostic implications in breast cancer: the relationship with VEGF expression and microvessel density. Oncol Rep. 2005;14:425–31.
40. Zhang J, Yan Y, Yang Y, Wang L, Li M, Wang J, Liu X, Duan X, Wang J. High infiltration of tumor-associated macrophages influences poor prognosis in human gastric cancer patients, associates with the phenomenon of EMT. Medicine (Baltimore). 2016;95:e2636.
41. Hanada T, Nakagawa M, Emoto A, Nomura T, Nasu N, Nomura Y. Prognostic value of tumor-associated macrophage count in human bladder cancer. Int J Urol. 2000;7:263–9.
42. Salvesen HB, Akslen LA. Significance of tumour-associated macrophages, vascular endothelial growth factor and thrombospondin-1 expression for tumour angiogenesis and prognosis in endometrial carcinomas. Int J Cancer. 1999;84:538–43.
43. Fujimoto J, Sakaguchi H, Aoki I, Tamaya T. Clinical implications of expression of interleukin 8 related to angiogenesis in uterine cervical cancers. Cancer Res. 2000;60:2632–5.
44. Shimura S, Yang G, Ebara S, Wheeler TM, Frolov A, Thompson TC. Reduced infiltration of tumor-associated macrophages in human prostate cancer: association with cancer progression. Cancer Res. 2000;60:5857–61.
45. Forssell J, Oberg A, Henriksson ML, Stenling R, Jung A, Palmqvist R. High macrophage infiltration along the tumor front correlates with improved survival in colon cancer. Clin Cancer Res. 2007;13:1472–9.
46. Fulkerson PC, Rothenberg ME. Targeting eosinophils in allergy, inflammation and beyond. Nat Rev Drug Discov. 2013;12:117–29.
47. Rothenberg ME, Hogan SP. The eosinophil. Annu Rev Immunol. 2006;24:147–74.
48. Kita H. Eosinophils: multifaceted biological properties and roles in health and disease. Immunol Rev. 2011;242:161–77.
49. Muniz VS, Weller PF, Neves JS. Eosinophil crystalloid granules: structure, function, and beyond. J Leukoc Biol. 2012;92:281–8.
50. Fernandez-Acenero MJ, Galindo-Gallego M, Sanz J, Aljama A. Prognostic influence of tumor-associated eosinophilic infiltrate in colorectal carcinoma. Cancer. 2000;88:1544–8.
51. Dorta RG, Landman G, Kowalski LP, Lauris JRP, Latorre MRDO, Oliveira DT. Tumour-associated tissue eosinophilia as a prognostic factor in oral squamous cell carcinomas. Histopathology. 2002;41:152–7.
52. Costello R, O'Callaghan T, Sebahoun G. [Eosinophils and antitumour response]. Rev Med Interne. 2005;26:479–84.
53. Ohkawara Y, Lim KG, Xing Z, Glibetic M, Nakano K, Dolovich J, Croitoru K, Weller PF, Jordana M. CD40 expression by human peripheral blood eosinophils. J Clin Invest. 1996;97:1761–6.
54. Woerly G, Roger N, Loiseau S, Dombrowicz D, Capron A, Capron M. Expression of CD28 and CD86 by human eosinophils and role in the secretion of type 1 cytokines (interleukin 2 and interferon gamma): inhibition by immunoglobulin a complexes. J Exp Med. 1999;190:487–95.
55. Shi HZ, Humbles A, Gerard C, Jin Z, Weller PF. Lymph node trafficking and antigen presentation by endobronchial eosinophils. J Clin Invest. 2000;105:945–53.
56. Lotfi R, Herzog GI, DeMarco RA, Beer-Stolz D, Lee JJ, Rubartelli A, Schrezenmeier H, Lotze MT. Eosinophils oxidize damage-associated molecular pattern molecules derived from stressed cells. J Immunol. 2009;183:5023–31.
57. Cormier SA, Taranova AG, Bedient C, Nguyen T, Protheroe C, Pero R, Dimina D, Ochkur SI, O'Neill K, Colbert D, Lombari TR, Constant S, McGarry MP, Lee JJ, Lee NA. Pivotal advance: eosinophil infiltration of solid tumors is an early and persistent inflammatory host response. J Leukoc Biol. 2006;79:1131–9.
58. Minton K. Granulocytes: eosinophils enable the antitumour T cell response. Nat Rev Immunol. 2015;15:333.
59. Carretero R, Sektioglu IM, Garbi N, Salgado OC, Beckhove P, Hammerling GJ. Eosinophils orchestrate cancer rejection by normalizing tumor vessels and enhancing infiltration of CD8(+) T cells. Nat Immunol. 2015;16:609–17.
60. Falcone FH, Zillikens D, Gibbs BF. The 21st century renaissance of the basophil? Current

insights into its role in allergic responses and innate immunity. Exp Dermatol. 2006;15:855–64.
61. Schroeder JT, DW MG Jr, Lichtenstein LM. Human basophils: mediator release and cytokine production. Adv Immunol. 2001;77:93–122.
62. Haas H, Falcone FH, Holland MJ, Schramm G, Haisch K, Gibbs BF, Bufe A, Schlaak M. Early interleukin-4: its role in the switch towards a Th2 response and IgE-mediated allergy. Int Arch Allergy Immunol. 1999;119:86–94.
63. Schroeder JT. Basophils beyond effector cells of allergic inflammation. Adv Immunol. 2009;101:123–61.
64. Prevete N, Staiano RI, Granata F, Detoraki A, Necchi V, Ricci V, Triggiani M, De Paulis A, Marone G, Genovese A. Expression and function of angiopoietins and their tie receptors in human basophils and mast cells. J Biol Regul Homeost Agents. 2013;27:827–39.
65. De Monte L, Wormann S, Brunetto E, Heltai S, Magliacane G, Reni M, Paganoni AM, Recalde H, Mondino A, Falconi M, Aleotti F, Balzano G, Ul HA, Doglioni C, Protti MP. Basophil recruitment into tumor-draining lymph nodes correlates with Th2 inflammation and reduced survival in pancreatic cancer patients. Cancer Res. 2016;76:1792–803.
66. Frossi B, De Carli M, Pucillo C. The mast cell: an antenna of the microenvironment that directs the immune response. J Leukoc Biol. 2004;75:579–85.
67. Qi X, Hong J, Chaves L, Zhuang Y, Chen Y, Wang D, Chabon J, Graham B, Ohmori K, Li Y, Huang H. Antagonistic regulation by the transcription factors C/EBPalpha and MITF specifies basophil and mast cell fates. Immunity. 2013;39:97–110.
68. Marone G, Galli SJ, Kitamura Y. Probing the roles of mast cells and basophils in natural and acquired immunity, physiology and disease. Trends Immunol. 2002;23:425–7.
69. Galli SJ, Franco CB. Basophils are back! Immunity. 2008;28:495–7.
70. Stone KD, Prussin C, Metcalfe DD. IgE, mast cells, basophils, and eosinophils. J Allergy Clin Immunol. 2010;125:S73–80.
71. Metcalfe DD. Mast cells and mastocytosis. Blood. 2008;112:946–56.
72. Nonomura N, Takayama H, Nishimura K, Oka D, Nakai Y, Shiba M, Tsujimura A, Nakayama M, Aozasa K, Okuyama A. Decreased number of mast cells infiltrating into needle biopsy specimens leads to a better prognosis of prostate cancer. Br J Cancer. 2007;97:952–6.
73. Rojas IG, Spencer ML, Martinez A, Maurelia MA, Rudolph MI. Characterization of mast cell subpopulations in lip cancer. J Oral Pathol Med. 2005;34:268–73.
74. Fukushima H, Ohsawa M, Ikura Y, Naruko T, Sugama Y, Suekane T, Kitabayashi C, Inoue T, Hino M, Ueda M. Mast cells in diffuse large B-cell lymphoma; their role in fibrosis. Histopathology. 2006;49:498–505.
75. Kormelink TG, Abudukelimu A, Redegeld FA. Mast cells as target in cancer therapy. Curr Pharm Des. 2009;15:1868–78.
76. Ribatti D, Vacca A, Nico B, Crivellato E, Roncali L, Dammacco F. The role of mast cells in tumour angiogenesis. Br J Haematol. 2001;115:514–21.
77. Rajput AB, Turbin DA, Cheang MC, Voduc DK, Leung S, Gelmon KA, Gilks CB, Huntsman DG. Stromal mast cells in invasive breast cancer are a marker of favourable prognosis: a study of 4,444 cases. Breast Cancer Res Treat. 2008;107:249–57.
78. Chan JK, Magistris A, Loizzi V, Lin F, Rutgers J, Osann K, DiSaia PJ, Samoszuk M. Mast cell density, angiogenesis, blood clotting, and prognosis in women with advanced ovarian cancer. Gynecol Oncol. 2005;99:20–5.
79. Welsh TJ, Green RH, Richardson D, Waller DA, O'Byrne KJ, Bradding P. Macrophage and mast-cell invasion of tumor cell islets confers a marked survival advantage in non-small-cell lung cancer. J Clin Oncol. 2005;23:8959–67.
80. Tan SY, Fan Y, Luo HS, Shen ZX, Guo Y, Zhao LJ. Prognostic significance of cell infiltrations of immunosurveillance in colorectal cancer. World J Gastroenterol. 2005;11:1210–4.
81. Latti S, Leskinen M, Shiota N, Wang YF, Kovanen PT, Lindstedt KA. Mast cell-mediated apoptosis of endothelial cells in vitro: a paracrine mechanism involving TNF-alpha-mediated down-regulation of bcl-2 expression. J Cell Physiol. 2003;195:130–8.
82. Leskinen MJ, Lindstedt KA, Wang YF, Kovanen PT. Mast cell chymase induces smooth muscle cell apoptosis by a mechanism involving fibronectin degradation and disruption of focal adhesions. Arterioscler Thromb Vasc Biol. 2003;23:238–43.

83. Hammer GE, Ma A. Molecular control of steady-state dendritic cell maturation and immune homeostasis. Annu Rev Immunol. 2013;31:743–91.
84. Liu K, Nussenzweig MC. Origin and development of dendritic cells. Immunol Rev. 2010;234:45–54.
85. Liu K, Victora GD, Schwickert TA, Guermonprez P, Meredith MM, Yao K, Chu FF, Randolph GJ, Rudensky AY, Nussenzweig M. In vivo analysis of dendritic cell development and homeostasis. Science. 2009;324:392–7.
86. Shortman K, Naik SH. Steady-state and inflammatory dendritic-cell development. Nat Rev Immunol. 2007;7:19–30.
87. Trombetta ES, Mellman I. Cell biology of antigen processing in vitro and in vivo. Annu Rev Immunol. 2005;23:975–1028.
88. Steinman RM. Decisions about dendritic cells: past, present, and future. Annu Rev Immunol. 2012;30(30):1–22.
89. Ljunggren HG, Karre K. In search of the missing self - Mhc molecules and Nk cell recognition. Immunol Today. 1990;11:237–44.
90. Vivier E, Nunes JA, Vely F. Natural killer cell signaling pathways. Science. 2004;306:1517–9.
91. Tomasello E, Blery M, Vely F, Vivier E. Signaling pathways engaged by NK cell receptors: double concerto for activating receptors, inhibitory receptors and NK cells. Semin Immunol. 2000;12:139–47.
92. Strengell M, Matikainen S, Siren J, Lehtonen A, Foster D, Julkunen I, Sareneva T. IL-21 in synergy with IL-15 or IL-18 enhances IFN-gamma production in human NK and T cells. J Immunol. 2003;170:5464–9.
93. Brady J, Carotta S, Thong RP, Chan CJ, Hayakawa Y, Smyth MJ, Nutt SL. The interactions of multiple cytokines control NK cell maturation. J Immunol. 2010;185:6679–88.
94. Lunemann A, Lunemann JD, Munz C. Regulatory NK-cell functions in inflammation and autoimmunity. Mol Med. 2009;15:352–8.
95. Becknell B, Caligiuri MA. Natural killer cells in innate immunity and cancer. J Immunother. 2008;31:685–92.
96. Kaiser BK, Yim D, Chow IT, Gonzalez S, Dai Z, Mann HH, Strong RK, Groh V, Spies T. Disulphide-isomerase-enabled shedding of tumour-associated NKG2D ligands. Nature. 2007;447:482–6.
97. Groh V, Wu J, Yee C, Spies T. Tumour-derived soluble MIC ligands impair expression of NKG2D and T-cell activation. Nature. 2002;419:734–8.
98. Castriconi R, Cantoni C, Della Chiesa M, Vitale M, Marcenaro E, Conte R, Biassoni R, Bottino C, Moretta L, Moretta A. Transforming growth factor beta 1 inhibits expression of NKp30 and NKG2D receptors: consequences for the NK-mediated killing of dendritic cells. Proc Natl Acad Sci U S A. 2003;100:4120–5.
99. Sconocchia G, Titus JA, Segal DM. Signaling pathways regulating CD44-dependent cytolysis in natural killer cells. Blood. 1997;90:716–25.
100. Wang W, Erbe AK, Hank JA, Morris ZS, Sondel PM. NK cell-mediated antibody-dependent cellular cytotoxicity in cancer immunotherapy. Front Immunol. 2015;6:368.
101. Ferlazzo G, Thomas D, Lin SL, Goodman K, Morandi B, Muller WA, Moretta A, Munz C. The abundant NK cells in human secondary lymphoid tissues require activation to express killer cell Ig-like receptors and become cytolytic. J Immunol. 2004;172:1455–62.
102. Sun JC, Beilke JN, Lanier LL. Adaptive immune features of natural killer cells. Nature. 2009;457:557–61.
103. Albertsson PA, Basse PH, Hokland M, Goldfarb RH, Nagelkerke JF, Nannmark U, Kuppen PJ. NK cells and the tumour microenvironment: implications for NK-cell function and anti-tumour activity. Trends Immunol. 2003;24:603–9.
104. Robey E, Fowlkes BJ. Selective events in T cell development. Annu Rev Immunol. 1994;12:675–705.
105. Germain RN. T-cell development and the CD4-CD8 lineage decision. Nat Rev Immunol. 2002;2:309–22.
106. Scollay R, Wilson A, D'Amico A, Kelly K, Egerton M, Pearse M, Wu L, Shortman K. Developmental status and reconstitution potential of subpopulations of murine thymocytes. Immunol Rev. 1988;104:81–120.

107. Blackburn CC, Manley NR. Developing a new paradigm for thymus organogenesis. Nat Rev Immunol. 2004;4:278–89.
108. Vonboehmer H, Teh HS, Kisielow P. The thymus selects the useful, neglects the useless and destroys the harmful. Immunol Today. 1989;10:57–61.
109. Leung RK, Thomson K, Gallimore A, Jones E, Van den Broek M, Sierro S, Alsheikhly AR, McMichael A, Rahemtulla A. Deletion of the CD4 silencer element supports a stochastic mechanism of thymocyte lineage commitment. Nat Immunol. 2001;2:1167–73.
110. Sharma P, Wagner K, Wolchok JD, Allison JP. Novel cancer immunotherapy agents with survival benefit: recent successes and next steps. Nat Rev Cancer. 2011;11:805–12.
111. Lugo-Villarino G, Maldonado-Lopez R, Possemato R, Penaranda C, Glimcher LH. T-bet is required for optimal production of IFN-gamma and antigen-specific T cell activation by dendritic cells. Proc Natl Acad Sci U S A. 2003;100:7749–54.
112. Zhu JF, Guo LY, Watson CJ, Hu-Li J, Paul WE. Stat6 is necessary and sufficient for IL-4's role in Th2 differentiation and cell expansion. J Immunol. 2001;166:7276–81.
113. Zhou L, Lopes JE, Chong MM, Ivanov II, Min R, Victora GD, Shen Y, Du J, Rubtsov YP, Rudensky AY, Ziegler SF, Littman DR. TGF-beta-induced Foxp3 inhibits T(H)17 cell differentiation by antagonizing RORgammat function. Nature. 2008;453:236–40.
114. Chen WJ, Jin WW, Hardegen N, Lei KJ, Li L, Marinos N, McGrady G, Wahl SM. Conversion of peripheral CD4(+)CD25(−) naive T cells to CD4(+)CD25(+) regulatory T cells by TGF-beta induction of transcription factor Foxp3. J Exp Med. 2003;198:1875–86.
115. Nurieva RI, Chung Y, Hwang D, Yang XO, Kang HS, Ma L, Wang YH, Watowich SS, Jetten AM, Tian Q, Dong C. Generation of T follicular helper cells is mediated by interleukin-21 but independent of T helper 1, 2, or 17 cell lineages. Immunity. 2008;29:138–49.
116. Staudt V, Bothur E, Klein M, Lingnau K, Reuter S, Grebe N, Gerlitzki B, Hoffmann M, Ulges A, Taube C, Dehzad N, Becker M, Stassen M, Steinborn A, Lohoff M, Schild H, Schmitt E, Bopp T. Interferon-regulatory factor 4 is essential for the developmental program of T helper 9 cells. Immunity. 2010;33:192–202.
117. Saule P, Trauet J, Dutriez V, Lekeux W, Dessaint JP, Labalette M. Accumulation of memory T cells from childhood to old age: central and effector memory cells in CD4(+) versus effector memory and terminally differentiated memory cells in CD8(+) compartment. Mech Ageing Dev. 2006;127:274–81.
118. Chen L, Flies DB. Molecular mechanisms of T cell co-stimulation and co-inhibition. Nat Rev Immunol. 2013;13:227–42.
119. Linsley PS, Clark EA, Ledbetter JA. T-cell antigen CD28 mediates adhesion with B cells by interacting with activation antigen B7/BB-1. Proc Natl Acad Sci U S A. 1990;87:5031–5.
120. Nam KO, Kang H, Shin SM, Cho KH, Kwon B, Kwon BS, Kim SJ, Lee HW. Cross-linking of 4-1BB activates TCR-signaling pathways in CD8+ T lymphocytes. J Immunol. 2005;174:1898–905.
121. Godfrey WR, Fagnoni FF, Harara MA, Buck D, Engleman EG. Identification of a human OX-40 ligand, a costimulator of CD4+ T cells with homology to tumor necrosis factor. J Exp Med. 1994;180:757–62.
122. Nocentini G, Riccardi C. GITR: a modulator of immune response and inflammation. Adv Exp Med Biol. 2009;647:156–73.
123. Linsley PS, Brady W, Urnes M, Grosmaire LS, Damle NK, Ledbetter JA. CTLA-4 is a second receptor for the B cell activation antigen B7. J Exp Med. 1991;174:561–9.
124. Freeman GJ, Long AJ, Iwai Y, Bourque K, Chernova T, Nishimura H, Fitz LJ, Malenkovich N, Okazaki T, Byrne MC, Horton HF, Fouser L, Carter L, Ling V, Bowman MR, Carreno BM, Collins M, Wood CR, Honjo T. Engagement of the PD-1 immunoinhibitory receptor by a novel B7 family member leads to negative regulation of lymphocyte activation. J Exp Med. 2000;192:1027–34.
125. Buchbinder EI, Desai A. CTLA-4 and PD-1 pathways similarities, differences, and implications of their inhibition. Am J Clin Oncol. 2016;39:98–106.
126. Liang SC, Latchman YE, Buhlmann JE, Tomczak MF, Horwitz BH, Freeman GJ, Sharpe AH. Regulation of PD-1, PD-L1, and PD-L2 expression during normal and autoimmune responses. Eur J Immunol. 2003;33:2706–16.

127. Okazaki T, Maeda A, Nishimura H, Kurosaki T, Honjo T. PD-1 immunoreceptor inhibits B cell receptor-mediated signaling by recruiting src homology 2-domain-containing tyrosine phosphatase 2 to phosphotyrosine. Proc Natl Acad Sci U S A. 2001;98:13866–71.
128. Anderson AC, Joller N, Kuchroo VK. Lag-3, Tim-3, and TIGIT: co-inhibitory receptors with specialized functions in immune regulation. Immunity. 2016;44:989–1004.
129. Joller N, Lozano E, Burkett PR, Patel B, Xiao S, Zhu C, Xia J, Tan TG, Sefik E, Yajnik V, Sharpe AH, Quintana FJ, Mathis D, Benoist C, Hafler DA, Kuchroo VK. Treg cells expressing the coinhibitory molecule TIGIT selectively inhibit proinflammatory Th1 and Th17 cell responses. Immunity. 2014;40:569–81.
130. Jordan MS, Boesteanu A, Reed AJ, Petrone AL, Holenbeck AE, Lerman MA, Naji A, Caton AJ. Thymic selection of CD4(+)CD25(+) regulatory T cells induced by an agonist self-peptide. Nat Immunol. 2001;2:301–6.
131. Croft M. The role of TNF superfamily members in T-cell function and diseases. Nat Rev Immunol. 2009;9:271–85.
132. Pardoll DM. The blockade of immune checkpoints in cancer immunotherapy. Nat Rev Cancer. 2012;12:252–64.
133. Nagasawa T. Microenvironmental niches in the bone marrow required for B-cell development. Nat Rev Immunol. 2006;6:107–16.
134. Hardy RR, Carmack CE, Shinton SA, Kemp JD, Hayakawa K. Resolution and characterization of pro-B and pre-pro-B cell stages in normal mouse bone marrow. J Exp Med. 1991;173:1213–25.
135. Tiegs SL, Russell DM, Nemazee D. Receptor editing in self-reactive bone marrow B cells. J Exp Med. 1993;177:1009–20.
136. Carsetti R, Kohler G, Lamers MC. Transitional B cells are the target of negative selection in the B cell compartment. J Exp Med. 1995;181:2129–40.
137. Pieper K, Grimbacher B, Eibel H. B-cell biology and development. J Allergy Clin Immunol. 2013;131:959–71.
138. Shlomchik MJ, Weisel F. Germinal center selection and the development of memory B and plasma cells. Immunol Rev. 2012;247:52–63.
139. Schroeder HW Jr, Cavacini L. Structure and function of immunoglobulins. J Allergy Clin Immunol. 2010;125:S41–52.
140. Lipman NS, Jackson LR, Trudel LJ, Weis-Garcia F. Monoclonal versus polyclonal antibodies: distinguishing characteristics, applications, and information resources. ILAR J. 2005;46:258–68.
141. Kung P, Goldstein G, Reinherz EL, Schlossman SF. Monoclonal antibodies defining distinctive human T cell surface antigens. Science. 1979;206:347–9.
142. Morrison SL, Johnson MJ, Herzenberg LA, Oi VT. Chimeric human antibody molecules: mouse antigen-binding domains with human constant region domains. Proc Natl Acad Sci U S A. 1984;81:6851–5.
143. Riechmann L, Clark M, Waldmann H, Winter G. Reshaping human antibodies for therapy. Nature. 1988;332:323–7.
144. Harding FA, Stickler MM, Razo J, DuBridge RB. The immunogenicity of humanized and fully human antibodies: residual immunogenicity resides in the CDR regions. MAbs. 2010;2:256–65.
145. Scott AM, Wolchok JD, Old LJ. Antibody therapy of cancer. Nat Rev Cancer. 2012;12:278–87.
146. Fridman WH, Pages F, Sautes-Fridman C, Galon J. The immune contexture in human tumours: impact on clinical outcome. Nat Rev Cancer. 2012;12:298–306.
147. Dunn GP, Old LJ, Schreiber RD. The three Es of cancer immunoediting. Annu Rev Immunol. 2004;22:329–60.
148. Dunn GP, Bruce AT, Ikeda H, Old LJ, Schreiber RD. Cancer immunoediting: from immunosurveillance to tumor escape. Nat Immunol. 2002;3:991–8.
149. Hanahan D, Weinberg RA. The hallmarks of cancer. Cell. 2000;100:57–70.
150. Teng MW, Galon J, Fridman WH, Smyth MJ. From mice to humans: developments in cancer immunoediting. J Clin Invest. 2015;125:3338–46.

151. Mellman I, Coukos G, Dranoff G. Cancer immunotherapy comes of age. Nature. 2011;480:480–9.
152. Gabrilovich DI, Ostrand-Rosenberg S, Bronte V. Coordinated regulation of myeloid cells by tumours. Nat Rev Immunol. 2012;12:253–68.
153. Huang B, Pan PY, Li QS, Sato AI, Levy DE, Bromberg J, Divino CM, Chen SH. Gr-1(+) CD115(+) immature myeloid suppressor cells mediate the development of tumor-induced T regulatory cells and T-cell anergy in tumor-bearing host. Cancer Res. 2006;66:1123–31.
154. Lindau D, Gielen P, Kroesen M, Wesseling P, Adema GJ. The immunosuppressive tumour network: myeloid-derived suppressor cells, regulatory T cells and natural killer T cells. Immunology. 2013;138:105–15.
155. Tangri S, LiCalsi C, Sidney J, Sette A. Rationally engineered proteins or antibodies with absent or reduced immunogenicity. Curr Med Chem. 2002;9:2191–9.
156. Weiner LM, Surana R, Wang SZ. Monoclonal antibodies: versatile platforms for cancer immunotherapy. Nat Rev Immunol. 2010;10:317–27.
157. Krummel MF, Allison JP. Cd28 and Ctla-4 have opposing effects on the response of T-cells to stimulation. J Exp Med. 1995;182:459–65.
158. Hodi FS, O'Day SJ, McDermott DF, Weber RW, Sosman JA, Haanen JB, Gonzalez R, Robert C, Schadendorf D, Hassel JC, Akerley W, van den Eertwegh AJM, Lutzky J, Lorigan P, Vaubel JM, Linette GP, Hogg D, Ottensmeier CH, Lebbe C, Peschel C, Quirt I, Clark JI, Wolchok JD, Weber JS, Tian J, Yellin MJ, Nichol GM, Hoos A, Urba WJ. Improved survival with ipilimumab in patients with metastatic melanoma. N Engl J Med. 2010;363:711–23.
159. Brahmer JR, Drake CG, Wollner I, Powderly JD, Picus J, Sharfman WH, Stankevich E, Pons A, Salay TM, McMiller TL, Gilson MM, Wang C, Selby M, Taube JM, Anders R, Chen L, Korman AJ, Pardoll DM, Lowy I, Topalian SL. Phase I study of single-agent anti-programmed death-1 (MDX-1106) in refractory solid tumors: safety, clinical activity, pharmacodynamics, and immunologic correlates. J Clin Oncol. 2010;28:3167–75.
160. Borghaei H, Paz-Ares L, Horn L, Spigel DR, Steins M, Ready NE, Chow LQ, Vokes EE, Felip E, Holgado E, Barlesi F, Kohlhaufl M, Arrieta O, Burgio MA, Fayette J, Lena H, Poddubskaya E, Gerber DE, Gettinger SN, Rudin CM, Rizvi N, Crino L, Blumenschein GR Jr, Antonia SJ, Dorange C, Harbison CT, Graf Finckenstein F, Brahmer JR. Nivolumab versus docetaxel in advanced nonsquamous non-small-cell lung cancer. N Engl J Med. 2015;373:1627–39.
161. Brahmer J, Reckamp KL, Baas P, Crino L, Eberhardt WE, Poddubskaya E, Antonia S, Pluzanski A, Vokes EE, Holgado E, Waterhouse D, Ready N, Gainor J, Aren Frontera O, Havel L, Steins M, Garassino MC, Aerts JG, Domine M, Paz-Ares L, Reck M, Baudelet C, Harbison CT, Lestini B, Spigel DR. Nivolumab versus docetaxel in advanced squamous-cell non-small-cell lung cancer. N Engl J Med. 2015;373:123–35.
162. Herbst RS, Baas P, Kim DW, Felip E, Perez-Gracia JL, Han JY, Molina J, Kim JH, Arvis CD, Ahn MJ, Majem M, Fidler MJ, de Castro G Jr, Garrido M, Lubiniecki GM, Shentu Y, Im E, Dolled-Filhart M, Garon EB. Pembrolizumab versus docetaxel for previously treated, PD-L1-positive, advanced non-small-cell lung cancer (KEYNOTE-010): a randomised controlled trial. Lancet. 2016;387:1540–50.
163. Rosenberg JE, Hoffman-Censits J, Powles T, van der Heijden MS, Balar AV, Necchi A, Dawson N, O'Donnell PH, Balmanoukian A, Loriot Y, Srinivas S, Retz MM, Grivas P, Joseph RW, Galsky MD, Fleming MT, Petrylak DP, Perez-Gracia JL, Burris HA, Castellano D, Canil C, Bellmunt J, Bajorin D, Nickles D, Bourgon R, Frampton GM, Cui N, Mariathasan S, Abidoye O, Fine GD, Dreicer R. Atezolizumab in patients with locally advanced and metastatic urothelial carcinoma who have progressed following treatment with platinum-based chemotherapy: a single-arm, multicentre, phase 2 trial. Lancet. 2016;387:1909–20.
164. U.S. Food and Drug Administration. Hematology/oncology (cancer) approvals & safety notifications. 2018.
165. Moon YW, Hajjar J, Hwu P, Naing A. Targeting the indoleamine 2,3-dioxygenase pathway in cancer. J Immunother Cancer. 2015;3:51.
166. Koblish HK, Hansbury MJ, Bowman KJ, Yang G, Neilan CL, Haley PJ, Burn TC, Waeltz P, Sparks RB, Yue EW, Combs AP, Scherle PA, Vaddi K, Fridman JS. [INCB preclin] Hydroxyamidine inhibitors of indoleamine-2,3-dioxygenase potently suppress systemic

tryptophan catabolism and the growth of IDO-expressing tumors. Mol Cancer Ther. 2010;9:489–98.
167. Liu X, Shin N, Koblish HK, Yang G, Wang Q, Wang K, Leffet L, Hansbury MJ, Thomas B, Rupar M, Waeltz P, Bowman KJ, Polam P, Sparks RB, Yue EW, Li Y, Wynn R, Fridman JS, Burn TC, Combs AP, Newton RC, Scherle PA. [INCB preclin] selective inhibition of IDO1 effectively regulates mediators of antitumor immunity. Blood. 2010;115:3520–30.
168. Metz R, Rust S, Duhadaway JB, Mautino MR, Munn DH, Vahanian NN, Link CJ, Prendergast GC. [Indoximod preclin] IDO inhibits a tryptophan sufficiency signal that stimulates mTOR: a novel IDO effector pathway targeted by D-1-methyl-tryptophan. Oncoimmunology. 2012;1:1460–8.
169. Iversen TZ, Engell-Noerregaard L, Ellebaek E, Andersen R, Larsen SK, Bjoern J, Zeyher C, Gouttefangeas C, Thomsen BM, Holm B, Straten PT, Mellemgaard A, Andersen MH, Svane IM. [IDO pep vac] Long-lasting disease stabilization in the absence of toxicity in metastatic lung cancer patients vaccinated with an epitope derived from indoleamine 2,3 dioxygenase. Clin Cancer Res. 2014;20:221–32.
170. Siu LL, Gelmon K, Chu Q, Pachynski R, Alese O, Basciano P, Walker J, Mitra P, Zhu L, Phillips P, Hunt J, Desai J. Abstract CT116: BMS-986205, an optimized indoleamine 2,3-dioxygenase 1 (IDO1) inhibitor, is well tolerated with potent pharmacodynamic (PD) activity, alone and in combination with nivolumab (nivo) in advanced cancers in a phase 1/2a trial. Cancer Res. 2017;77:CT116-CT.
171. Mautino MR, Jaipuri FA, Waldo J, Kumar S, Adams J, Allen CV, Marcinowicz-Flick A, Munn D, Vahanian N, Link CJJ. NLG919, a novel indoleamine-2,3-dioxygenase (IDO)-pathway inhibitor drug candidate for cancer therapy. AACR; 2013. p. 491.
172. Linch SN, McNamara MJ, Redmond WL. OX40 agonists and combination immunotherapy: putting the pedal to the metal. Front Oncol. 2015;5:34.
173. Aspeslagh S, Postel-Vinay S, Rusakiewicz S, Soria JC, Zitvogel L, Marabelle A. Rationale for anti-OX40 cancer immunotherapy. Eur J Cancer. 2016;52:50–66.
174. Topalian SL, Weiner GJ, Pardoll DM. Cancer immunotherapy comes of age. J Clin Oncol. 2011;29:4828–36.
175. Wargo JA, Cooper ZA, Flaherty KT. Universes collide: combining immunotherapy with targeted therapy for cancer. Cancer Discov. 2014;4:1377–86.
176. Sullivan RJ, Gonzalez R, Lewis KD, Hamid O, Infante JR, Patel MR, Hodi FS, Wallin J, Pitcher B, Cha E, Roberts L, Ballinger M, Hwu P. Atezolizumab (a) + cobimetinib (C) + vemurafenib (V) in BRAFV600-mutant metastatic melanoma (mel): updated safety and clinical activity. J Clin Oncol. 2017;35:3063.
177. Formenti SC, Demaria S. Combining radiotherapy and cancer immunotherapy: a paradigm shift. J Natl Cancer Inst. 2013;105:256–65.
178. Golden EB, Chachoua A, Fenton-Kerimian MB, Demaria S, Formenti SC. Abscopal responses in metastatic non-small cell lung cancer (NSCLC) patients treated on a phase 2 study of combined radiation therapy and ipilimumab: evidence for the in situ vaccination hypothesis of radiation. Int J Radiat Oncol. 2015;93:S66–S7.
179. Fiorica F, Belluomini L, Stefanelli A, Santini A, Urbini B, Giorgi C, Frassoldati A. Immune checkpoint inhibitor nivolumab and radiotherapy in pretreated lung cancer patients: efficacy and safety of combination. Am J Clin Oncol. 2018;41:1101–05.
180. Cai Z, Sanchez A, Shi Z, Zhang T, Liu M, Zhang D. Activation of toll-like receptor 5 on breast cancer cells by flagellin suppresses cell proliferation and tumor growth. Cancer Res. 2011;71:2466–75.
181. Wolska A, Lech-Maranda E, Robak T. Toll-like receptors and their role in carcinogenesis and anti-tumor treatment. Cell Mol Biol Lett. 2009;14:248–72.
182. Liu Y, Yan W, Tohme S, Chen M, Fu Y, Tian D, Lotze M, Tang DL, Tsung A. Hypoxia induced HMGB1 and mitochondrial DNA interactions mediate tumor growth in hepatocellular carcinoma through toll-like receptor 9. J Hepatol. 2015;63:114–21.
183. Shi M, Chen X, Ye K, Yao Y, Li Y. Application potential of toll-like receptors in cancer immunotherapy: systematic review. Medicine (Baltimore). 2016;95:e3951.
184. Li K, Qu S, Chen X, Wu Q, Shi M: Promising targets for cancer immunotherapy: TLRs,

RLRs, and STING-mediated innate immune pathways. Int J Mol Sci 2017;18. pii: E404.
185. Ishikawa H, Ma Z, Barber GN. STING regulates intracellular DNA-mediated, type I interferon-dependent innate immunity. Nature. 2009;461:788–92.
186. Fuertes MB, Kacha AK, Kline J, Woo SR, Kranz DM, Murphy KM, Gajewski TF. Host type I IFN signals are required for antitumor CD8+ T cell responses through CD8{alpha}+ dendritic cells. J Exp Med. 2011;208:2005–16.
187. Corrales L, Glickman LH, McWhirter SM, Kanne DB, Sivick KE, Katibah GE, Woo SR, Lemmens E, Banda T, Leong JJ, Metchette K, Dubensky TW Jr, Gajewski TF. Direct activation of STING in the tumor microenvironment leads to potent and systemic tumor regression and immunity. Cell Rep. 2015;11:1018–30.
188. Fu J, Kanne DB, Leong M, Glickman LH, McWhirter SM, Lemmens E, Mechette K, Leong JJ, Lauer P, Liu W, Sivick KE, Zeng Q, Soares KC, Zheng L, Portnoy DA, Woodward JJ, Pardoll DM, Dubensky TW, Kim Y. STING agonist formulated cancer vaccines can cure established tumors resistant to PD-1 blockade. Sci Transl Med. 2015;7:283ra52.
189. Deng LF, Liang H, Xu M, Yang XM, Burnette B, Arina A, Li XD, Mauceri H, Beckett M, Darga T, Huang XN, Gajewski TF, Chen ZJJ, Fu YX, Weichselbaum RR. STING-dependent cytosolic DNA sensing promotes radiation-induced type I interferon-dependent antitumor immunity in immunogenic tumors. Immunity. 2014;41:843–52.
190. Topalian SL, Taube JM, Anders RA, Pardoll DM. Mechanism-driven biomarkers to guide immune checkpoint blockade in cancer therapy. Nat Rev Cancer. 2016;16:275–87.
191. Topalian SL, Hodi FS, Brahmer JR, Gettinger SN, Smith DC, McDermott DF, Powderly JD, Carvajal RD, Sosman JA, Atkins MB, Leming PD, Spigel DR, Antonia SJ, Horn L, Drake CG, Pardoll DM, Chen L, Sharfman WH, Anders RA, Taube JM, McMiller TL, Xu H, Korman AJ, Jure-Kunkel M, Agrawal S, McDonald D, Kollia GD, Gupta A, Wigginton JM, Sznol M. Safety, activity, and immune correlates of anti-PD-1 antibody in cancer. N Engl J Med. 2012;366:2443–54.
192. U.S. Food and Drug Administration. FDA approves Keytruda for advanced non-small cell lung cancer. 2015. http://www.fda.gov/NewsEvents/Newsroom/PressAnnouncements/ucm465444.htm.
193. Herbst RS, Soria JC, Kowanetz M, Fine GD, Hamid O, Gordon MS, Sosman JA, McDermott DF, Powderly JD, Gettinger SN, Kohrt HE, Horn L, Lawrence DP, Rost S, Leabman M, Xiao Y, Mokatrin A, Koeppen H, Hegde PS, Mellman I, Chen DS, Hodi FS. Predictive correlates of response to the anti-PD-L1 antibody MPDL3280A in cancer patients. Nature. 2014;515:563–7.
194. Rittmeyer A, Barlesi F, Waterkamp D, Park K, Ciardiello F, von Pawel J, Gadgeel SM, Hida T, Kowalski DM, Dols MC, Cortinovis DL, Leach J, Polikoff J, Barrios C, Kabbinavar F, Frontera OA, De Marinis F, Turna H, Lee JS, Ballinger M, Kowanetz M, He P, Chen DS, Sandler A, Gandara DR, Grp OS. Atezolizumab versus docetaxel in patients with previously treated non-small-cell lung cancer (OAK): a phase 3, open-label, multicentre randomised controlled trial. Lancet. 2017;389:255–65.
195. Madore J, Vilain RE, Menzies AM, Kakavand H, Wilmott JS, Hyman J, Yearley JH, Kefford RF, Thompson JF, Long GV, Hersey P, Scolyer RA. PD-L1 expression in melanoma shows marked heterogeneity within and between patients: implications for anti-PD-1/PD-L1 clinical trials. Pigment Cell Melanoma Res. 2015;28:245–53.
196. Rosell R, Palmero R. PD-L1 expression associated with better response to EGFR tyrosine kinase inhibitors. Cancer Biol Med. 2015;12:71–3.
197. Sharma P, Allison JP. The future of immune checkpoint therapy. Science. 2015;348:56–61.
198. Hadrup S, Donia M, Thor Straten P. Effector CD4 and CD8 T cells and their role in the tumor microenvironment. Cancer Microenviron. 2013;6:123–33.
199. Zhang L, Conejo-Garcia JR, Katsaros D, Gimotty PA, Massobrio M, Regnani G, Makrigiannakis A, Gray H, Schlienger K, Liebman MN, Rubin SC, Coukos G. Intratumoral T cells, recurrence, and survival in epithelial ovarian cancer. N Engl J Med. 2003;348:203–13.
200. Ruffini E, Asioli S, Filosso PL, Lyberis P, Bruna MC, Macri L, Daniele L, Oliaro A. Clinical significance of tumor-infiltrating lymphocytes in lung neoplasms. Ann Thorac Surg. 2009;87:365–71; discussion 371–2.

201. Curiel TJ, Coukos G, Zou L, Alvarez X, Cheng P, Mottram P, Evdemon-Hogan M, Conejo-Garcia JR, Zhang L, Burow M, Zhu Y, Wei S, Kryczek I, Daniel B, Gordon A, Myers L, Lackner A, Disis ML, Knutson KL, Chen L, Zou W. Specific recruitment of regulatory T cells in ovarian carcinoma fosters immune privilege and predicts reduced survival. Nat Med. 2004;10:942–9.
202. Gobert M, Treilleux I, Bendriss-Vermare N, Bachelot T, Goddard-Leon S, Arfi V, Biota C, Doffin AC, Durand I, Olive D, Perez S, Pasqual N, Faure C, Coquard IR, Puisieux A, Caux C, Blay JY, Menetrier-Caux C. Regulatory T cells recruited through CCL22/CCR4 are selectively activated in lymphoid infiltrates surrounding primary breast tumors and lead to an adverse clinical outcome. Cancer Res. 2009;69:2000–9.
203. Fu JL, Xu DP, Liu ZW, Shi M, Zhao P, Fu BY, Zhang Z, Yang HY, Zhang H, Zhou CB, Ya JX, Jin L, Wang HF, Yang YP, Fu YX, Wang FS. Increased regulatory T cells correlate with CD8 T-cell impairment and poor survival in hepatocellular carcinoma patients. Gastroenterology. 2007;132:2328–39.
204. Llosa NJ, Cruise M, Tam A, Wicks EC, Hechenbleikner EM, Taube JM, Blosser RL, Fan HN, Wang H, Luber BS, Zhang M, Papadopoulos N, Kinzler KW, Vogelstein B, Sears CL, Anders RA, Pardoll DM, Housseau F. The vigorous immune microenvironment of microsatellite instable colon cancer is balanced by multiple counter-inhibitory checkpoints. Cancer Discov. 2015;5:43–51.
205. Galon J, Costes A, Sanchez-Cabo F, Kirilovsky A, Mlecnik B, Lagorce-Pages C, Tosolini M, Camus M, Berger A, Wind P, Zinzindohoue F, Bruneval P, Cugnenc PH, Trajanoski Z, Fridman WH, Pages F. Type, density, and location of immune cells within human colorectal tumors predict clinical outcome. Science. 2006;313:1960–4.
206. Tumeh PC, Harview CL, Yearley JH, Shintaku IP, Taylor EJ, Robert L, Chmielowski B, Spasic M, Henry G, Ciobanu V, West AN, Carmona M, Kivork C, Seja E, Cherry G, Gutierrez AJ, Grogan TR, Mateus C, Tomasic G, Glaspy JA, Emerson RO, Robins H, Pierce RH, Elashoff DA, Robert C, Ribas A. PD-1 blockade induces responses by inhibiting adaptive immune resistance. Nature. 2014;515:568–71.
207. Hamid O, Schmidt H, Nissan A, Ridolfi L, Aamdal S, Hansson J, Guida M, Hyams DM, Gomez H, Bastholt L, Chasalow SD, Berman D. A prospective phase II trial exploring the association between tumor microenvironment biomarkers and clinical activity of ipilimumab in advanced melanoma. J Transl Med. 2011;9:204.
208. Martens A, Wistuba-Hamprecht K, Yuan J, Postow MA, Wong P, Capone M, Madonna G, Khammari A, Schilling B, Sucker A, Schadendorf D, Martus P, Dreno B, Ascierto PA, Wolchok JD, Pawelec G, Garbe C, Weide B. Increases in absolute lymphocytes and circulating $CD4^+$ and $CD8^+$ T cells are associated with positive clinical outcome of melanoma patients treated with ipilimumab. Clin Cancer Res. 2016;22:4848–58.
209. Galon J, Mlecnik B, Bindea G, Angell HK, Berger A, Lagorce C, Lugli A, Zlobec I, Hartmann A, Bifulco C, Nagtegaal ID, Palmqvist R, Masucci GV, Botti G, Tatangelo F, Delrio P, Maio M, Laghi L, Grizzi F, Asslaber M, D'Arrigo C, Vidal-Vanaclocha F, Zavadova E, Chouchane L, Ohashi PS, Hafezi-Bakhtiari S, Wouters BG, Roehrl M, Nguyen L, Kawakami Y, Hazama S, Okuno K, Ogino S, Gibbs P, Waring P, Sato N, Torigoe T, Itoh K, Patel PS, Shukla SN, Wang YL, Kopetz S, Sinicrope FA, Scripcariu V, Ascierto PA, Marincola FM, Fox BA, Pages F. Towards the introduction of the 'Immunoscore' in the classification of malignant tumours. J Pathol. 2014;232:199–209.
210. Mlecnik B, Van den Eynde M, Bindea G, Church SE, Vasaturo A, Fredriksen T, Lafontaine L, Haicheur N, Marliot F, Debetancourt D, Pairet G, Jouret-Mourin A, Gigot JF, Hubert C, Danse E, Dragean C, Carrasco J, Humblet Y, Valge-Archer V, Berger A, Pages F, Machiels JP, Galon J. Comprehensive intrametastatic immune quantification and major impact of immunoscore on survival. J Natl Cancer Inst. 2018;110:97–108.
211. Pagès F, Mlecnik B, Marliot F, Bindea G, Ou F-S, Bifulco C, Lugli A, Zlobec I, Rau TT, Berger MD, Nagtegaal ID, Vink-Börger E, Hartmann A, Geppert C, Kolwelter J, Merkel S, Grützmann R, Van den Eynde M, Jouret-Mourin A, Kartheuser A, Léonard D, Remue C, Wang JY, Bavi P, MHA R, Ohashi PS, Nguyen LT, Han S, HL MG, Hafezi-Bakhtiari S, Wouters BG, Masucci GV, Andersson EK, Zavadova E, Vocka M, Spacek J, Petruzelka L,

Konopasek B, Dundr P, Skalova H, Nemejcova K, Botti G, Tatangelo F, Delrio P, Ciliberto G, Maio M, Laghi L, Grizzi F, Fredriksen T, Buttard B, Angelova M, Vasaturo A, Maby P, Church SE, Angell HK, Lafontaine L, Bruni D, El Sissy C, Haicheur N, Kirilovsky A, Berger A, Lagorce C, Meyers JP, Paustian C, Feng Z, Ballesteros-Merino C, Dijkstra J, van de Water C, van Lent-van Vliet S, Knijn N, Muşină A-M, Scripcariu D-V, Popivanova B, Xu M, Fujita T, Hazama S, Suzuki N, Nagano H, Okuno K, Torigoe T, Sato N, Furuhata T, Takemasa I, Itoh K, Patel PS, Vora HH, Shah B, Patel JB, Rajvik KN, Pandya SJ, Shukla SN, Wang Y, Zhang G, Kawakami Y, Marincola FM, Ascierto PA, Sargent DJ, Fox BA, Galon J. International validation of the consensus immunoscore for the classification of colon cancer: a prognostic and accuracy study. Lancet. 2018;391:2128–39.

212. Haymaker CL, Kim D, Uemura M, Vence LM, Phillip A, McQuail N, Brown PD, Fernandez I, Hudgens CW, Creasy C, Hwu WJ, Sharma P, Tetzlaff MT, Allison JP, Hwu P, Bernatchez C, Diab A. Metastatic melanoma patient had a complete response with clonal expansion after whole brain radiation and PD-1 blockade. Cancer Immunol Res. 2017;5:100–5.

213. Olugbile S, Park J-H, Hoffman P, Szeto L, Patel J, Vigneswaran WT, Vokes E, Nakamura Y, Kiyotani K. Sustained oligoclonal T cell expansion correlates with durable response to immune checkpoint blockade in lung cancer. J Cancer Sci Ther. 2017;9:717–22.

214. Inoue H, Park JH, Kiyotani K, Zewde M, Miyashita A, Jinnin M, Kiniwa Y, Okuyama R, Tanaka R, Fujisawa Y, Kato H, Morita A, Asai J, Katoh N, Yokota K, Akiyama M, Ihn H, Fukushima S, Nakamura Y. Intratumoral expression levels of PD-L1, GZMA, and HLA-A along with oligoclonal T cell expansion associate with response to nivolumab in metastatic melanoma. Oncoimmunology. 2016;5:e1204507.

215. Rizvi NA, Hellmann MD, Snyder A, Kvistborg P, Makarov V, Havel JJ, Lee W, Yuan JD, Wong P, Ho TS, Miller ML, Rekhtman N, Moreira AL, Ibrahim F, Bruggeman C, Gasmi B, Zappasodi R, Maeda Y, Sander C, Garon EB, Merghoub T, Wolchok JD, Schumacher TN, Chan TA. Mutational landscape determines sensitivity to PD-1 blockade in non-small cell lung cancer. Science. 2015;348:124–8.

216. Snyder A, Makarov V, Merghoub T, Yuan J, Zaretsky JM, Desrichard A, Walsh LA, Postow MA, Wong P, Ho TS, Hollmann TJ, Bruggeman C, Kannan K, Li Y, Elipenahli C, Liu C, Harbison CT, Wang L, Ribas A, Wolchok JD, Chan TA. Genetic basis for clinical response to CTLA-4 blockade in melanoma. N Engl J Med. 2014;371:2189–99.

217. Hugo W, Zaretsky JM, Sun L, Song C, Moreno BH, Hu-Lieskovan S, Berent-Maoz B, Pang J, Chmielowski B, Cherry G, Seja E, Lomeli S, Kong X, Kelley MC, Sosman JA, Johnson DB, Ribas A, Lo RS. Genomic and transcriptomic features of response to anti-PD-1 therapy in metastatic melanoma. Cell. 2016;165:35–44.

218. Le DT, Uram JN, Wang H, Bartlett BR, Kemberling H, Eyring AD, Skora AD, Luber BS, Azad NS, Laheru D, Biedrzycki B, Donehower RC, Zaheer A, Fisher GA, Crocenzi TS, Lee JJ, Duffy SM, Goldberg RM, de la Chapelle A, Koshiji M, Bhaijee F, Huebner T, Hruban RH, Wood LD, Cuka N, Pardoll DM, Papadopoulos N, Kinzler KW, Zhou S, Cornish TC, Taube JM, Anders RA, Eshleman JR, Vogelstein B, Diaz LA Jr. PD-1 blockade in tumors with mismatch-repair deficiency. N Engl J Med. 2015;372:2509–20.

219. Alexandrov LB, Nik-Zainal S, Wedge DC, Aparicio SA, Behjati S, Biankin AV, Bignell GR, Bolli N, Borg A, Borresen-Dale AL, Boyault S, Burkhardt B, Butler AP, Caldas C, Davies HR, Desmedt C, Eils R, Eyfjord JE, Foekens JA, Greaves M, Hosoda F, Hutter B, Ilicic T, Imbeaud S, Imielinski M, Jager N, Jones DT, Jones D, Knappskog S, Kool M, Lakhani SR, Lopez-Otin C, Martin S, Munshi NC, Nakamura H, Northcott PA, Pajic M, Papaemmanuil E, Paradiso A, Pearson JV, Puente XS, Raine K, Ramakrishna M, Richardson AL, Richter J, Rosenstiel P, Schlesner M, Schumacher TN, Span PN, Teague JW, Totoki Y, Tutt AN, Valdes-Mas R, van Buuren MM, van't Veer L, Vincent-Salomon A, Waddell N, Yates LR, Zucman-Rossi J, Futreal PA, McDermott U, Lichter P, Meyerson M, Grimmond SM, Siebert R, Campo E, Shibata T, Pfister SM, Campbell PJ, Stratton MR. Signatures of mutational processes in human cancer. Nature. 2013;500:415–21.

220. Lastwika KJ, Wilson W, Li QK, Norris J, Xu HY, Ghazarian SR, Kitagawa H, Kawabata S, Taube JM, Yao S, Liu LN, Gills JJ, Dennis PA. Control of PD-L1 expression by oncogenic activation of the AKT-mTOR pathway in non-small cell lung cancer. Cancer Res. 2016;76:227–38.

221. Ribas A, Robert C, Hodi FS, Wolchok JD, Joshua AM, Hwu WJ, Weber JS, Zarour HM, Kefford R, Loboda A, Albright A, Kang SP, Ebbinghaus S, Yearley J, Murphy E, Nebozhyn M, Lunceford JK, McClanahan T, Ayers M, Daud A. Association of response to programmed death receptor 1 (PD-1) blockade with pembrolizumab (MK-3475) with an interferon-inflammatory immune gene signature. J Clin Oncol. 2015:33.
222. Ayers M, Lunceford J, Nebozhyn M, Murphy E, Loboda A, Albright A, Cheng J, Kang SP, Ebbinghaus S, Yearley J, Shankaran V, Seiwert T, Ribas A, McClanahan T. Relationship between immune gene signatures and clinical response to PD-1 blockade with pembrolizumab (MK-3475) in patients with advanced solid tumors. J Immunother Cancer. 2015;3:P80.
223. Higgs BW, Morehouse C, Streicher K, Rebelatto MC, Steele K, Jin X, Pilataxi F, Brohawn PZ, Blake-Haskins JA, Gupta AK, Ranade K. Relationship of baseline tumoral IFNγ mRNA and PD-L1 protein expression to overall survival in durvalumab-treated NSCLC patients. J Clin Oncol. 2016;34:3036.
224. Fehrenbacher L, Spira A, Ballinger M, Kowanetz M, Vansteenkiste J, Mazieres J, Park K, Smith D, Artal-Cortes A, Lewanski C, Braiteh F, Waterkamp D, He P, Zou W, Chen DS, Yi J, Sandler A, Rittmeyer A, Group PS. Atezolizumab versus docetaxel for patients with previously treated non-small-cell lung cancer (POPLAR): a multicentre, open-label, phase 2 randomised controlled trial. Lancet. 2016;387:1837–46.
225. Blank CU, Haanen JB, Ribas A, Schumacher TN. Cancer immunology. The "cancer immunogram". Science. 2016;352:658–60.
226. Karasaki T, Nagayama K, Kuwano H, Nitadori JI, Sato M, Anraku M, Hosoi A, Matsushita H, Morishita Y, Kashiwabara K, Takazawa M, Ohara O, Kakimi K, Nakajima J. An immunogram for the cancer-immunity cycle: towards personalized immunotherapy of lung cancer. J Thorac Oncol. 2017;12:791–803.
227. Martens A, Wistuba-Hamprecht K, Geukes Foppen M, Yuan J, Postow MA, Wong P, Romano E, Khammari A, Dreno B, Capone M, Ascierto PA, Di Giacomo AM, Maio M, Schilling B, Sucker A, Schadendorf D, Hassel JC, Eigentler TK, Martus P, Wolchok JD, Blank C, Pawelec G, Garbe C, Weide B. Baseline peripheral blood biomarkers associated with clinical outcome of advanced melanoma patients treated with ipilimumab. Clin Cancer Res. 2016;22:2908–18.
228. Hopkins AM, Rowland A, Kichenadasse G, Wiese MD, Gurney H, McKinnon RA, Karapetis CS, Sorich MJ. Predicting response and toxicity to immune checkpoint inhibitors using routinely available blood and clinical markers. Br J Cancer. 2017;117:913–20.
229. Manson G, Norwood J, Marabelle A, Kohrt H, Houot R. Biomarkers associated with checkpoint inhibitors. Ann Oncol. 2016;27:1199–206.
230. Delyon J, Mateus C, Lefeuvre D, Lanoy E, Zitvogel L, Chaput N, Roy S, Eggermont AMM, Routier E, Robert C. Experience in daily practice with ipilimumab for the treatment of patients with metastatic melanoma: an early increase in lymphocyte and eosinophil counts is associated with improved survival. Ann Oncol. 2013;24:1697–703.
231. Ku GY, Yuan JD, Page DB, Schroeder SEA, Panageas KS, Carvajal RD, Chapman PB, Schwartz GK, Allison JP, Wolchok JD. Single-institution experience with ipilimumab in advanced melanoma patients in the compassionate use setting lymphocyte count after 2 doses correlates with survival. Cancer. 2010;116:1767–75.
232. Wilgenhof S, Du Four S, Vandenbroucke F, Everaert H, Salmon I, Lienard D, Marmol VD, Neyns B. Single-center experience with ipilimumab in an expanded access program for patients with pretreated advanced melanoma. J Immunother. 2013;36:215–22.
233. Di Giacomo AM, Danielli R, Calabro L, Bertocci E, Nannicini C, Giannarelli D, Balestrazzi A, Vigni F, Riversi V, Miracco C, Biagioli M, Altomonte M, Maio M. Ipilimumab experience in heavily pretreated patients with melanoma in an expanded access program at the University Hospital of Siena (Italy). Cancer Immunol Immunother. 2011;60:467–77.
234. Simeone E, Gentilcore G, Giannarelli D, Grimaldi AM, Caraco C, Curvietto M, Esposito A, Paone M, Palla M, Cavalcanti E, Sandomenico F, Petrillo A, Botti G, Fulciniti F, Palmieri G, Queirolo P, Marchetti P, Ferraresi V, Rinaldi G, Pistillo MP, Ciliberto G, Mozzillo N, Ascierto PA. Immunological and biological changes during ipilimumab treatment and their potential correlation with clinical response and survival in patients with advanced melanoma. Cancer Immunol Immunother. 2014;63:675–83.

235. Gebhardt C, Sevko A, Jiang HH, Lichtenberger R, Reith M, Tarnanidis K, Holland-Letz T, Umansky L, Beckhove P, Sucker A, Schadendorf D, Utikal J, Umansky V. Myeloid cells and related chronic inflammatory factors as novel predictive markers in melanoma treatment with ipilimumab. Clin Cancer Res. 2015;21:5453–9.
236. Kelderman S, Heemskerk B, van Tinteren H, van den Brom RR, Hospers GA, van den Eertwegh AJ, Kapiteijn EW, de Groot JW, Soetekouw P, Jansen RL, Fiets E, Furness AJ, Renn A, Krzystanek M, Szallasi Z, Lorigan P, Gore ME, Schumacher TN, Haanen JB, Larkin JM, Blank CU. Lactate dehydrogenase as a selection criterion for ipilimumab treatment in metastatic melanoma. Cancer Immunol Immunother. 2014;63:449–58.
237. Lee JH, Long GV, Boyd S, Lo S, Menzies AM, Tembe V, Guminski A, Jakrot V, Scolyer RA, Mann GJ, Kefford RF, Carlino MS, Rizos H. Circulating tumour DNA predicts response to anti-PD1 antibodies in metastatic melanoma. Ann Oncol. 2017;28:1130–6.
238. Kamphorst AO, Pillai RN, Yang S, Nasti TH, Akondy RS, Wieland A, Sica GL, Yu K, Koenig L, Patel NT, Behera M, Wu H, McCausland M, Chen ZJ, Zhang C, Khuri FR, Owonikoko TK, Ahmed R, Ramalingam SS. Proliferation of PD-1+CD8 T cells in peripheral blood after PD-1-targeted therapy in lung cancer patients. Proc Natl Acad Sci U S A. 2017;114:4993–8.
239. Gopalakrishnan V, Spencer CN, Nezi L, Reuben A, Andrews MC, Karpinets TV, Prieto PA, Vicente D, Hoffman K, Wei SC, Cogdill AP, Zhao L, Hudgens CW, Hutchinson DS, Manzo T, de Macedo MP, Cotechini T, Kumar T, Chen WS, Reddy SM, Sloane RS, Galloway-Pena J, Jiang H, Chen PL, Shpall EJ, Rezvani K, Alousi AM, Chemaly RF, Shelburne S, Vence LM, Okhuysen PC, Jensen VB, Swennes AG, McAllister F, Sanchez EMR, Zhang Y, Le Chatelier E, Zitvogel L, Pons N, Austin-Breneman JL, Haydu LE, Burton EM, Gardner JM, Sirmans E, Hu J, Lazar AJ, Tsujikawa T, Diab A, Tawbi H, Glitza IC, Hwu WJ, Patel SP, Woodman SE, Amaria RN, Davies MA, Gershenwald JE, Hwu P, Lee JE, Zhang J, Coussens LM, Cooper ZA, Futreal PA, Daniel CR, Ajami NJ, Petrosino JF, Tetzlaff MT, Sharma P, Allison JP, Jenq RR, Wargo JA. Gut microbiome modulates response to anti-PD-1 immunotherapy in melanoma patients. Science. 2018;359:97–103.
240. Topalian SL, Taube JM, Anders RA, Pardoll DM. Mechanism-driven biomarkers to guide immune checkpoint blockade in cancer therapy. Nat Rev Cancer. 2016;16:275–87.

第 2 章

黑色素瘤的免疫治疗

Isabella C. Glitza Oliva, Rana Alqusairi

译者：王 琪 赵 静

摘要 虽然黑色素瘤比其他皮肤癌更少见，但是仅在美国，每年黑色素瘤就造成近 10 000 人死亡。数十年来，对于转移性黑色素瘤患者，可用的治疗方案非常有限。然而，最近的突破为患者和供应商带来了新的希望。虽然 BRAF 和 MEK 抑制剂靶向治疗转移性黑色素瘤具有重要意义，但是本章回顾过去和当前可用的治疗选择，重点关注仍基于免疫治疗的方法。另外，我们综述了已切除的Ⅲ期和Ⅳ期黑色素瘤患者辅助治疗的最新进展结果，以及黑色素瘤脑转移患者辅助治疗的最新进展。最后，我们对免疫肿瘤学和黑色素瘤领域当前研究工作进行了简要概述。

关键词 黑色素瘤 免疫治疗 伊匹木单抗 帕博利珠单抗 纳武利尤单抗 CTLA-4 PD-1 PD-L1 辅助治疗 脑转移

引言

黑色素瘤是黑色素细胞恶性增殖的结果，主要在皮肤中可见，在葡萄膜、胃肠黏膜、泌尿生殖系统黏膜及脑膜或中枢神经系统中也可见[1]。尽管黑色素瘤仅占皮肤癌 1% 的比例，但它却是造成皮肤癌患者死亡的主要原因[1,2]，而且黑色素瘤年发病率在全世界范围内逐渐增加[3,4]。虽然发病率增加可能是由于人们对皮肤癌

I. C. Glitza Oliva (✉)
The University of Texas MD Anderson Cancer Center, Houston, TX, USA
e-mail: ICGlitza@mdanderson.org

R. Alqusairi
Baltimore, MD, USA

© Springer Nature Switzerland AG 2018
A. Naing, J. Hajjar (eds.), *Immunotherapy*, Advances in Experimental Medicine and Biology 995, https://doi.org/10.1007/978-3-030-02505-2_2

意识增强及早期检测引起的，但是日照相关行为如室内暴晒等导致了黑色素瘤发病率增加[2]。根据美国癌症协会的数据，2018年仅在美国有91 270例新发黑色素瘤患者，预计将有9320人死亡[5]。黑色素瘤可以影响任何人，但如皮肤白皙、紫外线辐射（日晒、晒黑床）、早期晒伤史、发育不良或非典型痣、50个或更多的小痣和家族性发育不良痣综合征等风险增加了黑色素瘤发生的可能性[6,7]。重要的是要注意到一点，虽然黑色素瘤可能与先前存在的痣相关，但约70%的病例可以从头发展（即不是从已有的色素病变中发展而来）[8][2]。黑色素瘤的预后与许多因素有关，如晚期、深度（厚度超过4mm）、高龄、男性及发病位置（胸部和背部）都与预后较差相关[3]。生存率主要取决于肿瘤分期，5年生存率：Ⅰ期和Ⅱ期98%，Ⅲ期62%，Ⅳ期18%[9,10]。

手术治疗是早期黑色素瘤治疗的主要手段，且有高度可能性通过手术治愈。基于原发黑色素瘤深度及存在溃疡，初次手术可能需要行前哨淋巴结活检以用于分期评估。对于晚期和不可切除的黑色素瘤患者，全身治疗为主要治疗方式。然而自2011年以来，我们已经看到转移性黑色素瘤治疗领域发生了重大变化，这种改变改善了大量患者的预后结果。

应该提到的是，我们也看到了黑色素瘤应用靶向治疗的显著成果，但本章的重点是总结转移性黑色素瘤免疫治疗方法的过去、现在和未来。

---

1 "Melanoma: Statistics   Cancer.Net." https://www.cancer.net/cancer-types/melanoma/statistics. Accessed 6 Feb. 2018.

2 "Cancer Facts & Figures 2017—American Cancer Society." https://www.cancer.org/content/dam/cancer-org/research/cancer-facts-and-statistics/annual-cancer-facts-and-figures/2017/cancerfacts-and-figures-2017.pdf. Accessed 6 Feb. 2018.

3 "Melanoma: Statistics   Cancer.Net." https://www.cancer.net/cancer-types/melanoma/statistics. Accessed 6 Feb. 2018.

4 "Skin Cancer Screening（PDQ®）—NCBI—NIH." 30 Nov. 2017，https://www.ncbi.nlm.nih.gov/books/NBK65861/. Accessed 6 Feb. 2018.

5 "Key Statistics for Melanoma Skin Cancer—American Cancer Society." 4 Jan. 2018，https://www.cancer.org/cancer/melanoma-skin-cancer/about/key-statistics.html. Accessed 6 Feb. 2018.

6 "Cancer Facts & Figures 2017—American Cancer Society." https://www.cancer.org/content/dam/ cancer-org/research/ cancer-facts-and-statistics/annual-cancer-facts-and-figures/2017/cancerfacts-and-figures-2017.pdf. Accessed 6 Feb. 2018.

7 "Meta-analysis of risk factors for cutaneous melanoma: I. Common and …" http://www.ejcancer.com/article/S0959-8049（04）00832-9/fulltext. Accessed 6 Feb. 2018.

8 "Skin Cancer Screening（PDQ®）—NCBI—NIH." 30 Nov. 2017，https://www.ncbi.nlm.nih.gov/books/NBK65861/. Accessed 6 Feb. 2018.

9 "Melanoma: Statistics | Cancer.Net." https://www.cancer.net/cancer-types/melanoma/statistics. Accessed 6 Feb. 2018.

10 "Cancer Facts & Figures 2017—American Cancer Society." https://www.cancer.org/content/dam/cancer-org/research/cancer-facts-and-statistics/annual-cancer-facts-and-figures/2017/cancerfacts-and-figures-2017.pdf. Accessed 6 Feb. 2018.

截至 2011 年的黑色素瘤治疗方案历史

高剂量白细胞介素-2

白细胞介素-2（IL-2）是一种 T 淋巴细胞生长因子，促进 T 淋巴细胞增殖和细胞毒活性[4]。这是第一个接受调节的免疫疗法，基于持久的客观缓解，于 1998 年被批准用于治疗转移性黑色素瘤。

1985~1993 年，对 270 例接受高剂量 IL-2（HD IL-2）治疗的黑色素瘤患者进行了汇总分析。整体客观缓解率（ORR）为 16%[CR6%，PR10%]。重要的是，30 个月仍存在持续缓解，治疗效果在患者中没有出现进展[5]。

45 例肾细胞癌患者和 245 例黑色素瘤患者接受 HD IL-2 治疗的回顾性分析得出中位 OS 为 16.8 个月[6]。具有良好治疗反应的患者没有达到中位 OS。与进展性疾病（PD）患者相比，稳定疾病（SD）患者中位 OS 为 38.2 个月，PD 患者中位 OS 为 7.9 个月。在达到 PR 或 CR 的患者中，3 年 OS 为 78%。

HD IL-2 的显著毒性需要密切监测并限制其特定中心的使用[7]。大多数患者发生的不良反应主要有低血压、肾功能损害、呼吸短促、肺部和全身水肿，以及被认为是由毛细血管引起的渗漏综合征和淋巴细胞渗透导致的神经精神改变。然而，毒副作用通常会在停止治疗之后消退。

化疗

1975~2011 年，达卡巴嗪（DTIC）是大多数黑色素瘤患者唯一可用的治疗方法，尽管其疗效有限。虽然报道 ORR 高达 20%，但 CR 很少见（3%~4%），缓解时间相当短（中位数 5~6 个月），只有 1%~2% 的患者长期存活[8,9]。不良反应通常是可控的，包括骨髓抑制、轻微恶心、呕吐、轻微脱发、疲劳，但大多数相关患者的报道表明他们能够维持可接受的生活质量[10,11]。

DTIC 的类似物替莫唑胺（TMZ）具有穿透脑屏障（BBB）的能力且具有一定的抗肿瘤活性[11-13]。一项随机临床Ⅲ期试验对 305 例单纯转移性黑色素瘤患者进行 DTIC 和 TMZ 的生存比较，两者的中位 OS 相似，TMZ 治疗组是 7.7 个月，DTIC 治疗组是 6.4 个月[危险比（HR）=1.18；95%置信区间（CI），0.92~1.52][14]。两组患者中位无进展生存期（PFS）均较短，TMZ 组（1.9 个月）或 DTIC 组（1.5 个月）间差异有统计学意义（P=0.012；HR=1.37；95%置信区间，1.07~1.75）。重要的是，TMZ 和 DTIC 具有相似的安全性，轻微至中度恶心呕吐、非累积性短暂的骨髓抑制是最常见的毒性之一。

卡铂与紫杉醇联合应用的 II 期临床试验结果表明，该方案对转移性黑色素瘤患者有一定的临床疗效。在 II 期试验初期，纳入 17 例没有接受过卡铂治疗或紫杉烷类化合物治疗的患者[15]。紫杉醇的剂量为 175mg/m^2，含卡铂[曲线下面积（AUC）7.5]。只有 15 例患者是可评估的，其中两例由于过敏反应被剔除研究。PR 率为 20%，该部分患者中 SD 占 47%。3 或 4 级血液毒性是常见的不良事件（AE）（$n=11$），但所有治疗相关毒性均为可逆的，无治疗相关死亡事件。

该方案作为二线治疗也显示出一定的疗效。既往治疗包括 TMZ 或 DTIC[16]。本回顾性研究对 31 例转移性黑色素瘤患者进行了评估。患者每周接受紫杉醇（100mg/m^2）和卡铂（AUC2）治疗，PR 率为 26%（$n=8$）和 SD 为 19%（$n=6$），病情稳定。中位缓解时间为 5.7 个月（范围为 2.5~7.3 个月）。未观察到意外毒性事件。

紫杉醇钠（Abraxane）是紫杉醇蛋白结合制剂。在一项 II 期临床试验中，评估了紫杉醇钠单一药物的疗效。该试验纳入了既往未接受治疗（$n=37$）或以前接受过治疗的患者（$n=37$）[17]。紫杉醇钠治疗方案：100mg/m^2，一周 3 次，共 4 周（以前治疗过的患者）或 150mg/m^2（初次化疗的患者）。既往未经治疗的患者反应率较高（21.6%vs.2.7%），然而，中位 PFS 分别为 4.5 个月和 3.5 个月，中位 OS 分别为 9.6 个月和 12.1 个月。3 级或 4 级毒性包括神经病变、脱发、中性粒细胞减少和疲劳。

在一个平行的 II 期试验中检测了紫杉醇钠（100mg/m^2）联合卡铂（AUC 2）的疗效。该试验纳入了之前治疗过的患者（$n=34$，超过 90%的患者曾接受过 DTIC 或 TMZ 治疗）和未接受过治疗的患者（$n=39$）[18]。在未接受过治疗的患者中，25.6%的患者有缓解（1 例 CR，9 例 PR；90% CI，16.7%~42.3%）。既往接受过化疗的患者中 8.8%达到部分缓解（3 例 PR；90% CI，2.5%~21.3%）。两组患者中位 PFS 相似（初次化疗组：4.5 个月；既往接受治疗组：4.1 个月），中位 OS 相似（分别为 11.1 个月和 10.9 个月）。毒性包括血小板减少、神经敏感问题、疲劳、恶心、呕吐。

在一项 II 期临床试验中[19]，顺铂、长春花碱、DTIC 三联化疗（CVD）显示出明显的抗肿瘤活性。转移性黑色素瘤患者接受长春花碱[1.6mg/（m^2·d），连续 5 天]、DTIC（800mg/m^2，第 1 天）和顺铂[20mg/（m^2·d），4 天]治疗。50 例可评估的患者中，4%（$n=2$）的患者达到 CR，36%（$n=18$）的患者达到 PR，平均缓解时间为 9 个月。对于有反应患者，中位 OS 为 12 个月。观察到显著的毒性，剂量限制毒性包括周围神经病变。

在 CVD 方案中添加 IL-2 和干扰素，该治疗被生物化学（BCT）标记。在 III 期试验中[20]，BCT 与 CVD 直接比较，入选的患者要么是未接受治疗的，要么是接受过辅助性干扰素治疗的，共评估 395 例患者（CVD，$n=195$；BCT，$n=200$）。

BCT 的反应率仅在数值上较高（19.5% vs.13.8%），但 BCT 组的中位 PFS 明显高于 CVD 组（4.8 个月 vs.2.9 个月；$P = 0.015$）。值得注意的是，PFS 的改善并没有转化为更长时间的 OS（9.0 个月 vs.8.7 个月），也没有转化为更高的 1 年生存率（41% vs.36.9%）。此外，3 级和 4 级毒性在 BCT 治疗组更常见（95% vs. 73%；$P = 0.001$）。

虽然目前很少在前线使用化疗，但许多试验正在探索化疗药物联合免疫治疗的有效性（如 NCT02617849、NCT01827111、NCT01676649）。

最后，作为孤立肢体灌注（ISP）的一部分，马法兰被用于局部转移的转移瘤患者已经数十年[21]。虽然在新的有效的靶向治疗和免疫治疗时代，它的使用已经显著减少，但需要指出的是，马法兰基础的 ILP（M-ILP）导致 40%～50%完全缓解，75%～80%的患者整体缓解[22]。当肿瘤坏死因子（TNF）加到马法兰方案中时，该方案的效果更佳（TM-ILP）[21]。

过继细胞疗法

过继细胞疗法（ACT）是一种使用患者自体衍生的 T 淋巴细胞为患者量身定制的治疗方法。虽然这种方法已经使用了数十年，但它的使用受到限制，需要专门的实验室和医院单位能够处理 HD IL-2 毒副作用，因为 HD IL-2 通常与 T 淋巴细胞产物联合使用[23]。

1994 年报道了一些使用自体 TIL 治疗转移性黑色素瘤的试验[24]。所有患者的 ORR 为 34%，而不良反应影响主要来自 HD-IL。另一项临床试验报道了 35 例转移性黑色素瘤患者的缓解率为 51%（9%CR）。治疗前接受 HD IL-2 联合化疗或两者单独均可。所有患者都在 T 淋巴细胞输注治疗前使用氟达拉滨和环磷酰胺进行了预处理，使淋巴细胞衰竭。平均反应时间为（11.5±2.2）个月[25]。自此，不同的方法被开发和检测以改善过继细胞疗法的疗效和毒性。目前正在进行多项临床试验（如 NCT02652455 和 NCT01955460）[26,27]。

免疫检查点抑制剂

检查点抑制剂（CPI）的发展已经彻底改变了转移性黑色素瘤的治疗方法，这些药物现在已成功地用于各种其他类型的癌症。然而，对 T 淋巴细胞信号转导机制的研究早在数十年前就开始了[28]。细胞毒性 T 淋巴细胞相关蛋白 4（CTLA-4）于 1987 年被发现，与 CD28 竞争性结合 CD80（B7-1）和 CD86（B7-2）[29]。CTLA-4 通过与 B7 蛋白（刺激 T 淋巴细胞所必需的蛋白）竞争性结合，下调 T 淋巴细胞活化的通路。最近，也有研究表明，抗 CTLA-4 诱导 ICOS⁺Th1 样 CD4 效应器细胞群的扩增意味着其与程序性细胞死亡蛋白 1（PD-1）抗体所参与的细胞通路不同，从而导致特异性肿瘤浸润耗竭样 CD8⁺T 淋巴细胞亚群的扩增[30]。与 CTLA-4 相似，PD-1 负调控抗肿瘤反应。

迄今为止，一种 CTLA-4 抗体（伊匹木单抗）和两种 PD-1 抗体已经获得了治疗黑色素瘤及其他类型癌症的监管批准。

伊匹木单抗

伊匹木单抗是一种完全人源的单克隆 IgG1 抗体，可抑制 CTLA-4。伊匹木单抗最初于 2011 年被 FDA 批准用于治疗无法切除的转移性黑色素瘤。

在一项随机、双盲、Ⅲ期研究中，676 例患者分别接受伊匹木单抗联合 gp100 肽疫苗、单独接受 gp100 或单独接受伊匹木单抗治疗，比例为 3∶1∶1[31]。伊匹木单抗联合 gp100 组的 OS（10.0 个月）明显长于单独接受 gp100 组（6.4 个月，$P<0.001$），且两个伊匹木单抗组间 OS 无差异（伊匹木单抗联合 gp100 组，HR=1.04；$P=0.76$）。单独接受伊匹木单抗组的 RR 为 10.9%，疾病控制率为 28.5%。在单独接受伊匹木单抗或伊匹木单抗联合 gp100 治疗的患者中，约 60% 发生了免疫相关的事件（相比之下，单独接受 gp100 组占 32%）。

在另一项Ⅲ期试验中，502 例未经治疗的转移性黑色素瘤患者被随机分配到伊匹木单抗（10mg/kg）+DTIC（850mg/m²）组（$n=250$）和 DTIC+安慰剂组（$n=252$）。伊匹木单抗+DTIC 组反应率（CR+PR）为 15.2%，而 DTIC+安慰剂组的反应率为 10.3%（$P=0.09$）。增加伊匹木单抗导致中位 OS 较 DTIC 安慰剂组显著延长，OS 分别为 11.2 个月和 9.1 个月（伊匹木单抗+DTIC 组死亡 HR 为 0.72；$P<0.001$）[32]。联合治疗导致更多的 3 级和 4 级毒性（56.3% vs.27.5%），最常见的 4 级毒性是肝酶升高。

此外，伊匹木单抗目前正在进行各种组合的临床试验，包括与化疗、放疗、疫苗和细胞因子（NCT02644967、NCT02259231、NCT02307149、NCT02203604、NCT02073123、NCT01940809、NCT03297463），以及与另一种 CPI（纳武利尤单抗，见下文）的组合。

一项回顾性研究试图在接受过 CPI 治疗的患者中确定 HD IL-2 是否有作用。作者发现 52 例转移性黑色素瘤患者接受过伊匹木单抗和 HD IL-2 治疗，272 例患者在接受 HD IL-2 治疗先前没有接受过 CPI 治疗[33]。先前使用伊匹木单抗与未使用 CPI 的患者的中位 OS 相似（19.3 个月 vs.19.4 个月），但是 HD IL-2 导致伊匹木单抗治疗患者的反应率更高（21% vs.12%）。两组之间的毒性相似，但 CTLA-4 诱发的结肠炎仍然是一个值得关注的问题。

PD-1 抑制剂

程序性细胞死亡蛋白 1（PD-1），是 T 淋巴细胞活性的负调控因子，通过过度暴露于肿瘤抗原的 T 淋巴细胞表达，其主要配体 PD-L1 常在癌细胞和 TIL 中表达[34]，另一种配体 PD-L2 主要由抗原提呈细胞（APC）表达。这两种配体都属于 B7 蛋白家族。PD-1 过表达、肿瘤细胞和 TIL 上的 PD-L1 的过表达，两者与某些肿瘤类型的疾病结局之间存在关联[35]。

纳武利尤单抗

纳武利尤单抗是一种针对 PD-1 的完全人源免疫球蛋白 IgG4 单克隆抗体，2014 年被批准用于转移性黑色素瘤的治疗。

在Ⅲ期随机双盲对照研究 Checkmate-066 中，418 例之前没有接受治疗且没有 *BRAF* 突变的转移性黑色素瘤患者被随机分配接受纳武利尤单抗（3mg/kg）和 DTIC 匹配的安慰剂治疗，或 DTIC（1000mg/m^2）和纳武利尤单抗匹配的安慰剂治疗[36]。纳武利尤单抗治疗组总有效率为 40%（95% CI，33.3~47.0），其中超过 7% 的患者达到完全缓解，而 DTIC 组总有效率为 13.9%（95% CI，9.5~19.4），以及 1% 的患者达到完全缓解。令人兴奋的是，纳武利尤单抗组 1 年 OS 为 72.9%，而 DTIC 组为 42.1%。纳武利尤单抗在 3 级和 4 级不良事件方面也优于 DTIC。

伊匹木单抗联合纳武利尤单抗

基于 CTLA-4 或 PD-1 免疫检查点抑制剂单药治疗的黑色素瘤患者的结果，以及对 T 淋巴细胞活化的更好理解，我们对伊匹木单抗和纳武利尤单抗联合和 CTLA-4 单药进行了试验。Checkmate-069 是一个双盲Ⅱ期研究，将 142 例以前未经治疗转移性黑色素瘤患者随机分配（以 2∶1 的比例），接受伊匹木单抗 3mg/kg 联合纳武利尤单抗 1mg/kg 或安慰剂，每 3 周 1 次，共 4 次，然后继续接受纳武利尤单抗 3mg/kg 或安慰剂治疗，每 2 周 1 次[37]。联合组总 RR 为 56%，22% 的患者达到 CR。与之前的报道相似，与纳武利尤单抗相比，伊匹木单抗患者的 RR 仅为 11%（$P<0.0001$），且没有患者达到完全缓解。中位随访时间为 24.5 个月（IQR 9.1~25.7），伊匹木单抗+纳武利尤单抗组未达到中位 PFS，仅 CTLA-4 组为 3.0 个月（95% CI，2.7~5.1）（HR=0.36，95% CI，0.22~0.56；$P<0.0001$）。在联合用药组中，49% 的患者因毒性而停止应用研究药物，而伊匹木单抗组这一比例为 22%。接受伊匹木单抗和纳武利尤单抗治疗的患者中，54% 的患者被报道了 3 级或 4 级

不良事件,而接受伊匹木单抗单药治疗的患者中,这一比例为 24%。

在一项大型、随机、双盲、Ⅲ期研究中(Checkmate-067),共有 945 例之前未接受治疗的患者以 1∶1∶1 比例被随机分配,接受纳武利尤单抗单药、纳武利尤单抗联合伊匹木单抗或伊匹木单抗单药治疗。纳武利尤单抗 3mg/kg,每 2 周 1 次(加上伊匹木单抗配伍的安慰剂),或纳武利尤单抗 1mg/kg 联合伊匹木单抗 3mg/kg,每 3 周 1 次,共 4 次(加上纳武利尤单抗配伍的安慰剂),然后继续接受 3mg/kg 纳武利尤单抗,每 2 周 1 次,进行至少 3 周期,或伊匹木单抗 3mg/kg 每 3 周 1 次,共 4 次剂量(加上纳武利尤单抗配伍安慰剂)[38]。总体反应率在伊匹木单抗组为 19%(2.2% CR),在纳武利尤单抗组为 43.7%(8.9% CR),在纳武利尤单抗和伊匹木单抗联合组为 57.6%(11.5%)。与伊匹木单抗组(2.9 个月)相比,联合用药组 PFS 明显延长(11.5 个月;死亡或疾病进展的 HR=0.42;99.5%CI,0.31~0.57;$P<0.001$),纳武利尤单抗组(6.9 个月;HR=0.74;95% CI,0.60~0.92)。与预期一样,联合用药组(55.0%)较单药组出现更多与治疗相关的 3 级和 4 级不良事件[纳武利尤单抗组(16.3%);伊匹木单抗组(27.3%)]。

帕博利珠单抗

帕博利珠单抗是第二种完全人源化的针对 PD-1 受体的 IgG4 抗体,目前已获得监管批准。它已经被 FDA 批准在多种不同的肿瘤类型中使用。在一个多中心Ⅱ期研究中(KEYNOTE-002),540 例曾接受过治疗的患者被随机分配(1∶1∶1)进入试验组,分别接受帕博利珠单抗 2mg/kg($n=180$)和 10mg/kg($n=181$),每 3 周 1 次,进行 4 次,或化疗(紫杉醇+卡铂、紫杉醇、卡铂、DTIC 或口服替莫唑胺;$n=179$)[39]。在帕博利珠单抗组观察到更高的有效率(2mg/kg 组:21%;10mg/kg 组:25%),而化疗组有效率为 4%。化疗组 3 级和 4 级不良事件发生率较高(26%),帕博利珠单抗组(2mg/kg 组:11%;10mg/kg 组:14%)。不出所料,在接受化疗的患者中观察到的最常见的 3 级或 4 级治疗相关不良事件为贫血、疲劳、中性粒细胞减少症和白细胞减少症,但在帕博利珠单抗组中,3 级或 4 级治疗相关不良事件极其罕见。

与伊匹木单抗相比,帕博利珠单抗显示出更好的客观结果。KEYNOTE-006 是一个Ⅲ期研究,该研究纳入了 834 例转移性黑色素瘤患者,患者随机(1∶1∶1)接受帕博利珠单抗(10mg/kg,每 2 周 1 次或每 3 周 1 次)或 4 倍剂量的伊匹木单抗(3mg/kg,每 3 周 1 次)治疗[40]。大多数患者是初次治疗。与伊匹木单抗组相比,帕博利珠单抗组的有效率更高(帕博利珠单抗组:每 2 周 1 次组为 33.7%,每 3 周 1 次组为 32.9%;伊匹木单抗组:11.9%)。帕博利珠单抗组 6 个月 PFS 接近 47%,而伊匹木单抗组 6 个月 PFS 为 26.5%。除了改善总体生存率外,帕博利珠单抗组 12 个月 OS 为 74.1%，而伊匹木单抗组 12 个月 OS 为 58.2%。没有发现罕见的毒性反应，常见的不良反应包括疲劳、腹泻、皮疹、瘙痒和免疫相关内分泌紊乱。与甲状腺相关的内分泌事件在帕博利珠单抗组更为常见，而在伊匹木单抗组结肠炎和垂体炎更为常见。帕博利珠单抗两组（每 2 周 1 次、每 3 周 1 次）、伊匹木单抗治疗的患者中发生 3~5 级不良事件概率分别是 13.3%、10.1%、19.9%。总体来说，帕博利珠单抗组比伊匹木单抗组具有更少的高级别不良事件。

KEYNOTE-029（Ib 期试验）报道了 153 例没有接受过 CPI 治疗的黑色素瘤患者的试验结果[41]。前期接受靶向治疗或化疗都是允许纳入的，但 87% 的患者是初次治疗。患者静脉常规剂量帕博利珠单抗（2mg/kg）联合伊匹木单抗（1mg/kg），4 个疗程后用帕博利珠单抗（2mg/kg）维持治疗。客观缓解率达到 61%（95% CI，53~69），完全缓解率为 15%，预估 1 年 PFS 为 69%（95%CI，60%~75%），预估 1 年总生存率为 89%（95% CI，83~93）。45% 的患者会出现 3 级和 4 级毒性反应，最常见的是皮肤反应（8%）、结肠炎（7%）和肝炎（6%）。但值得注意的是，当比较低剂量伊匹木单抗联合常规剂量帕博利珠单抗和低剂量纳武利尤单抗联合常规剂量伊匹木单抗的毒性数据时，低剂量伊匹木单抗联合常规剂量帕博利珠单抗的 3 级和 4 级毒性频率较低（Checkmate-069）。

PD-L1

针对 PD-L1 的抗体已在转移性黑色素瘤患者中进行了测试，这些抗体可以阻止 PD-L1 与其受体 PD-1 和 B7.1 结合。阿特珠单抗（或 MPDL3280A）是人类 IgG1 单克隆抗体，在 I 期试验中，对 45 例转移性黑色素瘤患者进行了不同剂量水平的阿特珠单抗治疗。近 2/3 的患者曾经接受过系统治疗（http：//ascopubs.org/doi/abs/10.1200/jco.2013.31.15_suppl.9010）。该试验结果显示总有效率为 26%，24 周的无进展生存为 35%。33% 的患者出现 3 级和 4 级毒副反应，包括高血糖（7%）和 ALT/AST 升高（7% 和 4%）。此外，MPDL3280A 也与靶向治疗联合进行了测试（http：//ascopubs.org/doi/abs/10.1200/jco.2013.31.15_suppl.9010）。虽然目前批准的三种 PD-L1 药物（阿特珠单抗、阿维鲁单抗和度伐鲁单抗）迄今还没有一种被批准用于治疗转移性黑色素瘤，但 PD-L1 抑制剂的多重联合试验正在进行中（NCT02535078、NCT02639026、NCT03273153、NCT03178851）。

肿瘤内疫苗接种

多种肿瘤内疫苗接种方法已在晚期黑色素瘤治疗方面进行了试验。这些疫苗的作用目的是引起对黑色素瘤肿瘤细胞表达抗原的免疫反应，如肿瘤相关抗原

(TAA)或突变源抗原(新抗原)。已经鉴定出多种 TAA,如黑色素瘤抗原 A1(MAGE-A1)、gp100 或 T 淋巴细胞识别的黑色素瘤抗原(mat-1/Melan-A)[42]。然而,单个方法获得的结果并不足以鼓舞人心,相比联合治疗方式可能更有希望。例如,联合高剂量 IL-2 检测到了一种合成多肽 gp100[43],它携带的免疫原性表位可被 T 淋巴细胞识别,从而诱导抗肿瘤活性。在本Ⅲ期试验中,185 例转移性黑色素瘤患者(允许既往接受过化疗、干扰素和低剂量 IL-2 治疗)随机分配接受 HD IL-2 单药或 gp100 和 HD IL-2 联合治疗。单纯接受 HD IL-2 治疗的患者有效率为 10%,联合应用 HD IL-2 治疗的患者有效率为 20%($P = 0.05$)。单纯接受 HD IL-2 的患者中位 OS 为 11.1 个月,联合治疗的患者中位 OS 为 17.8 个月($P = 0.06$)。两组毒副作用相似,然而与单纯 HD IL-2 组相比,疫苗/HD IL-2 组患者出现更多的心律失常、实验室检测结果异常和更多的神经事件。

PV-10 孟加拉玫瑰红

玫瑰红(RB)是一种水溶性可注射碘化荧光素衍生物。细胞内注射 PV-10 后,PV-10 在肿瘤溶酶体内蓄积,使肿瘤细胞快速裂解,暴露于电离辐射下可产生细胞毒性活性氧。PV-10 也可通过刺激抗肿瘤免疫反应对抗远处病灶[44]。在Ⅱ期研究中,80 例难治性Ⅲ期和Ⅳ期黑色素瘤患者接受病灶内 PV-10 治疗,总有效率为 51%(CR 率为 26%),其中 8%的患者在 52 周后无复发迹象[45]。重要的是,未注射性病变也表现出病灶消退。毒副反应良好,无治疗相关 4 级不良反应。最近发表的前瞻性Ⅱ期试验报告显示[46],45 例接受治疗的患者 ORR 为 87%(CR 率为 42%)。完全缓解与注射 PV-10 时少于 15 个转移病灶有关。PV-10 目前还没有被 FDA 批准用于转移性黑色素瘤的治疗,研究其与 CPI 联合治疗的有效性的临床试验也正在进行中(NCT02557321)。

T-VEC

T-VEC,一种基因修饰的单纯疱疹病毒(HSV)Ⅰ型,目前是唯一的经监管批准的黑色素瘤内溶瘤病毒治疗方法。它在受感染的黑色素瘤细胞内通过选择性肿瘤内复制和表达 GM-CSF(粒细胞巨噬细胞集落刺激因子),从而产生局部和全身抗肿瘤免疫效应[47]。该批准是基于对随机Ⅲ期临床试验中 436 例无法切除的Ⅲ期或Ⅳ期黑色素瘤患者的研究[48]。患者以 2∶1 比例被随机分配到病灶内 T-VEC 组(每次最多 4ml 治疗量)或皮下 GM-CSF 组(每天 125mg/m^2,连续 14 天,28 天一个周期)。与 GM-CSF 组比较,T-VEC 组的总有效率较高[26.4%(95%CI,21.4%~31.5%)vs.5.7%(95%CI,1.9%~9.5%)],反应更持久(16.3% vs. 2.1%,

$P<0.001$）。中位 OS 在 T-VEC 组比 GM-CSF 组更长（23.3 个月 vs.18.9 个月），但无统计学意义（$P=0.051$）。T-VEC 注射耐受性良好，据报道不良事件包括疲劳、寒战、发热、恶心、类流感样疾病，注射部位的反应，呕吐。发生 3 级和 4 级不良反应的发生率比较低，为 11%（GM-CSF 组为 5%）。

T-VEC 与 CPI 联合使用也显示出良好的效果。在 Ⅰb 阶段的试验中，T-VEC 联合伊匹木单抗治疗 19 例未经治疗的黑色素瘤患者（允许既往辅助治疗，距上次治疗时间≥6 个月）[49]。在第 1 周和第 4 周，T-VEC 在肿瘤内注射（总剂量高达 4ml），然后每两周 1 次。从第 6 周开始，每 3 周给药伊匹木单抗（3mg/kg）1 次，给药 4 次。客观缓解率为 50%，44% 的患者出现持久反应，持续≥6 个月。中位随访 20 个月（1.0~25.4 个月），18 个月的 PFS 为 50%，OS 为 67%，未观察到意外毒性事件。

T-VEC 联合帕博利珠单抗也进行了临床获益的试验评估。在 MASTERKEY-265 试验 Ⅰb 期研究中，21 例未接受系统治疗的晚期黑色素瘤患者在第 1 天、第 22 天，然后每 2 周接受 1 次 T-VEC（总体积高达 4ml）的体腔内（皮肤/皮下/淋巴结）治疗。第 36 天，然后每 2 周接受 1 次帕博利珠单抗（200mg）治疗[50]。相对危险度为 62%，CR 率为 33%，在未注射的非内脏和未注射的病变中分别有 43% 和 33% 的缓解。在本结果报道时，还未达到中位 PFS 和中位 OS。未记录到意外的不良事件，但作者描述了一些重叠的帕博利珠单抗相关毒性事件的发生。36% 的患者出现 3 级和 4 级毒副作用，包括皮疹（$n=2$）、肝酶升高（$n=2$）、高血糖（$n=2$）和鳞状细胞癌（$n=2$）。

目前正在进行多项关于 T-VEC 联合 CPI、靶向治疗和放疗疗效的临床试验（NCT02263508、NCT03088176、NCT02819843、NCT02965716）。由于 T-VEC 由活病毒组成，可能引起播散性疱疹性感染，因此在孕妇和免疫功能严重受损的患者中禁用（https：//www.fda.gov/downloads/BiologicsBloodVaccines/CellularGenetherapeuyproducts/ApprovedProducts/UCM469575.pdf）。因为已发现接受 T-VEC 治疗的患者可传播活病毒，因此，制订了严格的预防指南，特别是对婴儿、孕妇和免疫功能低下的患者。

黑色素瘤脑转移和免疫治疗

尽管免疫治疗和靶向治疗取得了进展，但仍有相当数量的患者在治疗过程中出现脑转移（MBM）[51]。

然而，最近一项针对黑色素瘤（$n=18$）或非小细胞肺癌（$n=34$）患者的 Ⅱ 期研究显示，单一药物帕博利珠单抗对 MBM 的有效率为 22%，达到持续缓解[52]。

没有意料之外的颅外毒性事件的报道,但黑色素瘤队列中的 3 例患者出现了短暂的神经系统不良事件。

重要的是,最近的两项研究表明,在未经治疗的 MBM 患者中,伊匹木单抗和纳武利尤单抗联合使用可以产生与 Checkmate-067 中观察到的颅外反应率相似的颅内反应率。在 Checkmate-204 中,75 例 MBM 患者接受伊匹木单抗(3mg/kg)联合纳武利尤单抗(1mg/kg)治疗,随后纳武利尤单抗(3mg/kg)维持治疗。在超过 9 个月的随访中,21%的患者达到了大脑 CR,而中位 PFS 没有达到。除了 33%的患者达到 PR 外,5%的患者达到 SD。重要的是,平均反应时间只有 2.8 个月(范围为 1~11 个月),在报道时尚未达到长期缓解。与 Checkmat-067 类似,52%的患者经历了 3 级或 4 级毒性反应,25%的患者不得不停止研究药物。重要的是,治疗相关的神经系统不良事件是罕见的,仅 8%患者发生了 3 级和 4 级毒性事件[53]。

由澳大利亚组(ABC 试验)发起的Ⅲ期临床试验第二阶段,将 MBM 患者随机分组,分别接受伊匹木单抗和纳武利尤单抗联合治疗(与 Checkmate-204 相同的剂量方案)或接受纳武利尤单抗单药治疗。与 Checkmate-204 相比,患者出现更多的脑转移例数,但在初治患者中,接受联合治疗的患者观察到的 RR 与 50%相似(CR 率 15%,PR 率 35%),而 SD 率为 10%。在本队列中接受治疗的 26 例患者中,46%的患者经历了 3 级和 4 级毒副反应,因而导致 27%的停药率。

由于这些结果带来了希望,因此目前正在进行多项临床试验,重点是针对 MBM 患者和需要使用皮质类固醇激素治疗的 MBM 患者,研究免疫治疗或联合治疗方法的有效性(NCT03175432、NCT02460068、NCT02621515、NCT02681549 和 NCT02716948)。

辅助治疗

全身辅助治疗的目的是降低术后高风险黑色素瘤复发的风险。传统上来说,这种方法主要针对Ⅲ期疾病患者,这类人群指有淋巴结和(或)转移的患者。淋巴结数目的增加,以及原发肿瘤深度的增加、有丝分裂率的增加及原发肿瘤溃疡的存在都与较差的预后相关[54]。

干扰素辅助治疗

在Ⅱ期或Ⅲ期黑色素瘤患者中,进行了不同剂量水平干扰素 α_2(INF-α_2)治疗的研究，以及多个综述对这些结果进行了总结[55]。

ECOG E1684 试验纳入了 287 例Ⅱ期/Ⅲ期黑色素瘤患者，随访时间最长，患者接受高剂量干扰素（HD INF）治疗或者仅观察[56]。HD INF 组中位无复发生存期（RFS）为 1.72 年观察组中位 RFS 为 0.98 年（$P = 0.0023$）。HD INF 组中位 OS 为 3.82 年，观察组中位 OS 为 2.78 年（$P = 0.0237$）。HD INF 组的 5 年生存率较观察组更高（46% vs.37%）。然而，中位随访时间 12.1 年，OS 获益不再被观察到，作者提出了老年队列中影响 OS 分析的相互竞争的死亡原因。

ECOG E1690 试验测试了两种不同的 INF 剂量水平，两种方案都没有显示 OS 的改善，但患者交叉分析可能改变了生存分析结果[57]。然而， 5 年 RFS 发生率 HD INF 组为 44%，低剂量 INF 组为 40%，观察组为 35%（$P = 0.3$）。E1684 和 E1690 的汇总分析显示确实存在 RFS 获益，但 HD INF 对 OS 生存无益处。其他汇总分析结果显示，溃疡性的原发性黑色素瘤患者的获益增加[58]。

聚乙二醇干扰素与 HD INF 相比，不良反应更少，并且具有更长的半衰期，每周需要注射更少量。然而，虽然 RFS 的改善与 HD INF 类似，但 OS 没有改善。此外，对 RFS 的积极影响随时间的推移而减少[59]。溃疡性原发性和微转移性结节病患者获得了最大的临床获益。

辅助生物化疗

为了提高辅助治疗的有效性，与标准的 HD INF 单药治疗相比，生物化疗疗程更短（最多 3 个周期）。在 SWOG S0008 Ⅲ期研究中，402 例Ⅲ期黑色素瘤患者接受了完全淋巴结清扫术，并被随机分配到生物化学治疗组（CVD，以 9MU/m^2 处方剂量，96 小时连续静脉输注，1～4 天；干扰素处方剂量：5MU/m^2，1～5 天。每 21 天重复 1 次治疗，共 3 个周期），或采用 HD INF 单药（每天 20MU/m^2 的 INF 静脉注射，连续 5 天，共 4 周，然后每周皮下注射 10MU/m^2，共 48 周）[60]。在 HDINF 组，43%的患者能够完成治疗，而在生物化疗组，80%的患者能够接受所有 3 个计划的治疗周期（$P<0.001$）。中位随访时间 7.2 年，生物化疗组和 HD INF 组中位 PFS 分别是 4.0 年和 1.9 年（$P =0.029$），5 年 RFS 分别为 48%和 39%。然而，尽管生物化疗组 OS 为 9.9 年，较 HD INF 组（6.7 年）长，但这一差距并没有统计学意义（HR=0.98；95% CI，0.74～1.31；两侧 P =0.55）。正如所期待的，两组患者的毒副反应不同，INF 治疗组肝功能异常发生率较高，生物化疗组患者低血压、血液、代谢、胃肠道毒副反应发生率较高。治疗组和对照组均未发现任何意外的新毒副反应。

辅助治疗中的检查点抑制剂

观察到伊匹木单抗对无法切除的晚期黑色素瘤患者的总体生存率和持久反应的改善，促进了伊匹木单抗在辅助治疗中有效性的研究。EORTC 18071 是一项Ⅲ期双盲随机研究，对完全切除的Ⅲ期黑色素瘤且没有接受过其他的系统治疗的患者，随机分配进入高剂量伊匹木单抗组（10mg/kg，每 3 周 1 次，共 4 次，然后每 3 个月 1 次，服用 1 次，最长可达 3 年）与安慰剂组。中位随访时间 2.74 年（IQR：2.28~3.22），伊匹木单抗组中位 RFS（26.1 个月）与安慰剂组比较明显改善（17.1 个月，$P=0.0013$）[61]。伊匹木单抗组 3 年 RFS 与安慰剂组比较也有改善[（46.5%；95% CI，41.5~51.3）vs.（34.8%；95% CI，30.1~39.5）]。与预期一样，治疗组的毒性更常见，包括肝脏和内分泌毒性。值得注意的是，在伊匹木单抗组中，5 例（1%）参与者发生了严重的与药物相关的不良事件并死亡。

本试验的最新进展，整体中位随访时间 5.3 年，伊匹木单抗组随访 5 年患者 65.4%（95% CI，60.8~69.6），而安慰剂组占 54.4%（95% CI，49.7~58.9）[62]。与安慰剂相比，接受伊匹木单抗治疗的患者的总生存率也有显著提高（因任何原因死亡的 HR=0.72；95% CI，0.58~0.88；$P=0.001$），所有亚组均观察到这一益处。

在随机双盲Ⅲ期试验（Checkmate-238）中，906 例经完全切除的ⅢB、ⅢC或Ⅳ期黑色素瘤患者被随机分配接受伊匹木单抗（10mg/kg）或纳武利尤单抗（3mg/kg），其主要终点为 RFS[63]。纳武利尤单抗组 12 个月 RFS（70.5%）明显高于伊匹木单抗组（60.8%）（$P<0.001$）。在分析时，两组试验均未达到 RFS 中值。与之前的报道相似，纳武利尤单抗具有良好的毒性谱，只有 14.4% 的患者发生了 3 级和 4 级毒性反应，而伊匹木单抗组的这一比例为 45.9%。基于 Checkmate 238，纳武利尤单抗于 2017 年 12 月获得监管部门批准，作为转移性黑色素瘤患者的辅助治疗方案。

最近公布的Ⅲ期试验结果表明，帕博利珠单抗可能成为一种很有前景的治疗选择（需要参考 SITC 2018，eggermont）。1019 例患者均为切除后Ⅲ期患者，术后均接受帕博利珠单抗（200mg，每 3 周 1 次）或安慰剂治疗，疗程长达 1 年（共13 次）或直至疾病复发。中位随访 15 个月，帕博利珠单抗组与安慰剂组比较，死亡或复发风险显著降低（43%；HR=0.57；95% CI，0.43~0.74；$P<0.0001$）。在辅助治疗中，不良事件与纳武利尤单抗相似。作为辅助治疗的第一次，该试验允许安慰剂组的患者在复发后交叉接受帕博利珠单抗，这将加深我们对复发后帕博利珠单抗疗效的理解。

黑色素瘤治疗未来

随着我们对肿瘤微环境和T淋巴细胞稳态认识的加深,许多新的靶点已经得到确认,并且正在临床试验中进行检测。

吲哚胺二氧合酶抑制剂

吲哚胺二氧合酶(IDO)抑制剂是近年来新兴的一类令人兴奋的抗癌药物。IDO是催化色氨酸合成犬尿氨酸的酶之一,它调控着第一步和限速步骤。T淋巴细胞的功能需要色氨酸,研究表明,肿瘤可以增加IDO水平,从而抑制细胞毒性T淋巴细胞的功能,从而激活Treg[64]。

艾卡哚司他是一种选择性的IDO1酶抑制剂,虽然它作为单一的抑制剂并没有显示出很大的作用,但是与CPI联合得以被研究[65]。艾卡哚司他基本上没有独立的抗肿瘤活性,然而,当它联合其他免疫检查点抑制剂时,如抗PD-1,可显示出极大的有效性。

最近一项Ⅰ期/Ⅱ期研究(ECHO-202/KEYNOTE-037)报道了黑色素瘤患者Ⅰ期/Ⅱ期研究得到的疗效和安全数据。Ⅰ期临床试验阶段患者接受艾卡哚司他(25mg、50mg、100mg、300mg口服,每天2次)联合帕博利珠单抗(2mg/kg或200mg)治疗,Ⅱ期临床试验接受艾卡哚司他(100mg,每天2次)联合帕博利珠单抗(200mg,每3周1次)(https://academic.oup.com/annonc/article/28/suppl_5/mdx377.001/4109288)。之前未接受过CPI治疗。54例有效评价患者的ORR为56%(CR率为11%),疾病控制率(CR+PR+SD)为78%。中位PFS为12.4个月,无进展生存率结果是鼓舞人心的(6个月:70%,12个月:54%,18个月:50%)。未发现明显增加的毒副作用,17.2%的患者出现3级和4级毒副反应。这些结果支持正在进行的艾卡哚司他联合帕博利珠单抗治疗晚期黑色素瘤的Ⅲ期临床试验(NCT02752074)。此外,艾卡哚司他与纳武利尤单抗联合使用疗效也正在评估中(NCT02327078)。

BMS-986205是另一种选择性IDO1抑制剂,与纳武利尤单抗和伊匹木单抗联合使用疗效正在进行评估(NCT02658890)。

淋巴细胞活化基因3(LAG-3)

LAG-3是一种免疫检查点受体(CD223),存在于活化的$CD4^+T$淋巴细胞和

CD8⁺T 淋巴细胞、NK 细胞、B 淋巴细胞和浆细胞样树突状细胞表面[66]。LAG-3 主要配体是 MHC Ⅱ类，对 T 淋巴细胞功能具有多种生物学效应，包括 T 淋巴细胞增殖、活化和稳态的负调控，在 T 淋巴细胞衰竭时 LAG-3 上调。近年来，其在树突状细胞成熟和活化中的作用也被报道[67]。LAG-3 抑制剂的研制现已进入临床试验阶段。在Ⅰ期/Ⅱa 临床试验中，43 例之前存在 PD-1/PD-L1 耐受且进展的黑色素瘤患者，联合 relatlimab（以前称为 BMS-986016）和纳武利尤单抗治疗（http://ascopubs.org/doi/abs/10.1200/jco.2017.35.15 _suppl.9520）。研究发现，31 例有效评估患者的疾病控制率为 45%，总有效率为 16%。甚至在之前对 PD-1 耐受的患者中观察到了疗效。重要的是，relatlimab 似乎没有增加毒性，因为 3 级或 4 级毒性仅在 9%的治疗患者中观察到。目前，多个临床试验正在评估抗-LAG-3 联合其他免疫疗法的疗效和抗-LAG-3 在其他肿瘤类型的疗效（NCT02676869、NCT01968109、NCT03250832、NCT03219268）。

T 淋巴细胞免疫球蛋白-3

T 淋巴细胞免疫球蛋白（TIM-3）是产生 IFN-γ 的特定细胞亚型 CD4⁺和 CD8⁺细胞及树突状细胞、NK 细胞、单核细胞表达的共抑制受体[68]。研究表明，晚期黑色素瘤患者的一部分 T 淋巴细胞上调了 Tim-3 的表达，并且 Tim-3 阳性的细胞似乎功能失调[69]。研究还表明，在联合 PD-1 单抗同时阻断的情况下，对逆转肿瘤诱导的 T 淋巴细胞衰竭和功能障碍方面具有协同作用。

目前,有少数 Tim-3 拮抗剂正处于早期临床开发阶段,或作为单药或联合 PD-1 或 PD-L1 单抗（NCT03099109、NCT03489343、NCT02817633、NCT02608268）。虽然这些试验大多集中在安全性上，但结果还是令人热切期待的。

OX40

OX40（或 CD134）是肿瘤坏死因子（TNF）受体超家族（TNFRSF）的成员之一、体外研究表明，通过刺激其配体，可以促进 T 淋巴细胞增殖，改善效应器功能，延长 T 淋巴细胞的存活时间，使用 OX40 激动剂治疗可以增强抗肿瘤免疫效果[70]。

在使用 OX40 激动剂小鼠单克隆抗体的第一阶段试验中，30 例患者中有 12 例出现转移病灶消退，其中 7 例为转移性黑色素瘤。7 例患者出现 3 级和 4 级淋巴细胞减少症，其他 1 级和 2 级毒副作用包括疲劳、恶心、呕吐、皮疹和类流感样症状。目前正在进行多项临床试验，包括联合阿特珠单抗（NCT02410512）、度伐鲁单抗（NCT02705482）或曲美木单抗（tremelimumab）（抗 CTLA-4；

NCT02705482）。在临床前模型中，人 OX40 配体融合蛋白 MEDI6383 可以启动细胞内信号通路，增强 T 淋巴细胞的存活、活性和增殖，目前正在与度伐鲁单抗联合使用进行评估（NCT02221960）[71]。

4-1BB

4-1BB（CD137）是 TNFRSF 的另一个成员，是一种可诱导的共刺激受体，表达于 T 淋巴细胞等免疫细胞上，可恢复效应器功能[72]。4-1BB 和 4-1BBL 相互作用导致细胞因子分泌和 $CD8^+T$ 淋巴细胞存活增加。乌瑞芦单抗（Urelumab）（BMS-663513）是一种完全人源化的 4-1BB 激动剂单抗，已在 I 期剂量递增研究中进行测试。54 例黑色素瘤患者中只有 3 例对单一治疗有反应（http://ascopubs.org/doi/abs/10.1200/jco.2008.26.15_suppl.3007）。然而，由于乌瑞芦单抗与纳武利尤单抗在临床前数据中的协同作用，这种联合目前正在 I 期剂量递增临床试验中评估。此外，在实体肿瘤患者中 PF-05082566（另一种 4-1BB 激动剂单抗）与帕博利珠单抗联合应用，并对其进行评价（NCT02253992、NCT02179918）。另一个有趣的组合正在研究中，在选择性的晚期或转移性癌中联合 PF-04518600（OX40 激动剂）和 PF-05082566（4-1BB 激动剂）（NCT02315066）。

PF-05082566（4-1BB 激动剂）也正在与阿维鲁单抗联合应用于晚期黑色素瘤患者（NCT02554812）。

Toll 样受体（TLR）

Toll 样受体是免疫识别受体家族成员之一，最初是通过其在固有免疫反应和适应性免疫反应中的作用被发现的[73]。此外，许多肿瘤类型表达功能性 TLR，导致肿瘤增殖、转移形成和对凋亡的抵抗。目前正在进行大量研究，以确定基于 TLR 的治疗方法是否可以提高抗癌免疫治疗的有效性（NCT02644967、NCT03052205、NCT00960752、NCT03445533）。

结论

过去十年在黑色素瘤治疗方面取得的许多突破性发现已经转化为其他类型肿瘤的成功治疗方法。虽然我们有理由保持乐观，但仍有许多未知之处，我们殷切期盼正在进行当中的试验的结果，希望能够指导治疗医生为每个患者选择最优的治疗方案。

参考文献

1. Tas F, Keskin S, Karadeniz A, et al. Noncutaneous melanoma have distinct features from each other and cutaneous melanoma. Oncology. 2011;81(5–6):353–8.
2. McCourt C, Dolan O, Gormley G. Malignant melanoma: a pictorial review. Ulster Med J. 2014;83(2):103–10.
3. Lideikaite A, Mozuraitiene J, Letautiene S. Analysis of prognostic factors for melanoma patients. Acta Med Litu. 2017;24(1):25–34.
4. Jiang T, Zhou C, Ren S. Role of IL-2 in cancer immunotherapy. Oncoimmunology. 2016;5(6):e1163462.
5. Atkins MB, Lotze MT, Dutcher JP, et al. High-dose recombinant interleukin 2 therapy for patients with metastatic melanoma: analysis of 270 patients treated between 1985 and 1993. J Clin Oncol. 1999;17(7):2105–16.
6. Hughes T, Klairmont M, Broucek J, Iodice G, Basu S, Kaufman HL. The prognostic significance of stable disease following high-dose interleukin-2 (IL-2) treatment in patients with metastatic melanoma and renal cell carcinoma. Cancer Immunol Immunother. 2015;64(4):459–65.
7. Schwartzentruber DJ. Guidelines for the safe administration of high-dose interleukin-2. J Immunother. 2001;24(4):287–93.
8. Serrone L, Zeuli M, Sega FM, Cognetti F. Dacarbazine-based chemotherapy for metastatic melanoma: thirty-year experience overview. J Exp Clin Cancer Res. 2000;19(1):21–34.
9. Hill GJ II, Krementz ET, Hill HZ. Dimethyl triazeno imidazole carboxamide and combination therapy for melanoma. IV. Late results after complete response to chemotherapy (Central Oncology Group protocols 7130, 7131, and 7131A). Cancer. 1984;53(6):1299–305.
10. Bajetta E, Del Vecchio M, Bernard-Marty C, et al. Metastatic melanoma: chemotherapy. Semin Oncol. 2002;29(5):427–45.
11. Bhatia S, Tykodi SS, Thompson JA. Treatment of metastatic melanoma: an overview. Oncology (Williston Park). 2009;23(6):488–96.
12. Li RH, Hou XY, Yang CS, et al. Temozolomide for treating malignant melanoma. J Coll Physicians Surg Pak. 2015;25(9):680–8.
13. Quirt I, Verma S, Petrella T, Bak K, Charette M. Temozolomide for the treatment of metastatic melanoma: a systematic review. Oncologist. 2007;12(9):1114–23.
14. Middleton MR, Grob JJ, Aaronson N, et al. Randomized phase III study of temozolomide versus dacarbazine in the treatment of patients with advanced metastatic malignant melanoma. J Clin Oncol. 2000;18(1):158–66.
15. Hodi FS, Soiffer RJ, Clark J, Finkelstein DM, Haluska FG. Phase II study of paclitaxel and carboplatin for malignant melanoma. Am J Clin Oncol. 2002;25(3):283–6.
16. Rao RD, Holtan SG, Ingle JN, et al. Combination of paclitaxel and carboplatin as second-line therapy for patients with metastatic melanoma. Cancer. 2006;106(2):375–82.
17. Hersh EM, O'Day SJ, Ribas A, et al. A phase 2 clinical trial of nab-paclitaxel in previously treated and chemotherapy-naive patients with metastatic melanoma. Cancer. 2010;116(1):155–63.
18. Kottschade LA, Suman VJ, Amatruda T III, et al. A phase II trial of nab-paclitaxel (ABI-007) and carboplatin in patients with unresectable stage IV melanoma: a North Central Cancer Treatment Group Study, N057E(1). Cancer. 2011;117(8):1704–10.
19. Legha SS, Ring S, Papadopoulos N, Plager C, Chawla S, Benjamin R. A prospective evaluation of a triple-drug regimen containing cisplatin, vinblastine, and dacarbazine (CVD) for metastatic melanoma. Cancer. 1989;64(10):2024–9.
20. Atkins MB, Hsu J, Lee S, et al. Phase III trial comparing concurrent biochemotherapy with cisplatin, vinblastine, dacarbazine, interleukin-2, and interferon alfa-2b with cisplatin, vinblastine, and dacarbazine alone in patients with metastatic malignant melanoma (E3695): a trial coordinated by the Eastern Cooperative Oncology Group. J Clin Oncol. 2008;26(35):5748–54.
21. Grunhagen DJ, Verhoef C. Isolated limb perfusion for stage III melanoma: does it still have a role in the present era of effective systemic therapy? Oncology (Williston Park).

2016;30(12):1045–52.
22. Eggermont AM, van Geel AN, de Wilt JH, ten Hagen TL. The role of isolated limb perfusion for melanoma confined to the extremities. Surg Clin North Am. 2003;83(2):371–84, ix.
23. Lotze MT, Rosenberg SA. Results of clinical trials with the administration of interleukin 2 and adoptive immunotherapy with activated cells in patients with cancer. Immunobiology. 1986;172(3–5):420–37.
24. Rosenberg SA, Yannelli JR, Yang JC, et al. Treatment of patients with metastatic melanoma with autologous tumor-infiltrating lymphocytes and interleukin 2. J Natl Cancer Inst. 1994;86(15):1159–66.
25. Dudley ME, Wunderlich JR, Yang JC, et al. Adoptive cell transfer therapy following non-myeloablative but lymphodepleting chemotherapy for the treatment of patients with refractory metastatic melanoma. J Clin Oncol. 2005;23(10):2346–57.
26. Baruch EN, Berg AL, Besser MJ, Schachter J, Markel G. Adoptive T cell therapy: an overview of obstacles and opportunities. Cancer. 2017;123(S11):2154–62.
27. Merhavi-Shoham E, Itzhaki O, Markel G, Schachter J, Besser MJ. Adoptive cell therapy for metastatic melanoma. Cancer J. 2017;23(1):48–53.
28. Page DM, Kane LP, Allison JP, Hedrick SM. Two signals are required for negative selection of CD4+CD8+ thymocytes. J Immunol. 1993;151(4):1868–80.
29. Brunet JF, Dosseto M, Denizot F, et al. The inducible cytotoxic T-lymphocyte-associated gene transcript CTLA-1 sequence and gene localization to mouse chromosome 14. Nature. 1986;322(6076):268–71.
30. Wei SC, Levine JH, Cogdill AP, et al. Distinct cellular mechanisms underlie anti-CTLA-4 and Anti-PD-1 checkpoint blockade. Cell. 2017;170(6):1120–33.e1117.
31. Hodi FS, O'Day SJ, McDermott DF, et al. Improved survival with ipilimumab in patients with metastatic melanoma. N Engl J Med. 2010;363(8):711–23.
32. Robert C, Thomas L, Bondarenko I, et al. Ipilimumab plus dacarbazine for previously untreated metastatic melanoma. N Engl J Med. 2011;364(26):2517–26.
33. Buchbinder EI, Gunturi A, Perritt J, et al. A retrospective analysis of high-dose interleukin-2 (HD IL-2) following ipilimumab in metastatic melanoma. J Immunother Cancer. 2016;4:52.
34. Pardoll DM. The blockade of immune checkpoints in cancer immunotherapy. Nat Rev Cancer. 2012;12(4):252–64.
35. Ohaegbulam KC, Assal A, Lazar-Molnar E, Yao Y, Zang X. Human cancer immunotherapy with antibodies to the PD-1 and PD-L1 pathway. Trends Mol Med. 2015;21(1):24–33.
36. Robert C, Long GV, Brady B, et al. Nivolumab in previously untreated melanoma without BRAF mutation. N Engl J Med. 2015;372(4):320–30.
37. Hodi FS, Chesney J, Pavlick AC, et al. Combined nivolumab and ipilimumab versus ipilimumab alone in patients with advanced melanoma: 2-year overall survival outcomes in a multicentre, randomised, controlled, phase 2 trial. Lancet Oncol. 2016;17(11):1558–68.
38. Larkin J, Hodi FS, Wolchok JD. Combined nivolumab and ipilimumab or monotherapy in untreated melanoma. N Engl J Med. 2015;373(13):1270–1.
39. Ribas A, Puzanov I, Dummer R, et al. Pembrolizumab versus investigator-choice chemotherapy for ipilimumab-refractory melanoma (KEYNOTE-002): a randomised, controlled, phase 2 trial. Lancet Oncol. 2015;16(8):908–18.
40. Robert C, Schachter J, Long GV, et al. Pembrolizumab versus ipilimumab in advanced melanoma. N Engl J Med. 2015;372(26):2521–32.
41. Long GV, Atkinson V, Cebon JS, et al. Standard-dose pembrolizumab in combination with reduced-dose ipilimumab for patients with advanced melanoma (KEYNOTE-029): an open-label, phase 1b trial. Lancet Oncol. 2017;18(9):1202–10.
42. Hirayama M, Nishimura Y. The present status and future prospects of peptide-based cancer vaccines. Int Immunol. 2016;28(7):319–28.
43. Schwartzentruber DJ, Lawson DH, Richards JM, et al. gp100 peptide vaccine and interleukin-2 in patients with advanced melanoma. N Engl J Med. 2011;364(22):2119–27.
44. Thompson JF, Hersey P, Wachter E. Chemoablation of metastatic melanoma using intralesional Rose Bengal. Melanoma Res. 2008;18(6):405–11.
45. Thompson JF, Agarwala SS, Smithers BM, et al. Phase 2 study of intralesional PV-10 in refrac-

tory metastatic melanoma. Ann Surg Oncol. 2015;22(7):2135–42.
46. Read TA, Smith A, Thomas J, et al. Intralesional PV-10 for the treatment of in-transit melanoma metastases-results of a prospective, non-randomized, single center study. J Surg Oncol. 2018;117(4):579–87.
47. Conry RM, Westbrook B, McKee S, Norwood TG. Talimogene laherparepvec: first in class oncolytic virotherapy. Hum Vaccin Immunother. 2018;14(4):839–46.
48. Andtbacka RH, Kaufman HL, Collichio F, et al. Talimogene laherparepvec improves durable response rate in patients with advanced melanoma. J Clin Oncol. 2015;33(25):2780–8.
49. Puzanov I, Milhem MM, Minor D, et al. Talimogene laherparepvec in combination with ipilimumab in previously untreated, unresectable stage IIIB-IV melanoma. J Clin Oncol. 2016;34(22):2619–26.
50. Ribas A, Dummer R, Puzanov I, et al. Oncolytic virotherapy promotes intratumoral T cell infiltration and improves anti-PD-1 immunotherapy. Cell. 2017;170(6):1109–19.e1110.
51. Cohen JV, Tawbi H, Margolin KA, et al. Melanoma central nervous system metastases: current approaches, challenges, and opportunities. Pigment Cell Melanoma Res. 2016;29(6):627–42.
52. Goldberg SB, Gettinger SN, Mahajan A, et al. Pembrolizumab for patients with melanoma or non-small-cell lung cancer and untreated brain metastases: early analysis of a non-randomised, open-label, phase 2 trial. Lancet Oncol. 2016;17(7):976–83.
53. Tawbi HA, Forsyth PAJ, Algazi PA, Hamid O, Hodi FS, Moschos S, Khushalani N, Margolin KA. Efficacy and safety of nivolumab (NIVO) plus ipilimumab (IPI) in patients with melanoma (MEL) metastatic to the brain: results of the phase II study CheckMate 204. J Clin Oncol. 2012;30 (Suppl; abstr 8584). 2017;35:(Suppl; abstr 9507).
54. Balch CM, Gershenwald JE, Soong SJ, et al. Final version of 2009 AJCC melanoma staging and classification. J Clin Oncol. 2009;27(36):6199–206.
55. Agha A, Tarhini AA. Adjuvant therapy for melanoma. Curr Oncol Rep. 2017;19(5):36.
56. Kirkwood JM, Resnick GD, Cole BF. Efficacy, safety, and risk-benefit analysis of adjuvant interferon alfa-2b in melanoma. Semin Oncol. 1997;24(1 Suppl 4):S16–23.
57. Kirkwood JM, Ibrahim JG, Sondak VK, et al. High- and low-dose interferon alfa-2b in high-risk melanoma: first analysis of intergroup trial E1690/S9111/C9190. J Clin Oncol. 2000;18(12):2444–58.
58. Ives NJ, Suciu S, Eggermont AMM, et al. Adjuvant interferon-alpha for the treatment of high-risk melanoma: an individual patient data meta-analysis. Eur J Cancer. 2017;82:171–83.
59. Eggermont AM, Suciu S, Testori A, et al. Long-term results of the randomized phase III trial EORTC 18991 of adjuvant therapy with pegylated interferon alfa-2b versus observation in resected stage III melanoma. J Clin Oncol. 2012;30(31):3810–8.
60. Flaherty LE, Othus M, Atkins MB, et al. Southwest Oncology Group S0008: a phase III trial of high-dose interferon Alfa-2b versus cisplatin, vinblastine, and dacarbazine, plus interleukin-2 and interferon in patients with high-risk melanoma--an intergroup study of cancer and leukemia Group B, Children's Oncology Group, Eastern Cooperative Oncology Group, and Southwest Oncology Group. J Clin Oncol. 2014;32(33):3771–8.
61. Eggermont AM, Chiarion-Sileni V, Grob JJ, et al. Adjuvant ipilimumab versus placebo after complete resection of high-risk stage III melanoma (EORTC 18071): a randomised, double-blind, phase 3 trial. Lancet Oncol. 2015;16(5):522–30.
62. Eggermont AM, Chiarion-Sileni V, Grob JJ, et al. Prolonged survival in stage III melanoma with ipilimumab adjuvant therapy. N Engl J Med. 2016;375(19):1845–55.
63. Weber J, Mandala M, Del Vecchio M, et al. Adjuvant nivolumab versus ipilimumab in resected stage III or IV melanoma. N Engl J Med. 2017;377(19):1824–35.
64. Muller AJ, DuHadaway JB, Donover PS, Sutanto-Ward E, Prendergast GC. Inhibition of indoleamine 2,3-dioxygenase, an immunoregulatory target of the cancer suppression gene Bin1, potentiates cancer chemotherapy. Nat Med. 2005;11(3):312–9.
65. Yue EW, Sparks R, Polam P, et al. INCB24360 (Epacadostat), a highly potent and selective Indoleamine-2,3-dioxygenase 1 (IDO1) inhibitor for immuno-oncology. ACS Med Chem Lett. 2017;8(5):486–91.
66. Goldberg MV, Drake CG. LAG-3 in cancer immunotherapy. Curr Top Microbiol Immunol. 2011;344:269–78.

67. Catakovic K, Klieser E, Neureiter D, Geisberger R. T cell exhaustion: from pathophysiological basics to tumor immunotherapy. Cell Commun Signal. 2017;15(1):1.
68. Hahn AW, Gill DM, Pal SK, Agarwal N. The future of immune checkpoint cancer therapy after PD-1 and CTLA-4. Immunotherapy. 2017;9(8):681–92.
69. Fourcade J, Sun Z, Benallaoua M, et al. Upregulation of Tim-3 and PD-1 expression is associated with tumor antigen-specific CD8+ T cell dysfunction in melanoma patients. J Exp Med. 2010;207(10):2175–86.
70. Buchan SL, Rogel A, Al-Shamkhani A. The immunobiology of CD27 and OX40 and their potential as targets for cancer immunotherapy. Blood. 2018;131(1):39–48.
71. Oberst MD, Auge C, Morris C, et al. Potent immune modulation by MEDI6383, an engineered human OX40 ligand IgG4P Fc fusion protein. Mol Cancer Ther. 2018;17(5):1024–38.
72. Chester C, Sanmamed MF, Wang J, Melero I. Immunotherapy targeting 4-1BB: mechanistic rationale, clinical results, and future strategies. Blood. 2018;131(1):49–57.
73. Huang B, Zhao J, Unkeless JC, Feng ZH, Xiong H. TLR signaling by tumor and immune cells: a double-edged sword. Oncogene. 2008;27(2):218–24.

第3章

肺癌的免疫治疗：肿瘤治疗的新时代

Luis Corrales，Katherine Scilla，Christian Caglevic，Ken Miller，
Julio Oliveira，Christian Rolfo

译者：赵 静 蔡修宇

摘要 在过去的10年里，随着新型、多种治疗方法的发展及对生物学的进一步了解，非小细胞肺癌（non-small cell lung cancer，NSCLC）的治疗策略发生了巨大的变化。化疗是第一个用于晚期疾病的全身治疗方法，相比姑息治疗更让患者获益。通过寻找致癌驱动基因，研究出了新型的靶向治疗方法，进而对某些患者的管理发生了重大变化，其中一些患者可以使用口服抑制剂作为一线治疗。而免疫疗法是一种潜在的选择，在肺癌的治疗中显示了有前景的结果。本章探讨了NSCLC研究中的两种细胞毒性T淋巴细胞相关抗原4（cytotoxic T lymphocyte associated antigen-4，CTLA-4）抑制剂：伊匹木单抗和曲美木单抗。免疫检查点抑制剂：程序性细胞死亡受体-1（programmed death-1，PD-1）（纳武利尤单抗，帕博利珠单抗）和程序性死亡配体-1（programmed death-ligand 1，PD-L1）（阿特珠单抗，度伐鲁单抗，阿维鲁单抗，BMS-936559）。并分析了上述药物应用于NSCLC治疗的研究、所涉及的证据及在管理患者中的潜在作用。免疫疗法已经改变了NSCLC的治疗模式，未来有望为患者带来更多获益。

关键词 NSCLC 免疫疗法 PD-L1/PD-1 精准肿瘤学 帕博利珠单抗 纳武利尤单抗 阿特珠单抗 免疫毒性

Luis Corrales 和 Katherine Scilla 对本章的贡献相同

L. Corrales
Medical Oncology Department，CIMCA/Hospital San Juan de Dios-CCSS，San José，Costa Rica

K. Scilla · K. Miller
Thoracic Oncology Program，University of Maryland Greenebaum Comprehensive Cancer Center，Baltimore，MD，USA

C. Caglevic
Medical Oncology Department，Clínica Alemana Santiago，Santiago，Chile

引言

在所有肺癌病例中，非小细胞肺癌（NSCLC）约占 85%。大多数 NSCLC 患者确诊时已属晚期，肺癌是全球癌症相关死亡的主要因素。烟草是该疾病最重要的危险因素，也可以解释其流行病学的地域差异[1]。环境污染和一些矿物质暴露也与 NSCLC 相关。例如，在智利的一些北方城市肺癌的发病率和死亡率非常高，可能与这些地区饮用水中的砷含量有关[2]。

几年前，转移性 NSCLC 还是一种不能治愈的恶性肿瘤，只有姑息治疗方式，治疗目的是提高患者的生活质量，延长生存期。20 世纪 80 年代末，加拿大的一项前瞻性随机试验表明，在转移性 NSCLC 患者中，与最佳支持治疗相比，以顺铂为基础的联合化疗使 OS 有一定提高。但是，这些治疗方法的毒性较高[3]。20 年后，一项荟萃分析显示，接受化疗和最佳支持治疗的晚期 NSCLC 患者与仅接受最佳支持治疗的患者相比，前者 1 年 OS 率提高 9%[4]。一项随机试验强调了组织学在晚期 NSCLC 患者治疗中的重要性，同组织学亚型患者接受不同的以顺铂为基础的联合化疗方案治疗，观察到 OS 的差异[5]。

转移性 NSCLC 一线细胞毒性化疗失败后，对于体能状态良好的患者，多西他赛（docetaxel）可作为二线治疗，与最佳支持治疗相比，OS 获益为 3 个月[6]。在一线未接受培美曲塞（pemetrexed）治疗的肺腺癌患者中，培美曲塞可作为二线治疗，与多西他赛相比，OS 结果类似，但毒性显著降低[7]。如果患者的病情在二线化疗中进展，但其体能状态没有明显恶化，则可以考虑后线治疗，但结果尚不明确，相关文献较少[8]。

在细胞毒性化疗基础上加入抗血管生成药物已成为提高转移性非鳞状

J. Oliveira
Medical Oncology Department, Portuguese Institute of Oncology of Porto, Porto, Portugal

C. Rolfo (✉)
Thoracic Oncology Program, University of Maryland Greenebaum Comprehensive Cancer Center, Baltimore, MD, USA

Marlene and Stewart Greenebaum Comprehensive Cancer Center, University of Maryland School of Medicine, Baltimore, MD, USA
e-mail: christian.rolfo@umm.edu

© Springer Nature Switzerland AG 2018
A. Naing, J. Hajjar (eds.), *Immunotherapy*, Advances in Experimental Medicine and Biology 995, https://doi.org/10.1007/978-3-030-02505-2_3

NSCLC 生存率的一种策略。几项临床试验的结果显示，FDA 批准贝伐珠单抗（bevacizumab）用于这类患者[9]。尼达尼布（nintedanib）是一种口服抗血管生成药物，能同时抑制血管内皮生长因子受体（vascular endothelial growth factor receptor，VEGFR）、成纤维生长因子受体（fibroblast growth factor receptor，FGFR）、血小板衍生生长因子（platelet derived growth factor，PDGF）及 RET[10]，已经在欧洲获批联合多西他赛用于非鳞状 NSCLC 二线治疗。在晚期肺腺癌患者中，多西他赛联合尼达尼布二线治疗相比多西他赛单药治疗，中位 OS 显著提高（12.6 个月 vs. 0.3 个月）[1,11]。

直至 21 世纪初，NSCLC 和小细胞肺癌的不同病理类型一直是指导肿瘤治疗决策的主要决定因素。在 NSCLC 患者中，区分鳞状和非鳞状组织也很重要，非鳞状组织主要由腺癌和大细胞癌亚型组成。转移性 NSCLC 患者根据组织学类型采用适当的化疗方案进行治疗。随后，主要在非鳞状细胞癌人群中发现了新的特异性基因和分子改变与潜在的靶向治疗药物，这进一步改变了晚期 NSCLC 的治疗策略。表皮生长因子（epidermal growth factor receptor，EGFR）突变和棘皮动物微管相关蛋白样 4-间变性淋巴瘤激酶（echinoderm microtubule-associated protein-like 4-anaplastic lymphoma kinase，EML4-ALK）融合基因[12]是临床上最常见的与靶向治疗疗效相关的基因改变。NSCLC 中其他不太常见的突变包括 ROS-1、BRAF、HER2、MEK、MET 和 RET。

癌症的特征是不同的基因和表观遗传的改变。肺癌中高频率的体细胞突变产生了肿瘤特异性抗原，并可能提高免疫原性[13]。但是，致癌过程的研究常独立于抗肿瘤免疫反应（immune response，IR），这是个悖论，因为免疫系统（immune system，IS）的一个基本功能就是区分自体和外来成分。具体地说，导致癌症发展的一个因素是旨在消除改变抗原的各种免疫机制的失败[14,15]。免疫系统以预防肿瘤发生为目的，有多种方式识别从内在抑制机制中逃逸的细胞，在癌变细胞生长和形成肿瘤前识别并破坏克隆，对已经形成的肿瘤进行识别和清除[16]。

固有免疫系统由 DC、巨噬细胞、NK 细胞、粒细胞（嗜碱性粒细胞、嗜酸性粒细胞和中性粒细胞）、补体蛋白、趋化因子和细胞因子等组成。固有免疫系统可对抗原产生快速的非特异性反应。相比之下，由 B 淋巴细胞、CD4$^+$T 淋巴细胞和 CD8$^+$T 淋巴细胞及抗体组成的适应性 IR 是针对特定抗原产生的缓慢特异性反应，并产生免疫记忆。抗肿瘤 IR 分为 7 个阶段 [14-17]，组成肿瘤免疫环：①肿瘤抗原释放（肿瘤细胞死亡）；②肿瘤抗原提呈[抗原提呈细胞（antigen-presenting cell，APC）]；③APC 和 T 淋巴细胞的启动和激活；④细胞毒性 T 淋巴细胞向肿瘤组织迁移；⑤T 淋巴细胞浸润肿瘤（细胞毒性 T 淋巴细胞、内皮细胞）；⑥T 淋巴细胞识别肿瘤细胞；⑦最终肿瘤细胞死亡。

在提呈阶段，APC 将抗原提呈给 T 淋巴细胞或 B 淋巴细胞，T 淋巴细胞或

B 淋巴细胞的细胞膜内分别有一个特定的识别受体：T 淋巴细胞受体（T cell receptor，TCR）或 B 淋巴细胞受体（B cell receptor，BCR）。然而，这种单一信号不足以激活淋巴细胞，需要同时有共刺激分子（CD80/CD28、CD40/CD4-配体、CD86/CTLA-4、ICOS/ICOS 配体等）相互作用。此外，我们必须考虑到，每一个正常 IR 都有防止其持久反应及过度反应的机制。在这个过程中，有一些重要机制：调节性 T 淋巴细胞（Treg）的参与，抑制性受体（称为检查点）的表达，细胞凋亡的激活及细胞的耗竭[18]。

与此同时，肿瘤发生逃逸或抑制 IR 的机制包括下调抗原提呈［下调主要组织相容性复合体（major histocompatibility complex，MHC）］、上调凋亡抑制剂（Bcl-XL、FLIP）及表达抑制性细胞表面分子[程序性细胞死亡配体 1（PD-L1）、FasL]。此外，肿瘤细胞分泌能够抑制效应免疫细胞功能的因子（TGF-β、IL-10、VEGF、LXR-L、神经节苷脂或可溶性 MICA）或者募集调节细胞产生免疫抑制微环境（IL-4、IL-13、GM-CS、IL-1β、VEGF 或 PGE$_2$）。一旦被募集，调节细胞可通过释放免疫抑制性细胞因子并改变微环境的营养成分来减弱抗肿瘤免疫。具体来说，分泌的 IL-4 和 IL-13 导致 M2 型巨噬细胞的募集和极化，表达 TGF-β、IL-10、PDGF，进而抑制 T 淋巴细胞。肿瘤细胞释放集落刺激因子 IL-1β、VEGF 或 PGE$_2$，导致的骨髓源性抑制细胞（myeloid-derived suppressor cell，MDSC）的积累，可以通过表达 TGR-β、ARG$_1$ 和 iNOS 来阻断 T 淋巴细胞的功能。Treg 也可以通过多种机制来抑制效应 T 淋巴细胞，包括表达 CTLA-4[16]。

基于这些理论，免疫疗法被认为是一种潜在治疗恶性肿瘤的选择。在 NSCLC 中，最初的疫苗试验没有提示临床获益[2]。最近，一些免疫治疗药物被证明对 NSCLC 患者有效。这些药物目前在 NSCLC 的管理中发挥了确定的作用。最初的免疫治疗研究评估了阻断 CTLA-4 通路的药物，但未能显示其对 NSCLC 患者的 OS 有益处。但是，抗 PD-1 和抗 PD-L1 单药治疗或与其他免疫治疗药物或化疗联合使用时，对 NSCLC 患者显示出令人印象深刻的阳性结果。

NSCLC 治疗的通路及免疫治疗药物

CTLA-4 通路

IS 具有负调节机制，可以限制 IR 潜在的有害扩增。具体来说，抗原暴露后，T 淋巴细胞表面会有不同分子的上调，目的是终止 IR。这些分子称为检查点。例如，CTLA-4、LAG-3、PD-1/2、TIM-3。在包括肺癌在内的一些肿瘤中，这些分子的表达发生了改变[19,20]。CTLA-4 在 Treg 上持续表达，但是仅在传统 T 淋巴细胞激活后表达上调。CTLA-4 发挥抑制细胞活化的功能。

在 APC 的 MHC 与 TCR 相互作用及共刺激分子（如 CD28 结合 CD80/86）的作用下，T 淋巴细胞被激活，CTLA-4 就会在细胞膜上表达。CD28 与 CTLA-4 有着相同的受体，CD80 和 CD86。但是 CTLA-4 与这两个受体的亲和力更高。这种相互作用可终止 IR。CTLA-4 的重要作用是维持自身耐受，该作用在敲除小鼠中被一种快速致死的系统免疫过度活化表型证实[21]。

CTLA-4 是临床上第一个针对癌症治疗的免疫检查点。抗 CTLA-4 抗体干预并阻断 CTLA-4 与其受体之间的相互作用，从而抑制 IR，使抗肿瘤 IR 得以维持。这与效应 T 细胞的增加和肿瘤内 Treg 的显著减少有关[22,23]。

CTLA-4 抑制剂

伊匹木单抗

目前，最成熟的 CTLA-4 抑制剂是伊匹木单抗。该药是一种完全人源化的 IgG1 抗细胞毒性 T 淋巴细胞抗原 CTLA-4 单克隆抗体，具有阻断 CTLA-4 与其配体结合的作用。通过阻断 T 淋巴细胞调节 CTLA-4 的调节机制，伊匹木单抗促使免疫系统攻击肿瘤细胞[24]。

伊匹木单抗最初是在加利福尼亚大学研发的，目前已获得百时美施贵宝（Bristol-Myers Squibb）的许可[25]。伊匹木单抗是第一个获批用于癌症治疗的检查点抑制剂。Hodi 等对比了伊匹木单抗单药或联合糖蛋白 100 肽疫苗（gp100）与 gp100 单药治疗不可切除和转移性黑色素瘤患者的效果，并公布了阳性总生存率结果[26]。尽管在不可切除或转移性黑色素瘤患者中有良好的结果，但接受伊匹木单抗单药治疗的 NSCLC 患者并没有获得相同的阳性结果。

卡铂联合紫杉醇双药化疗联合伊匹木单抗的理论基础是细胞毒性化疗引起肿瘤坏死并释放肿瘤抗原，可能增强免疫治疗的应答[27]。在一项 I 期临床试验中，Weber 在初治的黑色素瘤患者中检测了伊匹木单抗与细胞毒性化疗之间的相互作用。伊匹木单抗的静脉注射剂量为每 3 周 10mg/kg，最多 4 剂；卡铂的 AUC 为 6，紫杉醇为 175mg/m²，每 3 周给药 1 次。没有出现限制性毒性的患者可以从 24 周开始每 12 周接受 1 次伊匹木单抗维持治疗，直到出现限制性毒性或疾病进展。两组未发现相关药理学或药代动力学的研究结果[28]。

在一项 II 期临床试验中，针对不可根治性治疗的初治 IIIB 期/IV 期 NSCLC 患者，采用伊匹木单抗联合卡铂/紫杉醇双药化疗方案。该试验为一项三臂研究（1∶1∶1），纳入了 204 例患者。对照组为卡铂/紫杉醇双药化疗 6 个周期。实验组为伊匹木单抗 10mg/kg，同步卡铂/紫杉醇双药化疗 4 个周期，随后给予 2 个周期安慰剂治疗；或 2 个周期安慰剂+卡铂/紫杉醇之后伊匹木单抗+卡铂/紫杉醇 4 个周期。无限制性毒性和（或）无疾病进展的患者，可以在每 12 周的常规治疗结束后，接受伊匹木单抗/安慰剂作为维持治疗。患者反应的评估参照免疫相关疗效评价标准和修改的世界卫生组织（World Health Organization，WHO）标准。该研究的主要研究终点是免疫相关的无进展生存时间（immune-related progression-free survival，irPFS）；次要研究终点是无进展生存时间（progression-free survival，PFS）、OS、最佳总体有效率、免疫相关的最佳总体有效率及安全性。

主要研究终点 irPFS 的评估参照免疫相关实体瘤疗效评价标准（response evaluation criteria in solid tumors，RECIST），伊匹木单抗+双药化疗序贯治疗组（HR=0.72，P=0.05）达到主要研究终点，而伊匹木单抗联合双药化疗同步治疗组（HR=0.83，P=0.13）未能达到主要研究终点。卡铂+紫杉醇联合用药的中位 irPFS 为 4.6 个月，伊匹木单抗同步治疗组的中位 irPFS 为 5.5 个月，伊匹木单抗序贯治疗组的中位 irPFS 达到 5.7 个月。PFS 的评估参照修改后的 WHO 标准，伊匹木单抗序贯治疗组的 PFS 与对照组相比，获益具有统计学意义，但是伊匹木单抗同步治疗组的 PFS 无统计学意义。对照组的中位 OS 为 8.3 个月，序贯组中位 OS 为 12.2 个月（HR=0.87，P=0.23）；伊匹木单抗同步治疗组的总生存未获益（9.7 个月；HR=0.99，P=0.48）。亚组分析显示，在序贯治疗组中，病理类型为鳞癌的患者与非鳞癌的患者相比，前者 irPFS 和总生存率有获益趋势。关于毒性，3 组中的 3 级、4 级不良事件发生率相近：对照组 37%，同步组 41%，序贯组 39%。与卡铂/紫杉醇对照组相比，包含伊匹木单抗的试验组血液学不良事件发生率相近。非血液学、任何级别（>15%）的不良事件在对照组最为常见，包括疲劳、脱发、周围感觉神经病变、恶心、呕吐。伊匹木单抗组皮疹、腹泻和瘙痒的发生率高于对照组。与对照组相比，试验组的 3 级或 4 级免疫相关毒性发生率更高，如结肠炎、转氨酶升高和垂体炎（同步组 20%，序贯组 15%，对照组 6%）。报道了 2 例治疗相关的死亡病例，对照组和同步组各 1 例[29]。

最近发表的一项Ⅲ期研究评估了一线伊匹木单抗或安慰剂+紫杉醇和卡铂治疗晚期鳞状 NSCLC 的疗效和安全性。Ⅳ期或复发的未接受过化疗的鳞状 NSCLC 患者按 1∶1 分配，接受化疗（紫杉醇和卡铂）+伊匹木单抗 10mg/kg 治疗，或化疗+安慰剂治疗，每 3 周 1 个诱导治疗周期，包括 6 个周期化疗，在第 3~6 个周期联合伊匹木单抗或安慰剂治疗；在诱导治疗后，病情稳定或好转的患者每 12 周接受伊匹木单抗或安慰剂维持治疗。主要研究终点是 OS。入组 956 例患者，749 例患者接受至少 1 个周期的治疗（化疗+伊匹木单抗组，n= 388；化疗+安慰剂组，n= 361）。化疗+伊匹木单抗组的中位 OS 为 13.4 个月，化疗+安慰剂组的中位 OS 为 12.4 个月（HR=0.91；95%CI，0.77~1.07；P=0.25）[3]。另一项Ⅰ期临床研究（NCT01998126）也正在进行，该研究根据患者是否有 EGFR 或 ALK

突变，选择厄洛替尼（erlotinib）+伊匹木单抗治疗或克唑替尼（crizotinib）+伊匹木单抗治疗[30]。这两项研究的结果对于证实在鳞状 NSCLC 中伊匹木单抗联合细胞毒性化疗或在 EGFR 常见突变或 ALK 易位的 NSCLC 患者中伊匹木单抗联合靶向治疗的潜在益处将非常重要。

伊匹木单抗联合其他免疫治疗药物将在本章后面讨论。

曲美木单抗

曲美木单抗是一种抗 CTLA-4 IgG2 完全人源化单克隆抗体[31]。尽管与伊匹木单抗的作用机制相似，曲美木单抗作为单药治疗在 NSCLC 患者中并未显示出疗效。在一项针对 PS 评分良好的局部晚期或转移性 NSCLC 患者的Ⅱ期临床研究中，对已接受 4 个或 4 个以上周期以卡铂类为基础的化疗并有反应的患者，随机给予曲美木单抗或最佳支持治疗，结果显示，该研究未达到其主要研究终点 PFS，曲美木单抗治疗组的客观缓解率（objective response rate，ORR）仅为 4%。20% 的患者发生了 3 级或 4 级不良事件（包括 9% 的免疫相关毒性），最佳支持治疗组未发现不良事件[32]。

同时，一项针对既往接受过治疗的ⅢB 期和Ⅳ期 EGFR 突变阳性的 NSCLC 患者接受曲美木单抗联合吉非替尼（gefitinib）治疗的Ⅰ期临床研究正在进行（NCT02040064）[33]。

曲美木单抗联合其他免疫治疗药物将在本章后面讨论。

PD-1/PD-L1 通路

T 淋巴细胞、B 淋巴细胞，NK 细胞及骨髓源性抑制细胞（marrow-derived inhibitory cells，MDSC）激活后表面表达 PD-1 受体。其主要功能是限制 T 淋巴细胞在外周血发生效应时的活性（与之相反的是，抗 CTLA-4 抗体在 T 淋巴细胞的初始激活中发挥作用）。在慢性抗原暴露环境中过量诱导 PD-1 产生可导致 T 淋巴细胞功能耗尽或丧失[19-35]。组织中以干扰素-γ（interferon-γ，IFN-γ）为主的炎症因子引起 PD-1 的两种受体表达，即 PD-L1（programmed cell death ligand-1）和 PD-L2（programmed cell death ligand-2），进而下调 T 淋巴细胞的活性，抑制组织损伤并维持自身耐受。

包括 NSCLC 在内的很多肿瘤类型 PD-L1 高表达，提示 PD-1/PD-L1 通路激活是肿瘤逃避免疫监视和生长的常见机制[36,37]。

具体来说，PD-1/PD-L1 相互作用的功能包括抑制 T 淋巴细胞增殖、活化和效应（细胞因子释放和细胞毒性），促进 $CD4^+$ T 淋巴细胞分化为 Treg。PD-1 在大量的肿瘤浸润淋巴细胞（tumor-infiltrating lymphocytes，TIL）上表达，由于长期抗原刺激，TIL 几乎被耗尽，功能受到抑制。慢性病毒感染小鼠模型中，阻断 PD-1 通路可部分逆转这种衰竭状态[19]。

临床前研究证实，阻断 PD-1 信号通路可使 CD8$^+$ T 淋巴细胞功能和细胞毒性从衰竭表型恢复，并增强抗肿瘤免疫[38,39]。

抗 PD-1 药物

纳武利尤单抗

纳武利尤单抗（Opdivo$^®$，Bristol Mayer Squibb）是一种特异性针对人 PD-1 的基因编辑的完全人免疫球蛋白 G4（immunoglobulin G4，IgG4）单克隆抗体[40]。

设计 IgG4 同型是为了消除抗体依赖性细胞毒性（antibody-dependent cellular cytotoxicity，ADCC）。当 PD-1 在效应 T 淋巴细胞和其他免疫细胞上表达时，完整的 ADCC 有可能耗尽活化的 T 淋巴细胞和 TIL，并降低其活性。纳武利尤单抗与 PD-1 高亲和力结合，阻断其与 PD-L1 和 PD-L2 的相互作用[41]。

在 CA 209-003 研究中，一项针对 NSCLC、黑色素瘤、去势抵抗性前列腺癌、肾癌和结直肠癌患者的 I 期临床研究中，患者接受纳武利尤单抗单次剂量为每 2 周 0.1～10mg/kg，最多 12 个周期，直至完全缓解或出现限制性毒性、疾病进展或患者要求退出研究。该研究主要目的是评估纳武利尤单抗的安全性和耐受性。该试验设计为剂量递增和队列扩增，总共纳入 296 例患者，其中 122 例为 NSCLC 患者（鳞癌患者 47 例，非鳞癌患者 73 例，未知类型患者 2 例）。85%的 NSCLC 患者之前至少接受过二线治疗，其中 34%的患者接受过酪氨酸激酶抑制剂治疗，且未达到纳武利尤单抗的最大耐受剂量。在 NSCLC 扩增队列中，无论组织学亚型如何，患者均以 1mg/kg、3mg/kg 或 10mg/kg 的剂量使用纳武利尤单抗。据研究人员报告，有 11 例（4%）死亡与严重不良事件有关，均与纳武利尤单抗无关。14 例接受治疗的 NSCLC 患者有客观缓解，其中接受 1mg/kg 剂量的占 6%，3mg/kg 的占 32%，10mg/kg 的占 18%。鳞状和非鳞状 NSCLC 的总缓解率分别是 33%和 12%。8 例达到客观缓解的患者，其客观缓解时间持续了 24 周或更长时间。在病情稳定的患者中，有 7%的人在至少 24 周内没有病情进展。在考虑所入组患者的原发性肿瘤情况下，对 42 例样本进行 PD-L1 状态分析；17 例 PD-L1 阴性肿瘤无客观反应缓解，36%的 PD-L1 阳性肿瘤有客观缓解[42]。

2015 年发布的第二份 I 期临床试验报告只关注了 NSCLC 患者的 OS、缓解的持久性和长期安全性。入组的 NSCLC 患者总数为 129 例。患者每 2 周接受上述 3 种剂量中的 1 种，周期为 8 周，最长可达 96 周。中位年龄为 65 岁，42%的患者为鳞状细胞癌，57%的患者为非鳞状细胞癌，98%的患者的 ECOG 评分为 0～1，

54%的患者在首次使用纳武利尤单抗前接受过至少三线治疗。所有患者的中位 OS 为 9.9 个月，PFS 为 2.3 个月。纳入研究的患者 1 年生存率为 42%，2 年生存率为 24%，3 年生存率为 18%。进一步研究的剂量为 3mg/kg，每 2 周 1 次，该剂量的 1 年、2 年和 3 年生存率分别为 56%、42%和 27%，中位 OS 为 14.9 个月。总体缓解率为 17%，组织学亚型间无统计学差异，中位缓解持续时间（duration of response, DOR）为 17 个月，中位 PFS 为 20.6 个月。在所有患者中，71%的患者出现了各种级别的不良事件（最常见的是疲劳占 24%，食欲下降占 12%，腹泻占 10%），但只有 14%的患者出现了 3 级或 4 级毒性反应（最常见的是疲劳占 3%）。患者确定发生纳武利尤单抗相关的不良事件，则需要密切监测或使用免疫抑制治疗或激素替代治疗，41%的患者表现为"选择性不良事件"，但只有 4.7%的患者达到 3 级或 4 级。报道了 2 例 3 级或 4 级和 1 例 5 级肺炎，据报道与纳武利尤单抗有关。治疗相关的死亡事件有 3 例（2%），均与肺炎相关[43]。

Checkmate-063 是一项单臂、Ⅱ期临床试验，其中鳞状 NSCLC 患者使用纳武利尤单抗剂量为 3mg/kg，每 2 周 1 次，这些患者针对转移性或不可切除疾病曾经接受过至少二线治疗。共纳入 117 例患者。该研究的主要研究终点是客观缓解率（objective response rate, ORR），由独立的放射学审查委员会评估。ORR 为 14.5%，包括 1 例完全缓解的患者，平均缓解时间为 3.3 个月。中位 DOR 未达到。26%的患者达到影像学上最佳反应为病情稳定，中位持续时间为 6 个月。中位 PFS 为 1.9 个月，6 个月 PFS 率为 25.9%，1 年 PFS 率为 20%。中位 OS 为 8.2 个月，其中 1 年 OS 率为 40.8%。对患者提供的肿瘤样本进行评估，检测 PD-1 表达水平，临界值为 5%，PD-1 表达水平高于 5%的患者中，PR 患者占 24%，SD 患者占 5%，疾病进展（progressive disease, PD）患者占 44%；PD-1 低水平表达的患者有 14%达到 PR，20%达到 SD，49%达到 PD。17%的患者出现 3 级或 4 级不良事件，最常见的是疲乏（4%）、腹泻（3%）、肺炎（3%）、皮疹（1%）、瘙痒（1%）、肌肉痛（1%）和贫血（1%）。12%的治疗相关不良事件导致停药。研究者将 2 例死亡归因于使用纳武利尤单抗，一例死于肺炎，另一例死于缺血性脑卒中；然而，2 例患者都伴随多种疾病并出现病情进展[44]。在至少 11 个月的长期随访中，仍未达到中位缓解持续时间，也没有新发纳武利尤单抗治疗相关的死亡报告[45]。

Checkmate-017 是一项评估Ⅲ期或Ⅳ期鳞状 NSCLC 患者的Ⅲ期临床研究，入组患者为一线铂类双药化疗后疾病进展者。该研究比较了纳武利尤单抗每 2 周 3mg/kg 静脉注射和多西他赛每 3 周 75mg/m^2 静脉注射两种治疗方法，直到疾病进展或出现不可耐受的毒性反应。主要研究终点为 OS。对 260 例 ECOG 为 0～1 的患者进行随机分组。纳武利尤单抗组中位年龄为 62 岁，多西他赛组中位年龄为 64 岁，入组患者男性居多。纳武利尤单抗组和多西他赛组的中位 OS 分别为 9.2 个月和 6 个月；纳武利尤单抗组和多西他赛组的 1 年生存率分别为 42%和 24%。

纳武利尤单抗组 PFS 为 3.5 个月，ORR 为 20%，多西他赛组 PFS 为 2.8 个月，ORR 为 9%。中位缓解持续时间在多西他赛组为 8.4 个月，在纳武利尤单抗组未达到。采用免疫组化方法检测 PD-L1 表达水平，采用北美 Dako 公司的兔抗人单克隆抗体（Clone 28-8，epitomics）。任何水平的染色结果都被认为是阳性。将 PD-L1 阳性表达水平分为 3 类：1%、5% 和 10%。研究者的结论是 PD-L1 表达既不能预测纳武利尤单抗的预后，也不能预测其疗效。但在分析原始数据时发现，纳武利尤单抗治疗组中，与 PD-L1 表达水平低的患者相比，PD-L1 表达水平高于 10% 的患者有获益的趋势；以 5% 为临界值进行分析可能得到同样的结果。与纳武利尤单抗组相比，多西他赛组中所有级别和 3 级或 4 级不良事件发生率更高；所有级别不良事件发生率分别为 87% 和 59%，3 级或 4 级不良事件分别为 56% 和 8%。疲乏、食欲缺乏和腹泻是纳武利尤单抗组最常见的 3 级或 4 级不良反应。免疫介导的不良事件发生在胃肠道、肺和肾各 1 例[46]。

考虑到 OS 获益情况，独立数据监测委员会建议在 2015 年 1 月停止试验。2015 年 3 月，美国 FDA 批准纳武利尤单抗作为一线铂类双药化疗失败的鳞状 NSCLC 的二线治疗药物。

与 CheckMate 017 设计相似，CheckMate 057 是一项Ⅲ期临床试验，对比纳武利尤单抗与多西他赛用于接受铂类双药化疗期间或之后进展的非鳞状 NSCLC 患者。该研究次要终点包括 ORR，PFS 及参照 PD-L1 表达的疗效。582 例患者按 1：1 随机接受纳武利尤单抗或多西他赛治疗。纳武利尤单抗组的中位 OS 为 12.2 个月，12 个月 OS 率为 51%，18 个月 OS 率为 39%，多西他赛组中位 OS 为 9.4 个月，12 个月 OS 率为 39% 和 18 个月 OS 率为 23%。纳武利尤单抗和多西他赛的有效率中位 OS 为 19% 和 12%。多西他赛组的中位 PFS 比纳武利尤单抗组更高（4.2 个月 vs. 2.3 个月），但多西他赛组 1 年 PFS 率为 8%，纳武利尤单抗组为 19%。多西他赛组 3 级或 4 级不良事件发生率高于纳武利尤单抗组（54% vs. 10%）。纳武利尤单抗相关的最常见不良事件为疲乏、腹泻和恶心。与在 CheckMate017 中接受治疗的鳞状 NSCLC 患者相比，使用前面提到的相同免疫组织化学法检测的 PD-L1 表达情况可以预测所有研究终点的预后。亚组分析结果显示，与多西他赛组相比，当前或既往吸烟且有 KRAS 突变的患者，如果使用纳武利尤单抗治疗，也会受益。然而，与多西他赛组相比，有 EGFR 突变、年龄大于 75 岁或从未吸烟的患者采用纳武利尤单抗治疗未见明显获益[47]。基于这项试验的结果，FDA 于 2015 年 10 月批准纳武利尤单抗用于之前接受过治疗的非鳞状 NSCLC 患者。

最近更新了 CheckMate 017 和 CheckMate057 的 2 年生存率。在 CheckMate 017 中，鳞状 NSCLC 患者采用纳武利尤单抗治疗的 2 年生存率为 23%，多西他赛组 2 年生存率为 8%。在 CheckMate 057 中，非鳞状 NSCLC 患者采用纳武利尤单抗治疗的 2 年生存率为 29%，多西他赛组为 16%[48]。

CheckMate 026 评估了纳武利尤单抗作为一线治疗的情况。这项Ⅲ期临床试验将Ⅳ期或复发性非小细胞肺癌患者按1:1的比例随机分组:每2周接受3mg/kg剂量的纳武利尤单抗治疗,或每3周接受1次铂类为基础的化疗,疗程最长6个周期。允许化疗组患者交叉至纳武利尤单抗组。主要研究终点为PD-L1表达大于5%的患者的独立中心评估的PFS。纳入423例PD-L1表达水平在5%以上的患者。纳武利尤单抗组中位PFS为4.2个月,化疗组为5.9个月(HR=1.15;95%CI,0.91~1.45;P=0.25),纳武利尤单抗组中位OS为14.4个月,化疗组为13.2个月(HR=1.02;95%CI,0.80~1.30)。化疗组212例患者中有128例(60%)接受纳武利尤单抗作为后续治疗。接受纳武利尤单抗治疗的患者中3级或4级不良事件发生率为18%,化疗组为51%。因此,在这类人群中,纳武利尤单抗相比化疗在PFS或OS方面并没有更好的获益[4]。

一线治疗中也评估了联合治疗的情况。CheckMate012是一项Ⅰ期多臂试验,评估纳武利尤单抗与伊匹木单抗联合作为一线治疗应用于NSCLC患者。患者按1:1比例随机分组,接受纳武利尤单抗每2周1mg/kg+伊匹木单抗每6周1mg/kg,纳武利尤单抗每2周3mg/kg+伊匹木单抗每12周1mg/kg,或纳武利尤单抗每2周3mg/kg+伊匹木单抗每6周1mg/kg直至病情进展,出现不可耐受的毒性反应或患者拒绝接受治疗[49]。后面两组的结果显示,伊匹木单抗每12周治疗组中有18例患者获得客观缓解(objective response,OR)[47%(95% CI,31~64)],伊匹木单抗每6周治疗组有15例患者获得了OR[38%(95% CI,23~55)]。两组患者均未达到中位缓解持续时间,伊匹木单抗每12周治疗组的中位随访时间为12.8个月(IQR 9.3~15.5),伊匹木单抗每6周治疗组的中位随访时间为11.8个月(6.7~15.9)。在PD-L1大于或等于1%的患者中,每12周治疗组21例患者中有12例(57%)获得确定的客观缓解,每6周治疗组23例患者中为13例(57%)。伊匹木单抗每12周治疗组中,有14例患者(37%)出现3级、4级治疗相关的不良事件,伊匹木单抗每6周治疗组中,有13例患者(33%);最常见的3级、4级不良事件为脂肪酶升高[3例(8%)vs. 0例],肺炎[2例(5%)vs. 1例(3%)],肾上腺功能不全[1例(3%)vs. 2例(5%)]和结肠炎[1例(3%)vs. 2例(5%)][5]。

CheckMate227是一项开放标签的Ⅲ期试验,评估了纳武利尤单抗联合伊匹木单抗相比化疗用于肿瘤突变负荷高的患者(定义为每百万碱基对中有≥10个突变)。采用FoundationOne CDx检测既往未治疗的Ⅳ期或复发性NSCLC患者的肿瘤突变负荷。此外,PD-L1表达至少为1%的患者按1:1的比例随机接受纳武利尤单抗+伊匹木单抗、纳武利尤单抗单药治疗或化疗。肿瘤突变负荷高的患者,采用纳武利尤单抗+伊匹木单抗治疗的PFS较化疗组显著延长。纳武利尤单抗+伊匹木单抗治疗组的1年PFS率为42.6%,中位PFS为7.2个月(95% CI,5.5~13.2),化疗组的1年PFS率为13.2%,中位PFS为5.5个月(95% CI,4.4~5.8)。纳武利尤单抗+伊匹木单抗治疗组的 HR 为 0.58；97.5% CI，0.41~0.81；P<0.001，ORR 为 45.3%，而化疗组为 45.3%[6]。高肿瘤突变负荷已成为评价免疫治疗效果的一种可行的标志物，进而探寻对治疗反应更好的人群。

帕博利珠单抗

帕博利珠单抗（MK-3475，商品名 Keytruda®，美国默沙东公司 Merck Sharp & Dohme）是一种高选择性 IgG4κ 同型的抗 PD-1 单克隆抗体。这种高选择性抗体与 PD-1 结合而阻断 PD-1、PD-L1/PD-L2 通路，从而克服了这种主要的免疫检查点抑制[50]。该药于 2014 年获得批准适用于不可手术切除的转移性黑色素瘤。

晚期 NSCLC 患者作为 I 期 Keynote-001 临床试验的部分人群，被分配到多个扩展组中。患者入组标准为 ECOG PS 0-1，器官功能正常，无肺炎或自身免疫性疾病病史，目前未进行系统性免疫抑制治疗。该试验主要目的是评估帕博利珠单抗在 NSCLC 患者中的安全性、毒性和活性。经过修改后，该试验增加了一个共同主要研究终点，即 PD-L1 表达水平高的 NSCLC 患者的有效率。采用免疫组化 22C3 抗体药物 DX 检测 PD-L1 表达。患者随机分为 3 组：帕博利珠单抗每 3 周 2mg/kg，帕博利珠单抗每 3 周 10mg/kg 或帕博利珠单抗每 2 周 10mg/kg，均为静脉输注 30 分钟。

在 495 名随机接受至少 1 剂帕博利珠单抗的患者中，70%的患者出现了不良事件（包含所有级别），9.5%的患者出现 3 级或更高级别的不良事件。最常见的不良事件（包含所有级别）为疲乏、瘙痒和食欲下降。报道中最常见的治疗相关不良事件是输液反应（2%）、甲状腺功能减退（6.9%）及肺炎（3.6%），包括 1.8%的 3 级不良事件（肺炎）和 1 例因肺炎导致的死亡。三组患者的有效率相似，与剂量、时间和组织学无关。总体有效率为 19.4%（既往接受过治疗的占 18%，未接受过治疗的占 24.8%），总体疾病稳定率为 21.8%。目前或既往吸烟的患者（22.5%）相比从未吸烟的患者，前者治疗有效率更高（10.3%）。中位缓解持续时间为 12.5 个月（既往接受过治疗的为 10.4 个月，未接受过治疗的为 23.3 个月）。总体中位 PFS 为 3.7 个月（既往接受过治疗的为 3 个月，未接受过治疗的为 6 个月），总体中位 OS 为 12 个月（既往接受过治疗的为 9.3 个月，未接受过治疗的为 16.2 个月）。肿瘤标本评估显示，PD-L1 表达为 1%~49%的患者占 37.6%，高于 50%的患者占 23.2%。与 PD-L1 表达为 1%~49%或低于 1%的患者相比，PD-L1 过表达（50%或更高）的患者的客观缓解率更高（45.2%）。PD-L1 高表达组中位 PFS 为 6.3 个月，中位 OS 未达到[51]。

最近 Keynote-001 中更新的 PD-L1 表达为 1%~49%的患者的 OS 显示，既往接受治疗的患者的中位 OS 为 11.3 个月，而未接受治疗的患者的中位 OS 为 22.1 个月。PD-L1 表达为 50%或更高的患者，中位 OS 在既往接受过治疗的患者中为 15.4

个月，在未接受过治疗的患者中未达到[52]。

基于上述结果，美国食品药品监督管理局（FDA）于2015年10月批准帕博利珠单抗用于一线细胞毒性化疗失败PD-L1表达阳性的转移性NSCLC患者。

在24个国家进行的Keynote-010是一项开放标签的Ⅱ期或Ⅲ期临床试验，针对既往接受过至少一线铂类双药化疗的NSCLC，对比帕博利珠单抗与多西他赛治疗。所有患者肿瘤中PD-L1的表达必须至少达到1%，通过免疫组化试验（22C3抗体药物DX检测）进行评估，参照RECIST 1.1进行疗效评估。患者随机分组接受帕博利珠单抗每3周2mg/kg，每3周10mg/kg，或多西他赛每3周75mg/m^{2}治疗。主要研究终点为总体人群的OS和PFS及PD-L1高表达（50%或以上）患者的OS和PFS。991例NSCLC患者（鳞癌占22%）接受至少1剂帕博利珠单抗或多西他赛。28%的患者PD-L1表达50%及以上。总体人群中，两个剂量的帕博利珠单抗组的OS均较多西他赛组高，帕博利珠单抗2mg/kg组：HR=0.71，P=0.0008；帕博利珠单抗10mg/kg组：HR=0.61，P=0.0001。帕博利珠单抗2mg/kg组中位OS为10.4个月，1年生存率为43.2%；帕博利珠单抗10mg/kg组中位OS为12.7个月，1年生存率为52.3%；多西他赛组中位OS为8.5个月，1年生存率为34.6%。采用帕博利珠单抗治疗的两组在OS方面未见明显差异。亚组分析结果显示，腺癌患者明显获益，但鳞状NSCLC患者OS获益不明显。

PD-L1高表达（至少50%）的患者中，帕博利珠单抗相比多西他赛，前者OS更高。相比多西他赛组，帕博利珠单抗2mg/kg组HR=0.54（P=0.0002），帕博利珠单抗10mg/kg组HR=0.5（P=0.0001）。PD-L1高表达的患者中，帕博利珠单抗2mg/kg组中位OS为14.9个月，帕博利珠单抗10mg/kg组为17.3个月，多西他赛组为8.2个月。在总体人群中，相比多西他赛治疗，帕博利珠单抗组的PFS在统计学上并没有显著优势；但是采用帕博利珠单抗治疗的两组患者，PD-L1高表达患者的PFS显著延长（HR=0.59），帕博利珠单抗2mg/kg组中位PFS为5个月，帕博利珠单抗10mg/kg组为5.2个月，多西他赛组为4.1个月。采用帕博利珠单抗治疗的两组患者的客观缓解率明显高于多西他赛组。这在总体人群和PD-L1表达为50%或以上的患者中均可见。在总体人群中，帕博利珠单抗2mg/kg组有效率为18%，帕博利珠单抗10mg/kg组为18%，多西他赛组为9%；PD-L1表达50%或以上的患者中，帕博利珠单抗2mg/kg组有效率为30%，帕博利珠单抗10mg/kg组为29%，多西他赛组为8%。三组患者均无完全缓解。与多西他赛组相比，两组帕博利珠单抗治疗的毒性显著降低。因3级或4级不良事件而中断治疗的情况报告如下：帕博利珠单抗2mg/kg组有13例（4%），帕博利珠单抗10mg/kg组有16例（5%），多西他赛组有35例（10%）。帕博利珠单抗2mg/kg组与帕博利珠单抗10mg/kg组的免疫相关毒副反应发生率相近，分别为20%、19%。最常见的免疫相关不良事件为甲状腺功能减退、甲状腺功能亢进和肺炎。采用帕博利珠单抗治疗的两组患者中，超过1%的3～5级不良事件为肺炎和皮肤反应。帕博利珠单抗2mg/kg组有2例治疗相关的死亡（1例肺炎，1例肺部感染），帕博利珠单抗10mg/kg组有3例（1例心肌梗死，1例肺部感染，1例肺炎）[53]。

最近更新的Keynote-010报告显示，与低表达的亚组（PD-L1表达50%～74%、25%～49%和1%～24%）相比，PD-L1表达为75%或以上的患者OS、PFS和有效率获益在统计学上更明显。在多西他赛组中，无论PD-L1表达水平如何，均未见明显获益[54]。

在接受帕博利珠单抗治疗的患者中，PD-L1表达50%或以上并不能作为独立因素促使患者在OS方面获益。最近一份报告表明，Keynote-010的患者中，帕博利珠单抗组相比多西他赛组，前者OS获益较大（帕博利珠单抗2mg/kg组中位OS为9.4个月，HR=0.79；帕博利珠单抗10mg/kg组中位OS为10.8个月，HR=0.71；多西他赛组中位OS为8.6个月）[55]。

有关检测标本的重要性，用免疫组化的方法检测新鲜组织样本或存档样本的PD-L1表达水平，结果显示，两者的OS未见显著差异，且PD-L1表达50%或以上的情况也未见明显差异[56]。

Keynote-024是一项Ⅲ期临床试验，入组的305例肿瘤细胞PD-L1表达至少50%，表皮生长因子受体（EGFR）无敏感突变或ALK易位，未接受过治疗的晚期NSCLC患者，接受帕博利珠单抗治疗（每3周固定剂量200mg）或研究者选择的以铂类为基础的化疗。化疗组患者允许交叉至帕博利珠单抗治疗。主要研究终点PFS采用盲法，由独立的中心放射审查评估。次要研究终点是OS、ORR和安全性。帕博利珠单抗组的中位PFS为10.3个月（95% CI，6.7～未达到），化疗组为6.0个月（95% CI，4.2～6.2）（HR=0.50；95% CI，0.37～0.68；$P<0.001$）。6个月时的总生存率估计值，帕博利珠单抗组为80.2%，化疗组为72.4%（HR=0.60；95%CI，0.41～0.89；$P=0.005$）。帕博利珠单抗组的有效率高于化疗组（44.8% vs. 27.8%），且帕博利珠单抗组的中位缓解持续时间相比化疗组更长[未达到（1.9个月以上～14.5个月以上）vs.5个月（2.1个月以上～12.6个月以上）]。关于毒副反应，帕博利珠单抗组中任何级别的治疗相关不良事件发生率均低于化疗组，分别为73.4% vs.90.0%，3级、4级或5级治疗相关不良事件发生率分别为26.6% vs. 53.3%[7]。随访25个月后的更新分析显示，帕博利珠单抗治疗组OS为30.2个月，化疗组为14.2个月，死亡率降低37%（HR=0.63；95% CI，0.47～0.86；$P=0.002$）。帕博利珠单抗组24个月OS率为51.5%，化疗组为34.5%。帕博利珠单抗组12个月OS率为70.3%，化疗组为54.8%。帕博利珠单抗组ORR为45.5%（95%CI，37.4～53.7），化疗组为29.8%（95%CI，22.6～37.8）。帕博利珠单抗组的中位缓解持续时间未达到（范围为1.8个月以上～20.6个月以上），化疗组的中位缓解持续时间为7.1个月（范围为2.1个月以上～18.1个月以上）[8]。

Keynote-042 是一项针对一线转移或无法手术切除的 NSCLC 患者（鳞癌和非鳞癌）的Ⅲ期临床试验，患者无根治性治疗机会且 PD-L1 表达至少 1%。入组的患者分别接受帕博利珠单抗单药治疗或化疗（卡铂+紫杉醇或卡铂+培美曲塞）。通过肿瘤比例评分（tumor proportion score，TPS）评估 PD-L1 水平。主要研究终点为 TPS≥50%、TPS≥20%及 TPS≥1%的 OS。该研究达到了研究终点，其结果即将公布[57,58]。

同样也开展了研究评估帕博利珠单抗联合治疗。Keynote-189 是一项双盲、Ⅲ期临床试验，将 616 例既往未接受过治疗、无 EGFR 敏感突变或 ALK 突变的非鳞状 NSCLC 患者按 2∶1 比例分组，分别给予培美曲塞和一种铂类为基础的药物联合帕博利珠单抗 200mg 或安慰剂每 3 周 1 次，4 个周期后，给予培美曲塞联合帕博利珠单抗或安慰剂维持治疗，共维持 35 个周期。在安慰剂联合组中，确认疾病进展的患者可以采用帕博利珠单抗单药治疗。主要研究终点 OS 和 PFS 经由盲法、独立中心放射学审查评估。中位随访 10.5 个月时发现，联合帕博利珠单抗治疗组的 12 个月 OS 率为 69.2%（95%CI，64.1~73.8），安慰剂联合治疗组为 49.4%（95%CI，42.1~56.2）（HR=0.49；95%CI，0.38~0.64；$P<0.001$）。所有亚组帕博利珠单抗联合组均较安慰剂联合组有获益：PD-L1 TPS<1%（12 个月 OS 率，61.7% vs. 52.2%；HR=0.59；95%CI，0.38~0.92），TPS 1%~49%（12 个月 OS 率，71.5% vs. 50.9%；HR=0.55；95%CI，0.34~0.90），TPS 50%或以上（12 个月 OS 率，73.0% vs. 48.1%；HR=0.42；95%CI，0.26~0.68）。帕博利珠单抗联合组的中位 PFS 为 8.8 个月（95%CI，7.6~9.2），安慰剂联合组的中位 PFS 为 4.9 个月（95%CI，4.7~5.5）（HR=0.52；95%CI，0.43~0.64；$P<0.001$）。帕博利珠单抗联合组 3 级或以上不良事件发生率为 67.2%，安慰剂联合组为 65.8%。本试验中肺炎导致的死亡发生率与之前观察到的帕博利珠单抗单药治疗晚期 NSCLC 的发生率一致[9]。

PD-L1 抑制剂

类似于 PD-1 阻滞，另一个有趣的策略是通过单克隆抗体的结合来阻断 PD-L1。PD-L1 抗体不会阻断 PD-1 与 PD-L2/CD80 的相互作用。在免疫系统活化状态，PD-L1 抗体不阻断 PD-1 与 PD-L2/CD80 的相互作用在控制炎症，保护正常肺组织免受过度损伤方面有重要作用[59]。

与 PD-1 抑制剂相比，PD-L1 抑制剂不同的作用机制可以降低免疫相关的毒性，而且通过阻断 PD-L1 与 CD80 之间的相互作用，可以抑制 T 淋巴细胞的负向调控，理论上可以使单克隆抗体的活性最大化[60]，但临床上尚未证实。

目前有几种此类药物正在研究中。

度伐鲁单抗

度伐鲁单抗（MEDI4736）是高亲和性的人 IgG1 抗体，可以与 PD-1 和 CD80 结合但不与 PD-L2 结合，从而选择性地阻断 PD-L1 通路，降低因 PD-L2 通路的阻滞引起的免疫相关性毒性。

在一个剂量爬坡、队列扩大的Ⅰ期临床试验中，评估了度伐鲁单抗在经治或初治的 NSCLC 患者中的安全性和有效性。43%的患者出现了 1 级或 2 级的毒副反应，但没有报道 3～5 级的肺炎，经治的患者和初治的患者在毒性方面未见显著差异。在不同队列中接受治疗的 13 例患者的初步结果显示，用免疫 RECIST 标准评估，3 例出现部分缓解，2 例肿瘤缩小但未达到部分缓解。扩大队列招募了至少 300 例患者[61]。

最近报道了这项Ⅰ期和Ⅱ期临床试验的最新进展，198 例 NSCLC 患者（其中 116 例为非鳞状细胞癌，82 例为鳞状细胞癌）接受了度伐鲁单抗治疗：每 2 周静脉注射 10mg/kg，直至疾病进展或出现不可耐受的毒性或治疗满 1 年。如果患者在治疗 12 个月后失败了有机会重新接受度伐鲁单抗治疗。其客观缓解率为 14%，但 PD-L1 阳性患者的缓解率更高（23%）。从组织学上看，鳞状细胞癌的缓解率高于非鳞状细胞癌（分别为 21%和 10%）。缓解持续时间范围为 0.1～35 周。48%的患者出现治疗毒性，最常见的不良事件有疲劳（14%）、食欲缺乏（9%）和恶心（8%）。6%的患者发生了 3 级或 4 级毒性，只有 2%的患者因毒性而停止治疗。总体接受过治疗的人群中只报道了两例肺炎事件[62]。

最近一份基于初治人群的报告显示度伐鲁单抗的客观缓解率为 25%（鳞状和非鳞状 NSCLC 分别为 26%和 25%），12 周以上的疾病控制率为 56%。3 级以上的毒性发生率为 9%，7%的患者因毒性反应终止治疗，其中两例腹泻导致了治疗终止[63]。

度伐鲁单抗单药治疗在接受了放化疗的局部晚期的Ⅲ期患者中已显示出最有希望的结果。这项Ⅲ期临床研究以 2∶1 的比例分配患者接受每 2 周 1 次的度伐鲁单抗 10mg/kg 或安慰剂治疗，持续 1 年，患者在放化疗结束后 1～42 天内开始接受治疗。主要研究终点为 PFS 和 OS。这项研究纳入了 709 例患者，其中 473 例接受度伐鲁单抗治疗，236 例接受安慰剂治疗。研究结果显示，度伐鲁单抗治疗组和安慰剂组中位 PFS 分别为 16.8 个月（95% CI，13.0～18.1）和 5.6 个月（95% CI，4.6～7.8），且安慰剂组（HR=0.52，95%CI，0.42～0.65，$P<0.001$）；12 个月的 PFS 率分别为 55.9%和 35.3%，18 个月的 PFS 率分别是 44.2%和 27.0%。度伐鲁单抗治疗组中位缓解持续时间更长（18 个月的持续缓解率分别为 72.8% vs.46.8%）。度伐鲁单抗治疗组发生远处转移或死亡的中位时间比安慰剂组更长，为 23.2 个月 vs. 14.6 个月（$P<0.001$）。鉴于这项临床研究的性质，即在确切的治疗管理之后没有后续治疗的建议，因此不良事件的评估在此项临床研究中也很重

要。3级或4级的不良事件发生率在度伐鲁单抗治疗组为29.9%，而在安慰剂治疗组为26.1%。最常见的3级或4级不良事件是肺炎（分别为4.4%和3.8%）。同时，有15.4%的度伐鲁单抗治疗组患者和9.8%的安慰剂组患者因不良事件停止了研究药物治疗[10]。此项研究的意义可能是近十年来在局部晚期疾病方面最重要的进展。

抗PD-L1和抗CTLA-4抗体的联合是目前正在评估的NSCLC患者的一个很有前途的治疗选择。一项多中心、非随机、开放的Ⅰb期临床研究评估了102例局部晚期或转移性NSCLC患者联合使用度伐鲁单抗和曲美木单抗的安全性和抗肿瘤活性。度伐鲁单抗的剂量为每4周3mg/kg、10mg/kg、15mg/kg或20mg/kg，或每2周10mg/kg；曲美木单抗的剂量为1mg/kg、3mg/kg或10mg/kg，每4周给药，共6次，然后每12周给药，共3次。剂量限制性毒性发生在每4周接受度伐鲁单抗20mg/kg+曲美木单抗3mg/kg的队列中，6例中有2例发生剂量限制性毒性（1例转氨酶3级升高，1例脂肪酶4级升高）。26%的患者因毒性反应而停止治疗，最常见的不良事件是腹泻（32%）、疲劳（24%）和瘙痒（21%）。最常见的3级或以上毒性为腹泻（11%）、结肠炎（9%）和脂肪酶增高（8%）。在研究期间的22例死亡事件中，有3例由治疗所致。安全性数据显示最大的可选择的剂量为度伐鲁单抗20mg/kg+曲美木单抗1mg/kg。63例可评估肿瘤反应的患者中，客观反应率为17%（PD-L1阴性患者5%），疾病控制率为29%。基于此，该研究的作者得出结论，PD-L1状态可能无法预测度伐鲁单抗+曲美木单抗联合用药的疗效[64]。

度伐鲁单抗由阿斯利康（AstraZeneca）授权，目前正在进行针对NSCLC患者的不同临床试验，包括评估度伐鲁单抗联合奥斯替尼治疗的TATTON研究，以及度伐鲁单抗单药或联合曲美木单抗治疗等研究。

阿特珠单抗

阿特珠单抗（MPDL3280A）是另一种抗PD-L1的药物，这是一种人源化IgG1单克隆抗体，含有突变的Fc区域，旨在避免Fc受体结合，从而避免PD-L1导致的抗体依赖的细胞毒作用（antibody-dependent cell-mediated cytotoxicity，ADCC）[65]。

在一项扩大的Ⅰ期研究中，经治的鳞状和非鳞状NSCLC患者接受阿特珠单抗治疗，剂量为1～20mg/kg。据报道，3级或4级不良事件包括心包积液（6%）、脱水（4%）、呼吸困难（4%）和疲劳（4%）。没有发生与治疗相关的死亡，按RECIST 1.1评估的客观缓解率为24%。24周PFS率为48%。PD-L1阳性的患者达到了100%的客观缓解率（4/4），而PD-L1阴性的患者总体缓解率达15%（4/26），疾病进展率为58%[66]。

在一项包含了黑色素瘤和肾细胞癌等其他癌种的研究的扩大队列中纳入了85例鳞状或非鳞状NSCLC患者，NSCLC患者接受每3周1次阿特珠单抗治疗，客观缓解率达到21%。目前或既往吸烟者比从不吸烟者有更高的缓解率（42% vs.

10%）。PD-L1 表达水平较高的患者比未表达 PD-L1 的患者缓解率更高。对于在这个试验中接受治疗的所有患者，包括 NSCLC 和其他肿瘤类型患者，据报道，毒性发生率（包含所有级别）为 70%，最常见不良事件是疲劳（24%）、食欲缺乏（11%）、恶心（11%）、发热（11%）、腹泻（10%）和皮疹（10%）；39%的患者出现 3 级或 4 级毒性反应，包括呼吸困难（4%）、贫血（3.6%）、疲劳（3.2%）和高血糖（2.5%）[67]。

针对 PD-L2 高表达的不同癌症类型的临床结果也显示了阿特珠单抗治疗的优越性[68]。

阿特珠单抗联合化疗在 NSCLC 患者一线治疗中已经进行了 Ⅰb 期试验。患者每 3 周静脉注射 15mg/kg 的阿特珠单抗和 4~6 周期的铂类为基础化疗后用阿特珠单抗维持治疗。结果显示 3 级或 4 级毒性发生率高达 13%，大部分为化疗相关的血液毒性，有 1 例长期中性粒细胞减少后因念珠菌感染死亡。联合不同化疗方案的总有效率有差异，在 60%~75%，客观反应与 PD-L1 的表达状态无关[69]。

Ⅱ期临床研究 BIRCH 是一个开放的多中心研究，旨在评估阿特珠单抗在 PD-L1 表达的 NSCLC 患者中的安全性和有效性。该研究纳入了 667 例经治或初治患者。PD-L1 状态采用罗氏诊断公司开发的免疫组化方法对肿瘤细胞（TC）和肿瘤浸润免疫细胞（IC）进行评估，因此最终结果根据两者的评分来综合判定：TC 0（TC0＜1%），TC1（1%≤TC1＜5%），TC2（5%≤TC2＜50%）或 TC3（TC3≥50%）和 IC 0（IC0＜1%），IC 1（1%≤IC1＜5%），IC 2（5%≤IC2＜10%）或 IC 3（IC3≥10%）。符合试验条件的是评分为 TC 2/3 或 IC 2/3 的患者。患者接受每 3 周 1 次 1200mg 的阿特珠单抗静脉注射治疗。主要终点为客观应答率。得分为 TC3/IC3 的患者缓解率高于 TC 2/3 或 IC 2/3 患者：一线治疗为 26% vs.19%，二线治疗为 24% vs.17%，三线以上治疗为 27% vs. 17%[70]。

POPLAR 研究是一项 Ⅱ 期研究，对比了阿特珠单抗和多西他赛在二线治疗，无论 PD-L1 的表达状态的局部晚期或转移性 NSCLC 的疗效，PD-L1 的表达采用罗氏诊断公司开发的免疫组化方法来评估。287 例患者每 3 周给予阿特珠单抗 1200mg 的固定剂量。POPLAR 的主要终点是 OS。PD-L1 阳性的所有亚组中，阿特珠单抗组患者的 OS 均高于多西他赛，任何 PD-L1 表达的患者中阿特珠单抗组和多西他赛的中位 OS 为 15.5 个月 vs. 9.2 个月（HR=0.59，$P=0.005$），PD-L1 中度表达的患者（TC2/3 或 IC2/3）为 15.1 月 vs.7.4 个月（HR=0.54，$P=0.014$），PD-L1 高表达的患者（TC3 或 IC3）为 15.5 个月 vs. 11.1 个月（HR=0.49，$P=0.068$）。PD-L1 阴性表达患者（TC 0 且 IC 0）两组 OS 无差异（均为 9.7 个月）[71]。

POPLAR 研究的最新数据表明，与多西他赛相比，阿特珠单抗延长了 OS，两条生存曲线分开（中位 OS 为 12.6 个月 vs. 9.7 个月，$P=0.011$）；TC3 或 IC3 亚组的中位 OS 为未达到 vs. 11.1 个月（$P=0.033$）。在组织学上，两种组织学亚型（鳞状 vs. 非鳞状）无明显差异，阿特珠单抗组 OS 均优于多西他赛组[72]。

OAK 研究是一项Ⅲ期、开放的、二线及以后的国际临床研究。纳入了既往接受过 1 或 2 种化疗但未接受过抗 CTLA-4、抗-PD-L1 或抗-PD-L1 治疗的ⅢB 期或Ⅳ期鳞状或非鳞状 NSCLC 患者。以 1∶1 的比例随机分组：每 3 周给予阿特珠单抗 1200mg 或多西他赛 75mg/m^2。共同主要终点为意向治疗（intention-to-treat, ITT）人群和 PD-L1 表达状态为 TC1/2/3 或 IC1/2/3（PD-L1≥1%的肿瘤细胞或 tumor-inflträting 免疫细胞）人群中的 OS。研究共纳入 1225 例患者，其中 425 例患者被随机分到阿特珠单抗治疗组，另 425 例患者被随机分到多西他赛治疗组。在两组目标人群中，与多西他赛治疗组相比，阿特珠单抗治疗组患者的 OS 明显延长。在 ITT 人群中，中位 OS 为 13.8 个月（95% CI, 11.8～15.7）vs. 9.6 个月（95% CI, 8.6～11.2）；HR=0.73（95% CI, 0.62～0.87）；P = 0.0003，在 TC1/2/3 或 IC1/2/3 人群中，中位 OS 为 15.7 个月（95% CI, 12.6～18.0）vs. 10.3 个月（95% CI, 8.8～12.0）；HR=0.74（95% CI, 0.58～0.93）；P=0.0102。PD-L1 表达为 TC0 和 IC0 的患者也有阳性结果，中位 OS 为 12.6 个月 vs. 8.9 个月；HR=0.75（95% CI, 0.59～0.96）。鳞癌和非鳞癌 NSCLC 患者的 OS 改善相似。在毒副反应方面，阿特珠单抗组和多西他赛组治疗相关的 3 级或 4 级不良事件的发生率分别为 15% 和 43%，多西他赛组出现 1 例死于呼吸道感染的与治疗相关的死亡事件[11]。

阿特珠单抗联合贝伐珠单抗的治疗在不考虑 PD-L1 的表达的初治的转移性非鳞状 NSCLC 患者中进行了评估。IMpower 150 研究是国际性、开放的、Ⅲ期临床研究，共纳入 1202 名患者，以 1∶1∶1 的比例随机分为三个治疗组：阿特珠单抗+卡铂+紫杉醇（ACP），阿特珠单抗+贝伐珠单抗+卡铂+紫杉醇（ABCP）和贝伐珠单抗+卡铂+紫杉醇（BCP），各组给药 4～6 周期。诱导化疗后，患者继续接受阿特珠单抗或贝伐珠单抗，或同时接受这两种药物维持治疗直至疾病进展或出现无法耐受的毒性。主要的终点为野生型（wild type，WT）（无 EGFR 突变或 ALK 重排）ITT 人群的 PFS、效应 T 淋巴细胞相关基因信号（Teff）高表达的 WT 人群的 PFS 及 WT 总体人群的 OS。Teff 定义为 PD-L1，CXCL9 和 IFN-γ 信使 RNA（mRNA）。在 WT 人群中，ABCP 组较 BCP 组中位 PFS 显著延长（8.3 个月 vs. 6.8 个月，HR=0.62，95% CI, 0.52～0.74，P<0.001）。在 Teff 高表达的 WT 人群中，与 BCP 组相比，ABCP 组的 PFS 明显延长（11.3 个月 vs. 6.8 个月，HR 0.51, 95% CI, 0.38～0.68, P<0.001）。亚组分析显示无论 PD-L1 表达状态如何，PFS 均得到延长，包括无 PD-L1 表达、PD-L1 低表达、Teff 低表达的人群。值得注意的是，在对 EGFR 突变或 ALK 重排患者的分析中（n=108），ABCP 组较 BCP 组 PFS 也更长（9.7 个月 vs. 6.1 个月，HR=0.59, 95% CI, 0.37～0.94）。在 WT 人群中，与 BCP 组相比，ABCP 组 OS 明显延长（19.2 个月 vs. 14.7 个月，HR=0.78, 95% CI, 0.64～0.96，P = 0.02）。ABCP 组和 BCP 组的 3 级或 4 级治疗相关不良事件发生率分别为 55.7%和 47.7%。ABCP 组的毒性谱与每种药物已知的毒性谱是一致的[73]。

本研究数据表明，在免疫检查点抑制剂中加入细胞毒性化疗可能会增强免疫检查点抑制剂对 PD-1/PD-L1 的抑制作用。

阿维鲁单抗

阿维鲁单抗（MSB0010718C）是一种完全人源化 PD-L1 的 IgG1 单克隆抗体，保留了天然 Fc 段，可诱导 ADCC 作用[74]。

在一项开放性、平行队列扩增的Ⅰ期临床研究中，在包括 NSCLC、胃癌、卵巢癌、黑色素瘤和乳腺癌患者在内的局部晚期或转移性实体瘤中评估了阿维鲁单抗的安全性和耐受性。阿维鲁单抗按 10mg/kg 每 2 周给药 1 次。共 480 例患者接受了治疗，其中 68% 的患者出现不良事件，最常见的是疲劳（20%）、恶心（13%）、输液相关反应（9%）、腹泻（7%）、发冷（7%）、食欲缺乏（6%）、发热（5%）、流感样疾病（5%）和关节痛（5%）。34 例患者因不良事件停止治疗，包括 8 例出现输液反应的患者。与药物相关的 3 级或以上的不良事件发生率为 12%，其中，最常见的毒性为贫血（5 例），疲劳（5 例），GGT 增加（4 例），输液反应（4 例），脂肪酶升高（4 例），淋巴细胞减少（3 例）。11.7% 的患者发生免疫相关的毒性反应，最常见的是甲状腺功能减退（4.0%）及肺炎（1.5%）[75]。

在本研究中，对接受过含铂类双药化疗的ⅢB 期或Ⅳ期 NSCLC 患者，阿维鲁单抗按 10mg/kg 每 2 周给药 1 次，直到完全缓解或疾病进展或出现不可耐受的毒性。共纳入 184 例 NSCLC 患者（62% 为腺癌，29% 为鳞癌）。70% 的患者发生至少一例任何级别的不良事件。最常见的毒性是疲劳、恶心、输液相关反应、发冷、食欲减退和腹泻。12% 的患者存在 3 级或 4 级药物毒性，包括 4 例输液反应。报告了 3 例与药物相关的死亡（放射性肺炎、急性呼吸衰竭和疾病进展）。缓解率和疾病稳定率分别为 12% 和 38%（PD-L1 阳性患者的缓解率为 14.4%，PD-L1 阴性患者缓解率为 10%）。总体 PFS 为 11.6 周（PD-L1 阳性患者为 11.7 周，PD-L1 阴性患者为 5.9 周）[76]。

在一项Ⅰb 期临床研究中，在 145 例无 EGFR 或 ALK 突变的晚期或转移性 NSCLC 患者（63% 为腺癌，27% 为鳞状细胞癌）中评估了阿维鲁单抗一线治疗的应用，无论 PD-L1 状态如何。

患者每 2 周静脉注射阿维鲁单抗 10mg/kg，直至疾病进展或毒性无法耐受。56% 的患者发生了任何级别的毒性反应，最常见的不良事件是输液反应（16%）和疲劳（14%）。9% 的患者发生了 3 级或 4 级毒性反应。没有观察到与治疗相关的死亡事件。按 RECIST 1.1 评估的总体缓解率为 18.7%（1 例完全缓解，13 例部分缓解），45% 的患者获得了病情稳定。所有的缓解病例均发生在 PD-L1 阳性患者中，所有 PD-L1 阴性患者均未出现缓解。所有接受治疗的患者 PFS 为 11.6 周[77]。目前，一项评估阿维鲁单抗和多西他赛二线治疗 PD-L1 阳性表达的 NSCLC 患者的临床研究正在进行中[78]。

BMS-936559

BMS-936559 是一种完全人源化 IgG4 抗体，抑制 PD-L1 与 PD-1 和 CD80 的结合，不仅与 PD-L1 结合，而且与 CTLA-4、CD28 也具有高亲和性[59]。在该药物剂量爬坡和队列扩大的 I 期临床试验中纳入了黑色素瘤、NSCLC、肾细胞癌及其他肿瘤（卵巢、胰腺癌、直肠癌）患者。3 级或 4 级毒性发生率为 8.6%，未观察到治疗相关的死亡事件。不良事件包括甲状腺功能减退、肝炎、结节病、眼内炎和重症肌无力。在多线治疗后的患者中观察到客观缓解，包括持续 1 年以上的缓解[79]。这种药物尽管目前没有在癌症患者中进行研究，但是正在进行一些脓毒症治疗的临床试验。

免疫治疗和非小细胞肺癌：里程碑、担忧、恐惧和挑战

NSCLC 是世界上最常见的恶性肿瘤。Globocan 的官方数据显示，2012 年全球新增病例 1 824 701 例，死亡病例 158 925 例。换句话说，每 100 个人被诊断为肺癌，将有 87 人在 12 个月内死于肺癌。总体人群和男性群体中，NSCLC 都是癌症死亡的首要原因，而女性群体中，NSCLC 是癌症死亡的第二大原因[80]。在美国，自 2012 年以来 NSCLC 的发病率和死亡率有下降的趋势。反烟草法律法规可能在这一曲线的改善趋势中发挥了重要作用。然而，据报道，在美国 2006~2012 年间肺癌患者的 5 年生存率仅为 17.7%。2016 年，预计新增病例为 224 390 例，同年死亡病例为 158 080 例，占该国癌症死亡病例的 26.5%[81]。

20 世纪 80 年代至 21 世纪前 5 年，不可切除或转移性 NSCLC 患者的治疗上几乎没有能真正影响预后的进步：一些新的化疗方案（一线治疗总是以铂类为基础的两药化疗）；尝试在化疗方案中添加抗血管生成药物；二线细胞毒性化疗的发展。然而，这些进步对提高总生存率并没有取得很大的成效，对 5 年生存率的影响明显较小。21 世纪一开始是针对 EGFR 基因突变，数年后针对 ALK 基因易位，靶向治疗已经在这种恶性肿瘤的治疗中占据了一席之地，对这类患者的总体生存率产生了很大的影响，这类患者大约占到全世界 NSCLC 总体人群的 1/5~1/4，地区之间存在差异可能是基因和烟草消费的缘故。

我们见证了系统性癌症治疗最具革命性的里程碑——免疫疗法的出现。2010 年发表了黑色素瘤患者的第一个意想不到的结果，改变了这种恶性肿瘤的治疗方式。荟萃分析显示，接受过伊匹木单抗治疗的患者中，有 1/4 的人活了 3 年以上，生存曲线上有一个明显的平稳期。现在谈论"治愈癌症"还为时过早，尽管如此，免疫疗法

似乎是解决这一问题的方法。我们目前正处于一场信息风暴之中，它的能力远远超过我们的分析能力和理解。新药正在出现，评估药物的临床试验正在进行中。

NSCLC 免疫治疗药物的首次报道和批准相对较新，需要时间来评估长期疗效；然而，根据目前的信息，我们已经可以说，必定可以改变治疗不可治愈的 NSCLC 患者的治疗模式。

肺癌细胞具有多种免疫抑制机制，这些机制对其免疫逃逸和生存至关重要。抗 CTLA-4 的药物，如伊匹木单抗，改变了黑色素瘤治疗的模式，在临床试验中没有显示出对 NSCLC 患者的预期疗效。尽管如此，其他检查点抑制剂如抗 PD-1 和抗 PD-L1 正在涌现。这些药物不像细胞毒性化疗那样直接攻击肿瘤细胞，它们通过抑制参与免疫耐受和肿瘤逃避免疫反应的主要机制来发挥作用。

在 NSCLC 中，抗 PD-1 和抗 PD-L1 单克隆抗体与细胞毒性化疗相比，具有显著的活性、显著的生存结局、持久的应答和良好的安全性，包括未经治疗的鳞状和非鳞状组织学患者（表 3.1 和表 3.2）。此外，不表达 PD-L1 的肿瘤患者使用抗 PD-1 药物治疗时，与化疗患者的疗效相似，但与标准治疗相比，PD-L1 表达水平高的患者效果要好得多。

表 3.1 晚期 NSCLC 关键的二线Ⅲ期免疫治疗临床试验

临床试验	病理类型，PD-L1 表达的要求	药物	样本量	中位 PFS（月）	中位 OS（月）
Checkmate-017	鳞癌	纳武利尤单抗	135	3.5	9.2
		多西他赛	137	2.8	6.0
Checkmate-057	非鳞癌	纳武利尤单抗	292	2.3	12.2
		多西他赛	290	4.2	9.4
Keynote-010	NSCLC，≥1%	帕博利珠单抗 2 mg/kg	344	3.9	10.4
		帕博利珠单抗 10 mg/kg	346	4.0	12.7
		多西他赛	343	4.0	8.5
OAK	NSCLC	阿特珠单抗	425	2.8	13.8
		多西他赛	425	4.0	9.6

表 3.2 晚期 NSCLC 中关键的一线Ⅲ期免疫治疗临床试验

临床试验	病理类型，PD-L1 表达的要求	药物	样本量	中位 PFS（月）	中位 OS（月）
Keynote -024	NSCLC，≥50%	帕博利珠单抗	154	10.3	30.2
		含铂化疗	151	6.0	14.2
Keynote -189	非鳞癌	帕博利珠单抗+铂+培美曲塞	410	8.8	NR
		安慰剂+铂+培美曲塞	206	4.9	11.3

续表

临床试验	病理类型, PD-L1 表达的要求	药物	样本量	中位 PFS（月）	中位 OS（月）
IMpower-150	非鳞癌	阿特珠单抗+卡铂+紫杉醇	348	N/A	N/A
		阿特珠单抗+贝伐珠单抗+卡铂+紫杉醇	356	8.3	19.2
		贝伐珠单抗+卡铂+紫杉醇	336	6.8	14.7

注: NR. 未达到; N/A. 无数据。

目前正在研究如何通过预测生物标志物来选择最有可能对免疫治疗产生反应的患者。由于 PD-1/PD-L1 通路激活在下调 T 淋巴细胞活性中发挥重要作用, 目前已有多项研究在关注肿瘤微环境成分[23-88]。PD-L1 在特定的实体肿瘤, 包括鳞状和非鳞状 NSCLC 中表达上调, 其表达可通过 TC 和 IC 的免疫组化检测。

抗 PD-1 抗体帕博利珠单抗和抗 PD-L1 抗体阿特珠单抗对 PD-L1 阳性患者的预后均有较大影响。然而, 纳武利尤单抗在不需要 PD-L1 阳性证明的情况下获得了批准, 尽管 PD-L1 阳性患者有获益的趋势, 主要是在腺癌中。一个大问题是如何将不同试验的结果转化为对 PD-L1 阳性的定义、界值, 以及如何确定每例患者的最佳治疗方式[89], 这是令人困惑的问题。只是根据不同试验的公布结果, 我们不能确定一种抗 PD-1 药物是否比其他抗 PD-1 药物更有效。所有已批准的抗 PD-1 药物和在研发中的抗 PD-1 和抗 PD-L1 药物均采用不同的检测方法检测 PD-L1 表达水平[90]。可能在短时间内, 一些正在开发的免疫治疗药物将获得批准, 到时将更难以决定治疗方式。PD-L1 似乎是一种预测标志物, 然而, 当一种生物标志物有几种免疫组化检测方法时, 很难决定使用哪一种, 同样重要的是要了解目前的每一种检测方法都与一种特定的药物相关联问题。在大多数临床试验中均检测了 PD-L1 在肿瘤细胞中的表达, 然而, 阿特珠单抗的试验也包含了免疫细胞中 PD-L1 的检测。但是不可能提供一个患者不同的组织样本来寻找最佳治疗方案。为了使制药行业能够找到一种通用的检测 PD-L1 表达的方法, 并且能够找到相似的界值点来比较不同药物对同一适应证的疗效, 监管机构的参与非常必要。

除了 PD-L1 表达外, 其他生物标志物也在研究中。独立于 PD-L1 的表达状态, 肺癌的肿瘤异质性和突变密度及肿瘤微环境在免疫治疗患者的反应和结果的差异性中起着重要作用。PD-L1 的表达可能是预测疗效的第一个生物标志物, 然而, 目前尚不清楚药物耐药的几种机制, 也不清楚 PD-L1 阴性患者为何能对治疗产生反应。

将抗 PD-1 或抗 PD-L1 与抗 CTLA-4 药物联合使用似乎是一种有效的方法来改善 NSCLC 预后。相关临床试验正在进行, 初步的数据是乐观的。其他与免疫相关的治疗策略也正在研究中，包括免疫治疗联合化疗、抗血管生成治疗和特定突变的靶向治疗（如抗 EGFR 或抗 ALK 突变）。免疫疗法作为局部晚期疾病患者放化疗后辅助治疗也在研究中。

众所周知，免疫治疗的毒性与化疗不同。免疫疗法的不良事件发生率较低，但在某些情况下可能会很严重，难以预测，且表现形式不寻常。这种情况需要肿瘤学家接受与免疫相关的不良事件识别及其特殊治疗方面的培训[91]。

全球许多接受免疫治疗的 NSCLC 患者之所以能够获得这些药物，是因为他们参与了临床试验，或者他们得到了一种特殊药物的慈善支持。然而，这些治疗方法的商业价值有伦理问题。毫无疑问，制药公司在药物开发上投入了大量资金，然而，目前这些药物的费用将限制患者接受治疗的可能性，并且这些药物在合法供应的情况下，将影响若干国家的经济。更重要的是，目前免疫治疗的联合方式如果将来被批准用于 NSCLC，每个患者每年可能要花费 100 万美元。这一经济问题和伦理问题将迫使我们希望很好地选择真正从免疫治疗获益的患者，并且希望寻找到能够确保对治疗产生良好和长期反应的生物标志物。

在一个短暂的时期内，免疫治疗已经成为 NSLCL 及其他一些恶性肿瘤的主要治疗手段，并且免疫治疗将为未来癌症的治愈提供有力的帮助。

参考文献

1. Molina J, Yang P, Cassivi S, et al. Non-small cell lung cancer: epidemiology, risk factors, treatment, and survivorship. Mayo Clin Proc. 2008;83(5):584–94.
2. Ferreccio C, González C, Milosavjlevic V, et al. Lung cancer and arsenic concentrations in drinking water in Chile. Epidemiology. 2000;11(6):673–9.
3. Rapp E, Pater JL, Willan A, et al. Chemotherapy can prolong survival in patients with advanced non-small-cell lung cancer—report of a Canadian multicenter randomized trial. J Clin Oncol. 1988;6(4):633–41.
4. NSCLC Meta-Analyses Collaborative Group. Chemotherapy in addition to supportive care improves survival in advanced non-small-cell lung cancer: a systematic review and meta-analysis of individual patient data from 16 randomized controlled trials. J Clin Oncol. 2008;26:4617–25.
5. Scagliotti GV, Parikh P, von Pawel J, et al. Phase III study comparing cisplatin plus gemcitabine with cisplatin plus pemetrexed in chemotherapy-naive patients with advanced-stage non-small-cell lung cancer. J Clin Oncol. 2008;26(21):3543–51.
6. Fossella FV, Lynch T, Shepherd FA. Second line chemotherapy for NSCLC: establishing a gold standard. Lung Cancer. 2002;38(Suppl 4):5–12.
7. Hanna N, Shepherd FA, Fossella FV, et al. Randomized phase III trial of pemetrexed versus docetaxel in patients with non-small-cell lung cancer previously treated with chemotherapy. J Clin Oncol. 2004;22(9):1589–97.
8. Rolfo C, Caglevic C, Mahave M, Bustamante E, Castañon E, Gil Bazo I, Marquez-Medina D. Chapter 14. Chemotherapy beyond the second line of treatment in non-small cell lung cancer: new drug development. In: Fighting lung cancer with conventional therapies. Hauppauge, NY: Nova Science Publishers; 2015. p. 229–40.
9. Vokes E, Salgia R, Karrison R. Evidence-based role of bevacizumab in non-small cell lung cancer. Ann Oncol. 2013;24(1):6–9.

10. Caglevic C, Grassi M, Raez L, Listi A, Giallombardo M, Bustamante E, Gil-Bazo I, Rolfo C. Nintedanib in non-small cell lung cancer: from preclinical to approval. Ther Adv Respir Dis. 2015;9(4):164–72.
11. Reck M, Kaiser R, Mellemgaard A, et al. Docetaxel plus nintedanib versus docetaxel plus placebo in patients with previously treated non-small-cell lung cancer (LUME-Lung 1): a phase 3, double-blind, randomised controlled trial. Lancet Oncol. 2014;15(2):143–55.
12. Horn L, Pao W. EML4-ALK: honing in on a new target in non-small-cell lung cancer. J Clin Oncol. 2009;27(26):4232–5.
13. Lawrence MS, Stojanov P, Polak P, et al. Mutational heterogeneity in cancer and the search for new cancer-associated genes. Nature. 2013;499(7457):214–8.
14. Györki D, Callahan M, Wolchock J, Ariyan C. The delicate balance of melanoma immunotherapy. Clin Transl Immunol. 2013;2:e5.
15. Yu H, Kortylewski M, Pardoll D. Crosstalk between cancer and immune cells: role of STAT3 in the tumour microenvironment. Nat Immunol Rev. 2007;7:41–51.
16. Vesely M, Kershaw M, Schreiber R, Smyth M. Natural innate and adaptive immunity to cancer. Annu Rev Immunol. 2011;29:235–71.
17. Chen D, Mellman I. Oncology meets immunology: "The Cancer-Immunity Cycle". Immunity. 2013;39(25):1–10.
18. Abbas A, Lichtman A, Pillai S. Immunity to tumors. In: Cellular and molecular immunology. Philadelphia: Elsevier; 2015. p. 383–97.
19. Pardoll D. The blockade of immune checkpoints in cancer immunotherapy. Nat Rev Cancer. 2012;12:252–64.
20. Cebon J, Behren A. Evolving role of tumor antigens for future melanoma therapies. Future Oncol. 2014;10:1457–68.
21. Topalian SL, Drake CG, Pardoll DM. Immune checkpoint blockade: a common denominator approach to cancer therapy. Cancer Cell. 2015;27(4):450–61.
22. Boussiotis V. Somatic mutations and immunotherapy outcome with CTLA-4 blockade in melanoma. N Engl J Med. 2014;371(23):30–2.
23. Postow MA, Callahan MK, Wolchok JD. Immune checkpoint blockade in cancer therapy. J Clin Oncol. 2015;33:1974–82.
24. Weber J. Anti–CTLA-4 antibody ipilimumab: case studies of clinical response and immune-related adverse events. Oncologist. 2007;12:864–72.
25. Cameron F, Whiteside G, Perry C. Ipilimumab: first global approval. Drugs. 2011;71(8):1093–104.
26. Hodi F, O'Day S, McDermott D, et al. Improved survival with ipilimumab in patients with metastatic melanoma. N Engl J Med. 2010;363(8):711–23.
27. Tomasini P, Khobta N, Greillier L, Barlesi F. Ipilimumab: its potential in non-small cell lung cancer. Ther Adv Med Oncol. 2012;4(2):43–50.
28. Weber J, Hamid O, Amin A, et al. Randomized phase I pharmacokinetic study of ipilimumab with or without one of two different chemotherapy regimens in patients with untreated advanced melanoma. Cancer Immun. 2013;13:7.
29. Lynch T, Bondarenko I, Luft A. Ipilimumab in combination with paclitaxel and carboplatin as first-line treatment in stage IIIB/IV non-small-cell lung cancer: results from a randomized, double-blind, multicenter phase II study. J Clin Oncol. 2012;30(17):2046–54.
30. https://clinicaltrials.gov/ct2/show/NCT01998126.
31. Ribas A, Hanson D, Noe D, et al. Tremelimumab (CP-675,206), a cytotoxic T lymphocyte-associated antigen 4 blocking monoclonal antibody in clinical development for patients with cancer. Oncologist. 2007;12(7):873–83.
32. Zatloukal P, Heo DS, Park K, et al. Randomized phase II clinical trial comparing tremelimumab (CP-675,206) with best supportive care (BSC) following first-line platinum-based therapy in patients (pts) with advanced non-small cell lung cancer (NSCLC). J Clin Oncol (Meeting Abstracts). 2009;27(15S):8071.
33. https://clinicaltrials.gov/ct2/show/NCT02040064.
34. https://clinicaltrials.gov/show/NCT01285609.
35. Nguyen L, Ohashi P. Clinical blockade of PD1 and LAG3-potencial mechanisms of action. Nat Immunol Rev. 2015;15:45–56.

36. Zou W, Chen L. Inhibitory B7-family molecules in the tumor microenvironment. Nat Rev Immunol. 2008;8(6):467–77.
37. Konishi J, Yamazaki K, Azuma M, et al. B7-H1 expression on non small cell lung cancer cells and its relationship with tumor-infiltrating lymphocytes and their PD-1 expression. Clin Cancer Res. 2004;10(15):5094–100.
38. Pauken KE, Wherry EJ. Overcoming T cell exhaustion in infection and cancer. Trends Immunol. 2015;36(4):265–76.
39. Chinai JM, Janakiram M, Chen F, et al. New immunotherapies targeting the PD-1 pathway. Trends Pharmacol Sci. 2015;36(9):587–95.
40. Wang C, Thudium K, Han M, et al. In vitro characterization of the anti-PD-1 antibody nivolumab, BMS-936558, and in vivo toxicology in non-human primates. Cancer Immunol Res. 2014;2:846.
41. Sundar R, Cho B-C, Brahmer JR, Soo RA. Nivolumab in NSCLC: latest evidence and clinical potential. Ther Adv Med Oncol. 2015;7(2):85–96.
42. Topalian SL, et al. Safety, activity, and immune correlates of anti-PD-1 antibody in cancer. N Engl J Med. 2012;366:2443–54.
43. Gettinger SN, et al. Overall survival and long-term safety of nivolumab (anti-programmed death 1 antibody, BMS-936558, ONO-4538) in patients with previously treated advanced non-small-cell lung cancer. J Clin Oncol. 2015;33:2004–12.
44. Rizvi NA, Mazieres J, Planchard D, et al. Activity and safety of nivolumab, an anti-PD-1 immune checkpoint inhibitor, for patients with advanced, refractory squamous non-small-cell lung cancer (CheckMate 063): a phase 2, single-arm trial. Lancet Oncol. 2015;16:257–65.
45. Horn L, Rizvi N, Mazieres J, et al. Longer-term follow-up of a phase 2 study (CheckMate 063) of nivolumab in patients with advanced refractory squamous (SQ) non-small cell lung cancer (NSCLC). J Thor Oncol. 2015;10(9 Suppl 2), abstract 02.03.
46. Brahmer J, Reckamp KL, Baas P, et al. Nivolumab versus docetaxel in advanced squamous-cell non-small-cell lung cancer. N Engl J Med. 2015;373:123–35.
47. Borghaei H, Paz-Ares L, Horn L, et al. Nivolumab versus docetaxel in advanced non-squamous non-small-cell lung cancer. N Engl J Med. 2015;373(17):1627–39.
48. Borghaei H, Brahmer J, Horn L, et al. Nivolumab vs docetaxel in patients with advanced NSCLC: CheckMate 017/057 2-y update and exploratory cytokine profile analyses. J Clin Oncol. 2016;34(Suppl), abstr 9025.
49. https://clinicaltrials.gov/ct2/show/NCT01454102.
50. Najjar Y, Kirkwood J. Pembrolizumab: pharmacology and therapeutics. Am J Hematol Oncol. 2014;10(5):17–9.
51. Garon E, Rizvi N, Hui R, et al. Pembrolizumab for the treatment of non-small-cell lung cancer. N Engl J Med. 2015;372:2018–28.
52. Hui R, Gandhi L, Carcereny Costa E, et al. Long-term OS for patients with advanced NSCLC enrolled in the KEYNOTE-001 study of pembrolizumab. J Clin Oncol. 2016;34(Suppl), abstr 9026.
53. Herbst R, Baas P, Kim DW, et al. Pembrolizumab versus docetaxel for previously treated, PD-L1-positive, advanced non-small-cell lung cancer (KEYNOTE-010): a randomised controlled trial. Lancet. 2016;387(10027):1540–50.
54. Baas P, Garon E, Herbst R, et al. Relationship between level of PD-L1 expression and outcomes in the KEYNOTE-010 study of pembrolizumab vs docetaxel for previously treated, PD-L1-Positive NSCLC. J Clin Oncol. 2016;34(Suppl), abstr 9015.
55. Garon E, Herbst R, Kim DW, et al. Pembrolizumab vs docetaxel for previously treated advanced NSCLC with a PD-L1 tumor proportion score (TPS) 1%–49%: results from KEYNOTE-010. J Clin Oncol. 2016;34(Suppl), abstr 9024.
56. Herbst R, Baas P, Perez-Gracia JL, et al. Archival vs new tumor samples for assessing PD-L1 expression in the KEYNOTE-010 study of pembrolizumab vs docetaxel for previously treated advanced NSCLC. J Clin Oncol. 2016;34(Suppl), abstr 3030.
57. https://clinicaltrials.gov/ct2/show/NCT02220894.
58. https://clinicaltrials.gov/ct2/show/NCT02343952.
59. Philips GK, Atkins M. Therapeutic uses of anti-PD-1 and anti-PD-L1 antibodies. Int Immunol. 2015;27(1):39–46.

60. Haile S, Dalal S, Clements V. Soluble CD80 restores T cell activation and overcomes tumor cell programmed death ligand-1-mediated immune suppression. J Immunol. 2013;191(5): 2829–36.
61. Brahmer J, Rizvi N, Lutzky J, et al. Clinical activity and biomarkers of MEDI4736, an anti-PD-L1 antibody, in patients with NSCLC. J Clin Oncol. 2014;32(Suppl):5s, abstr 8021.
62. Rizvi N, Brahmer J, Ou SH, et al. Safety and clinical activity of MEDI4736, an anti-programmed cell death-ligand 1 (PD-L1) antibody, in patients with non-small cell lung cancer (NSCLC). J Clin Oncol. 2015;33(15_Suppl, May 20 Supplement):8032.
63. Antonia S, Kim SW, Spira A, et al. Safety and clinical activity of durvalumab (MEDI4736), an anti-PD-L1 antibody, in treatment-naïve patients with advanced non–small-cell lung cancer. J Clin Oncol. 2016;34(Suppl), abstr 9029.
64. Antonia S, Goldberg S, Balmanoukian A, et al. Safety and antitumour activity of durvalumab plus tremelimumab in non-small cell lung cancer: a multicentre, phase 1b study. Lancet Oncol. 2016;17(3):299–308.
65. Reichert J. Antibodies to watch in 2016. MAbs. 2016;8(2):197–204.
66. Spigel D, Gettinger S, Horn L, et al. Clinical activity, safety, and biomarkers of MPDL3280A, an engineered PD-L1 antibody in patients with locally advanced or metastatic non-small cell lung cancer (NSCLC). J Clin Oncol. 2013;31(Suppl), abstr 8008.
67. Herbst R, Soria J-C, Kowanetz M, et al. Predictive correlates of response to the anti-PD-L1 antibody MPDL3280A in cancer patients. Nature. 2014;515(7528):563–7.
68. Schmid P, Hegde P, Zou W, et al. Association of PD-L2 expression in human tumors with atezolizumab activity. J Clin Oncol. 2016;34(Suppl), abstr 11506.
69. Liu S, Powderly J, Camidge R, et al. Safety and efficacy of MPDL3280A (anti-PDL1) in combination with platinum-based doublet chemotherapy in patients with advanced non-small cell lung cancer (NSCLC). J Clin Oncol. 2015;33(Suppl), abstr 8030.
70. Besse B, Johnson M, Jänne PA, et al. Phase II, single-arm trial (BIRCH) of atezolizumab as first-line or subsequent therapy for locally advanced or metastatic PD-L1-selected non-small cell lung cancer (NSCLC). Presented at 2015 European Cancer Congress, 25–29 Sept, Vienna, Austria. Abstract 16LBA.
71. Fehrenbacher L, Spira A, Ballinger M, et al. Atezolizumab versus docetaxel for patients with previously treated non-small-cell lung cancer (POPLAR): a multicentre, open-label, phase 2 randomised controlled trial. Lancet. 2016;387(10030):1837–46.
72. Smith D, Vansteenkiste J, Fehrenbacher L, et al. Updated survival and biomarker analyses of a randomized phase II study of atezolizumab vs docetaxel in 2L/3L NSCLC (POPLAR). J Clin Oncol. 2016;34(Suppl), abstr 9028.
73. Socinski MA, Jotte RM, Cappusso F, et al. Atezolizumab for first-line treatment of metastatic nonsquamous NSCLC. N Engl J Med. 378(24):2288–301.
74. Hamanishi J, Mandai M, Konishi I. Immune checkpoint inhibition in ovarian cancer. Int Immunol. 2016;7. pii: dxw020.
75. Kelly K, Patel M, Infante J, et al. Avelumab (MSB0010718C), an anti-PD-L1 antibody, in patients with metastatic or locally advanced solid tumors: assessment of safety and tolerability in a phase I, open-label expansion study. J Clin Oncol. 2015;33(Suppl), abstr 3044.
76. Gulley J, Spigel D, Kelly K, et al. Avelumab (MSB0010718C), an anti-PD-L1 antibody, in advanced NSCLC patients: a phase 1b, open-label expansion trial in patients progressing after platinum-based chemotherapy. J Clin Oncol (Meeting Abstracts). 2015;33(15_Suppl):8034.
77. Verschraegen C, Chen F, Spigel D, et al. Avelumab (MSB0010718C; anti-PD-L1) as a first-line treatment for patients with advanced NSCLC from the JAVELIN Solid Tumor phase 1b trial: safety, clinical activity, and PD-L1 expression. J Clin Oncol. 2016;34(Suppl) abstr 9036.
78. https://clinicaltrials.gov/ct2/show/NCT02395172.
79. Brahmer J, Tykodi S, Chow L, et al. Safety and activity of anti-PD-L1 antibody in patients with advanced cancer. N Engl J Med. 2012;366:2455–65.
80. Globocan. Estimated cancer incidence, mortality and prevalence worldwide 2012. 2012. http://globocan.iarc.fr/Pages/fact_sheets_population.aspx.
81. NIH, National Cancer Institute: surveillance, epidemiology and end results. http://seer.cancer.gov/statfacts/html/lungb.html.

82. Antonia S, Brahmer J, Gettinger S, et al. Nivolumab (anti-PD-1; BMS-936558, ONO-4538) in combination with platinum-based doublet chemotherapy in advanced non-small cell lung cancer (NSCLC). J Clin Oncol. 2014;32(Suppl):5s, abstr 8113.
83. Gettinger S, Shepherd F, Antonia S, et al. First-line nivolumab (anti-PD-1; BMS-936558, ONO-4538) monotherapy in advanced NSCLC: safety, efficacy, and correlation of outcomes with PD-L1 status. J Clin Oncol. 2014;32(Suppl):5s, abstr 8024.
84. Gettinger SN. Presented at European Society for Medical Oncology (ESMO), 25–29 Sept 2015, Vienna, Austria.
85. Antonia S, Gettinger S, Quan Man Chow L, et al. Nivolumab (anti-PD-1; BMS-936558, ONO-4538) and ipilimumab in first-line NSCLC: interim phase I results. J Clin Oncol. 2014;32(Suppl):5s, abstr 8023.
86. Rizvi NA, Gettinger SN, Goldman JW, et al. Safety and efficacy of first-line nivolumab and in non-small cell lung cancer. In: 16th World Conference on Lung Cancer. Abstract ORAL02.05. Presented 7 Sept 2015.
87. Hellmann M, Gettinger S, Goldman J, et al. CheckMate 012: safety and efficacy of first-line nivolumab and ipilimumab in advanced NSCLC. J Clin Oncol. 2016;34(Suppl), abstr 3001.
88. Santarpia M, Karachaliou N. Tumor immune microenvironment characterization and response to anti-PD-1 therapy. Cancer Biol Med. 2015;12(2):74–8.
89. Carbognin L, Pilotto S, Milella M, et al. Differential activity of nivolumab, pembrolizumab and MPDL3280A according to the tumor expression of programmed death-ligand-1 (PD-L1): sensitivity analysis of trials in melanoma, lung and genitourinary cancers. PLoS One. 10(6):e0130142. https://doi.org/10.1371/journal.pone.0130142.
90. Kerr K, Hirsch F. Programmed death ligand-1 immunohistochemistry. Friend or Foe? Arch Pathol Lab Med. 2016;140:326–31.
91. Michot JM, Bigenwald C, Champiat S, et al. Immune-related adverse events with immune checkpoint blockade: a comprehensive review. Eur J Cancer. 2016;54:139–48.

第 4 章

急性髓系白血病和骨髓增生异常综合征免疫治疗的更新：单克隆抗体和检查点抑制剂即将进入临床实践

Lucia Masarova，Hagop Kantarjian，Farhad Ravandi，Padmanee Sharma，Guillermo Garcia-Manero，Naval Daver

译者：赵 沙 陈 健

摘要 在过去的几年中，我们对急性髓系白血病（AML）和骨髓增生异常综合征（MDS）发病机制的理解不断加深，使这些疾病的治疗得到了长足发展。本章总结了 AML 和 MDS 中免疫治疗已有的临床数据，并聚焦于单克隆抗体、T 淋巴细胞偶联抗体、嵌合抗原受体（CAR）-T 淋巴细胞治疗和 PD-1/PD-L1 或细胞毒性 T 淋巴细胞相关蛋白 4（CTLA-4）介导的免疫检查点抑制治疗。目前，在初治和复发/难治 AML 和 MDS 中，均有大量临床试验正在进行。由于白血病原始细胞具有较强的异质性，因此需要免疫治疗、分子靶向治疗和化疗联合应用，才能达到最好的疗效。有多个这类 AML 组合疗法相关的临床试验都正在招募患者，不同临床阶段的试验都有，对单例患者来说，找到相关的分子生物学指标对于选择最适合的组合方案尤为关键。

关键词 急性髓系白血病 免疫治疗 单克隆抗体 免疫检测点抑制

Lucia Masarova and Naval Daver collected and reviewed the data and wrote the paper. All authors participated in the discussion, have reviewed and approved the current version of the manuscript.

Naval Daver is responsible for the overall content as guarantor.

L. Masarova · H. Kantarjian · F. Ravandi · G. Garcia-Manero · N. Daver (*)
Department of Leukemia, MD Anderson Cancer Center, Houston, TX, USA
e-mail: ndaver@mdanderson.org

P. Sharma
Department of Immunotherapy Platform, MD Anderson Cancer Center, Houston, TX, USA

© Springer Nature Switzerland AG 2018
A. Naing, J. Hajjar (eds.), *Immunotherapy*, Advances in Experimental Medicine and Biology 995, https://doi.org/10.1007/978-3-030-02505-2_4

引言

急性髓系白血病（AML）是一种具有遗传学异质性的疾病，其特点是髓系祖细胞的克隆性扩增。尽管对 AML 生物学行为的理解在不断加深，但对于 AML 的治疗，过去 40 多年一直没有实质性的进展。标准的一线治疗方案为 20 世纪 70 年代引入的 3+7 诱导方案[1]，然后根据患者复发的风险进行巩固治疗或进行异基因干细胞移植（alloSCT）。然而 AML 长期的患者 OS 仍然不良，在年轻患者约为 40%，在老年患者（年龄>65 岁）仅为 10%~15%[2]。大多数患者对诱导方案原发耐药，或短期缓解后复发，可能是由于化疗耐药的白血病干细胞持续存在，或存在小体积的微小残留病灶。

近年来，靶向肿瘤特异性抗原利用相应的抗体促使患者自身免疫系统攻击肿瘤细胞来达到治疗目的，已成为多种血液系统恶性肿瘤临床研究的新领域，其包括 AML 和 MDS。

在本章中，重点关注 AML 中正在进行临床试验的、基于上述理论的"免疫治疗"药物，具体包括单克隆抗体、T 淋巴细胞治疗。表 4.1 和表 4.2 汇总了目前正在进行的临床试验，本章论述的重点是 AML 及 MDS 中免疫治疗的最新进展。

单克隆抗体

单克隆抗体（MoAb）治疗已成为肿瘤治疗中必不可少的组成部分，这种疗法对白血病同样适用，因为单克隆抗体可以很容易接触到血液和骨髓里面的白血病细胞。理想的靶点需要在白血病细胞上高表达而在普通造血干细胞上不表达。在 AML 中，可能作为靶向治疗抗体靶点的抗原包括 CD33、CD123、CD32、CD25、CD44、CD96、CLL-1 和 TIM-3 等[3]。

在目前 AML 相关单克隆抗体的临床研发中，大部分研究都聚焦在 CD33 和 CD123 上。由于单纯的单克隆抗体疗效有限，近期大部分研究的中心转移到了偶联细胞毒性物质的单克隆抗体上（又称抗体-药物偶联，ADC）。另外，单克隆抗体研发中还有新的方向，可以将细胞毒性 T 淋巴细胞（通过 CD3）与白血病细胞（通过与白血病特异性抗原结合）结合，激活 T 淋巴细胞，杀伤白血病细胞，这类药物包括双向特异性 T 淋巴细胞衔接子（BiTE）、靶向 NK 细胞表面 CD16 的双向特异性和三向特异性杀伤细胞衔接子及双向亲和重复靶向双特异性分子（DART）。

表 4.1 AML 和 MDS 单克隆抗体的临床试验

分期	靶向	治疗	主要终点	适应证
II	CD33	GO	ORR,毒性	R/R AML(市场批准)
II/III		GO + 阿糖胞苷 vs."7+3"	ORR, OS,毒性	一线,老年 AML
II		GO + 白消安 + 咖啡酸片 → alloSCT	ORR, OS	第一次完全缓解高危 AML, HR MDS, R/R MDS
III[a]		全反式维 A 酸±GO 化疗	OS	新发 AML, NPM1 突变
I/II[a]		GO 和 AZA	毒性—MTD, ORR	R/R AML
II		alloSCT 后合并 GO	移植物衰竭发生率, OS, 毒性	第 1/2 次完全缓解 AML, MDS<5%原始细胞
OBS		GO 和 CHT(MYLOR 方案)	ORR,毒性	R/R AML
I b/II		GO/PF-04518600/阿维鲁单抗/AZA/utomilumab/glasdegib	毒性, ORR	R/R AML
III		GO/柔红霉素/克拉屈滨/AC220	OS, ORR,毒性	一线,老年患者;R/R AML
I b[a]		SGN-CD33A+"7+3," SGN-CD33A+HDAC; SGN-CD33A 单用	毒性—MTD	所有 AML
III[a]		SGN-CD33A + DAC/AZA	OS	AML 一线治疗
I/II[a]		SGN-CD33A + AZA	毒性, ORR	中危-2/高危 MDS 一线治疗
I/II[a]		SGN-CD33A 和 FluMel → autoSCT;SGN-CD33A	毒性, ORR, OS	R/R AML ASCT 前 ASCT 后维持治疗
I		AMG330	毒性	R/R AML
I		AMG673	毒性—MTD	R/R AML
II		BI 836858 和 DAC	毒性—MTD, ORR	R/R AML,不适合一线治疗的 AML 老年患者
		BI 836858 和 F16IL2	毒性—MTD	R/R AML 后用 SCT
I/II		BI 836858	毒性—MTD;第一次输注 PRBC	低/中危-1 MDS±PRBC 依赖
I[a]		BI 836858	毒性	R/R AML 或在第一次完全缓解,复发高危型
I	CD123	SL-401 和 AZA	毒性—MTD	不适合一线治疗的 AML;R/R AML, HR MDS
I/II		SL-401	毒性, OS	HR AML,第一次完全缓解时微小残留病变(巩固治疗)

续表

分期	靶向	治疗	主要终点	适应证
Ⅰ		XmAb14045	毒性—MTD	R/R AML
Ⅰ		IMGN779	毒性—MTD	R/R AML，
Ⅰ	CD123×CD3	JNJ-63709178	毒性	R/R AML
Ⅰ		MGD006	毒性	R/R AML，中危-2 和高危 MDS
Ⅱ	CD38	达雷木单抗	ORR	R/R AML，HR MDS
Ⅰ	CD25	ADCT-301	ORR	R/R AML
Ⅰ	CD47	Hu5F9-G4	毒性—MTD	R/R AML，HR MDS
Ⅰ		CC-90002	毒性—MTD	R/R AML，HR MDS
Ⅰ		TTI-621/SIRPαFc±纳武利尤单抗±rituximab	毒性	R/R AML，MDS
Ⅰ/Ⅱ	CXCR4	乌洛鲁单抗 + LD Ara-C	毒性—MTD，ORR	一线治疗 AML

注：R/R.难治/复发；AML. 急性髓系白血病；MDS. 骨髓增生异常综合征；ORR. 总有效率；OS. 总体生存期；PFS. 无进展生存；alloSCT. 异基因干细胞移植；autoSCT. 自体干细胞移植；GO. 吉妥珠单抗；FluMel. 氟达拉滨和马法兰；MTD. 最大耐受剂量；HR. 高风险；PRBC.血细胞比容；DAC. 地西他滨；AZA. 阿扎胞苷；HiDAC. 高剂量阿糖胞苷；CHT. 化疗。

数据来源于 ClinicalTrials.gov（https：//clinicaltrials.gov）assessed on 6/1/2018

a 开放，当还没有招募中

表 4.2　AML 和 MDS 中免疫检查点抑制剂和 CAR-T/NK 细胞的临床试验

分期	靶向	药物	主要终点	适应证
Ⅰ	CTLA4	伊匹木单抗	毒性	R/R AML，HR MDS
Ⅰ		伊匹木单抗和 DAC	毒性	一线，老年患者，R/R AML
Ⅱ	PD-1	Pidilizumab + DC 疫苗	毒性	在采取 DC 细胞前处于完全缓解的 AML
Ⅱ		纳武利尤单抗+"7＋3"	无病生存	一线治疗 AML，<60 岁
Ⅱ		纳武利尤单抗	无病生存	AML 在 CR
Ⅱ		纳武利尤单抗 vs. OBS	PFS	有微小残留病变完全缓解的 AML
Ⅱ		帕博利珠单抗和 AZA	毒性—MTD	R/R AML，一线，老年 AML
Ⅰ/Ⅱ		帕博利珠单抗和 DAC	可行性	R/R AML
Ⅱ		帕博利珠单抗	CR 的整合，ORR	老年 AML 完全缓解的巩固治疗
0/试验Ⅰ		帕博利珠单抗	ORR，OS	R/R AML 诱导后
Ⅱ		帕博利珠单抗和 HiDAC	ORR	R/R AML
Ⅱ		帕博利珠单抗	可行性	R/R AML SCT 后
0/试验		帕博利珠单抗	毒性—MTD	R/R AML SCT 后

续表

分期	靶向	药物	主要终点	适应证
I/II		帕博利珠单抗和 FluMel → autoSCT	ORR/2 年	完全缓解的 HR AML
I		恩替司他和帕博利珠单抗	毒性—MTD	去甲基化药物治疗失败的 MDS
I/II	PD-1 和 CTLA4	伊匹木单抗/纳武利尤单抗/两药联合	ORR，完全缓解	完全缓解后的 AML，复发高危型
I/Ib		伊匹木单抗/纳武利尤单抗	毒性—MTD	SCT 后 R/R AML
II		伊匹木单抗和纳武利尤单抗和硫唑嘌呤	ORR	去甲基化药物治疗失败，HR MDS
II		伊匹木单抗±纳武利尤单抗+硫唑嘌呤	ORR	R/R AML；一线，老年 AML
I	CLL1 和 CD3	MCLA-117	毒性—MTD	一线，老年 AML，R/R AML
I	PD-L1 和 TIM-3	PDR001/MBG453 + DAC	毒性—MTD	R/R AML，一线，老年 AML，HR MDS
I/II	PD-L1	阿特珠单抗和 SGI-110	毒性—MTD，ORR	去甲基化药物治疗失败 MDS
I		度伐鲁单抗±AZA 和曲美木单抗	毒性—MTD	去甲基化药物治疗失败 MDS
II		度伐鲁单抗伴随 AZA	ORR	老年 AML 患者，HRMDS 一线治疗
I/II		阿维鲁单抗伴随 AZA	毒性—MTD	R/R AML
I		阿维鲁单抗伴随 DAC	毒性—MTD	一线，老年 AML
II	KIR	Lirilumab 和 AZA	ORR	R/R AML
II		Lirilumab 和 AZA and 纳武利尤单抗	ORR	所有 MDS 的一线治疗
I/II	CD33	CAR-T	毒性	R/R AML
I	CD33	CAR-T	毒性	R/R AML
I	CD123	CAR-T	毒性	R/R AML
0/试验 I	CD123	CAR-T	毒性	R/R AML
I	CD133	CAR-T	毒性	R/R AML
I	CD33/CD56	CAR-NK	毒性	R/R AML
I/II	CD7	CAR-NK	毒性	R/R AML
I	CIK	激活的 CIK 细胞 IL-2	毒性	R/R AML，MDS
I	CD123	UCAR-T（同种异体细胞）	毒性	R/R AML

注：R/R.难治/复发；AML. 急性髓系白血病；MDS. 骨髓增生异常综合征；ORR. 总有效率；OS. 总体生存期；PFS. 无进展生存；alloSCT. 异基因干细胞移植；autoSCT. 自体干细胞移植；GO. 吉妥珠单抗 FluMel. 氟达拉滨和马法兰；MTD. 最大耐受剂量；HR. 高风险；DC.树突状细胞；DAC. 地西他滨；数据来源于 ClinicalTrials.gov（https：//clinicaltrials.gov）assessed on 6/1/2018

抗 CD-33 抗体

CD33 是髓系分化抗原，主要表达在非常早期的髓系祖细胞表面和大于 90% 的 AML 原始细胞表面[4]。

吉妥珠单抗

AML 中最有名的单克隆抗体为吉妥珠单抗（Gemtuzumab Ozogamicin，GO）是一种人源化的抗 CD33 单克隆抗体，与破坏 DNA 的毒素——卡里奇霉素相偶联的药物，其研发过程有成功也有失败。在 2000 年的一项大型 Ⅱ 期临床试验中，对于首次复发的老年 AML 患者，吉妥珠单抗的 ORR 为 30%（即 CR+CRi，完全缓解+血象未完全恢复的完全缓解），基于这样的结果，FDA 当年加速批准吉妥珠单抗在这类患者中的临床应用[5,6]。后来 Ⅲ 期临床试验——SWOG S0106 的结果表明，该药并不能带来生存获益，反而增加了早期死亡率，增加了筛窦阻塞综合征和静脉闭塞症（VOD）的发生率[7]，因此在上市 10 年后，主动从美国市场退市。在该项研究中，吉妥珠单抗的剂量是非分次的 $6mg/m^2$。接下来的 4 项大型随机试验显示，将吉妥珠单抗分次加入标准诱导化疗方案，患者 OS 得到改善，而早期死亡率和 VOD 发生率并无增加，在低危和中危患者中尤其明显[8-10]。

近期，另有一项多中心、Ⅲ 期随机研究（实验组：对照组=1：1）入组 237 例老年初发 AML 患者，比较了吉妥珠单抗与最佳支持治疗（BSC, best supportive care）的疗效，结果显示，GO 组患者有更好的生存获益，两组患者中位 OS 分别为吉妥珠单抗组 4.9 个月，BSC 组 3.6 个月（P=0.005，HR=0.69，95%CI，0.53～0.9），一年的 OS 率分别为吉妥珠单抗组 24.3%，BSC 组 9.7%。更重要的是，吉妥珠单抗对多个亚组都显示出一致的疗效，而在 CD33 高表达的患者组、低危/中危核型组合中，女性患者疗效最好。在吉妥珠单抗组中，整体有效率（CR/CRi）为 27%（30 例患者中 111 例有效）[11]。另有一项 Ⅱ 期研究表明，一个疗程的吉妥珠单抗在复发 AML 患者中就可以达到 26% 的 CR 率[12]，至此吉妥珠单抗的疗效已经是毋庸置疑。

最终，在 2017 年 9 月，FDA 重新批准吉妥珠单抗用于治疗 CD33 阳性的成人 AML 患者，以及单药或与化疗联合治疗 2 岁以上的复发或难治 AML 患者。目前，有多项临床研究正在开展，来探索吉妥珠单抗在初治和复发 AML 患者中的疗效、安全性和最优用法（表 4.1）。

SGN33A

SGN33A（Vadastuximab Talirine）的临床前研究表明，该药物对 AML 细胞系有很强的杀伤作用（比吉妥珠单抗高 30%以上）[13,14]，目前大量的 I 期和 II 期临床研究正在评估该药在初发、复发或难治及老年 CD33 阳性 AML 患者中，作为单药或与化疗、去甲基化药物[如阿扎胞苷（AZA）及地西他滨（DAC）]联合应用的疗效。

这些 I 期或 II 期临床试验的初步结果表明，SGN33A 疗效确切，起效快，患者可达到深度缓解，安全性方面可耐受。单药使用时，40μg/kg 剂量的 SGN33A 在复发或难治 AML 患者和老年初发的 AML 患者（共 131 例）中整体缓解率（CR/CRi）可达 28%，原始细胞清除率可达 47%。最常见的不良反应为骨髓抑制（>3 级中性粒细胞减少发生率 15%，贫血发生率 25%，血小板减少发生率 31%）。8 周死亡率为 8%[15]。

SGN33A 在与诱导化疗方案或 HMA 联用时显示出更好的疗效，在初发 AML 患者中，（CR/CRi）分别达到 78%[16]和 73%[17]。在 II 期临床研究中，SGN33A 的早期死亡率与标准化疗及 HMA 单药的早期死亡率类似。以上这些结果令人鼓舞，促进了一项全球双盲、安慰剂对照的后续 III 期临床研究的开展，来研究 SGN33A 加和不加 HMA 在不适合诱导化疗的初发 AML 患者中的疗效和安全性。

然而，SGN33A 接下来的发展令人失望，FDA 在 2016 年 12 月至 2017 年 3 月间，由于该药在造血干细胞移植前使用出现肝毒性或 VOD，将部分 SGN33A 的临床试验调整为"间歇性临床暂停"状态。最终根据某独立委员会的评估，III 期 CASCADE 临床试验中，SGN33A 组患者具有更高的死亡率（包括致死性感染）[18]，鉴于这样的结果，FDA 在 2017 年 6 月搁置了所有 SGN33A 的临床试验。目前，CASCADE 临试验的相关数据正在分析中，但是 SGN33A 在 AML 中的研究应该不太可能继续了。

IMGN779

IMGN779（ImmunoGen）是另外一种具有很好初步临床疗效的抗-CD33 抗体，由人源性的抗体与新型 DNA 烷化剂 DGN462 偶联而成，其中 DGN462 包含吲哚啉-苯二氮䓬二联体[19]。

在临床前的研究中，IMGN779 对 AML 细胞系显示出强大的杀伤力，包括对 FLT3 突变的细胞系也是如此[20]。而且，近期的研究显示，阿糖胞苷可能会通过增加 AML 细胞表面 CD33 的表达来增敏 IMGN779 的疗效，引起更强烈的 DNA 损伤、细胞周期阻滞和凋亡。这项结果也提示在临床试验中将以上两种药物组合，可能发挥更好的作用[21]。

IMNG779 初步的 I 期临床结果表明，在 26 例复发或难治 AML 患者中（包括 19%异基因造血干细胞移植后复发的患者）疗效显著。该药物安全性好，在 0.7mg/kg 剂量下无药物限制毒性。在 10%以上的患者中观察到的 3 级以上不良反应包括中性粒细胞缺乏引起的发热（39%）、肺炎（19%）、贫血（19%）、呼吸衰竭（15%）和低磷酸盐血症（12%）。在剂量为 0.39～0.70mg/kg 时，9 例患者全部出现外周血原始细胞减少，中位减少量为 67%（范围：15%～100%）。另外，有 3 例患者在治疗的前 3 个周期内出现骨髓原始细胞大量减少，减少量分别为 96%、90%和 48%[22]。

抗 CD123 抗体

CD123，即人白介素-3 受体 α 链，IL-3Rα，可与白介素-3 结合。在 AML 患者中研究数量其次多的单抗是 CD123 单抗，CD123 可与 IL-3α 结合，促进细胞生存和增殖[23]，促进白血病复发和对化疗耐药[24]。

JNJ-56022473

JNJ-56022473（Talacotuzumab，之前 CSL-362 的变异体）是第二种抗 CD123 单抗，为完全人源化的细胞毒性增强版单抗，可与 NK 细胞表面的 CD16 结合发挥作用，I 期临床研究结果显示，该药对 CD123 阳性、初次或再次 CR/CRi、具有复发高风险 AML 患者的维持治疗具有较好的疗效和安全性。在该项试验中，50% 的患者（10/20）表现为持续 CR，中位 CR 持续时间为 34^+ 周，最常见的治疗相关和剂量限制性不良反应为高血压和输注反应[25]。一项评估 DAC 加或不加 talacotuzumab 治疗不适合强化疗初发 AML 患者的 II 期/III 期临床研究已经启动（$n=326$）。但在 2017 年 10 月，J&J 公司决定终止该药物的进一步研发，具体原因未公布。

SL-401

目前，SL-401 是前景最好的抗 CD123 抗体之一（又名 DT388IL3），并在 2017 年 10 月被 FDA 和 EU 批准为治疗浆细胞性母细胞样树突状细胞肿瘤（BPDCN）的突破性药物。SL-401 是一种重组融合蛋白，由减毒白喉毒素和人类 IL-3 配体组成[26]，在与 CD123 结合以后被内化，引起蛋白质合成受阻和细胞死亡。

针对 BPDCN 患者的 II 期临床试验显示，SL-401 具有很优良的疗效，整体缓解率（ORR）达到 84%（其中在初治患者中 ORR 为 95%）[27]。

而在 AML 患者中 SL-401 的效果就没有那么振奋人心。在一项纳入了 74 例 AML/MDS（其中 56 例为复发/难治 AML）患者的 I 期临床研究中，使用该药物仅有 2 例患者完全缓解，4 例部分缓解，另有 4 例骨髓原始细胞减少大于 50%。中位生存期和 12 个月的 OS 率分别为 3.2 个月和 22%，均比历史数据要好。所有 ≥3 级的不良反应均为一过性，包括转氨酶升高（20%）和毛细血管渗漏综合征（4%）[28,29]。评估 SL-401 在复发或难治 AML 中疗效的 II 期临床试验正在进行中，到目前为止，6 例患者中有 3 例病情稳定超过 12 个周期，6 例患者中有 3 例为疾病稳定状态[30]。该药物也正在进行一项 II 期、多中心、两步法研究，评估在首次或二次 CR、具有高复发风险的 AML 患者中进行维持治疗的疗效。第一步剂量确定阶段在 9 例患者中顺利完成，未发现药物限制性毒性，推荐 II 期临床在维持治疗中的剂量为 12μg/kg。最常见 ≥3 级的不良反应包括 ALT/AST 升高（31%）、血小板减少（19%）和细胞因子释放综合征（CRS，13%）。其中 5 例患者无复发生存至少为 5 个月[31]。来源于既往研究的转化医学数据表明，DPH1 酶的表达量降低是 SL-401 耐药可能的机制，该酶可将组氨酸转化为白喉酰胺，后者为 ADP 核糖基化的直接靶点，而这种耐药可通过 SL-401 与阿扎胞苷（AZA）联用克服[32]。基于这些数据，一项多中心的、探索 SL-401 联合 AZA 治疗 AML/MDS 患者的 I 期临床研究已经启动，目前正在招募患者中（表 4.1）。

抗-KIR 抗体

AML 的免疫治疗中，另一种有趣的药物是靶向 NK 细胞表面杀伤细胞免疫球蛋白受体（KIR）的抗体，即 lirilumab。AML 患者中 NK 细胞介导抗肿瘤效应的增强与 KIR 和 I 类 HLA 结合减少相关[33]。

一项初次 CR 后老年 AML 患者的 II 期、随机、双盲、安慰剂对照、维持治疗的研究显示，lirilumab 安全性好（n=153）。在该项研究中，患者被随机分为安慰剂组（n=51）、lirilumab 间歇性治疗组（0.1mg/kg，n=50）或 lirilumab 持续输注组（1mg/kg，n=51），共治疗 2 年时间。从随机分组至 CR 的中位时间为 3.3 个月。由于多例患者早期复发，持续输注组（1mg/mg）在中期分析的时候终止了治疗，剩下两组患者继续治疗，最终结果显示，中位治疗周期数在 lirilumab（0.1mg/kg）和安慰剂组分别为 14.7 个和 13.8 个。中位随访 36.6 个月后，lirilumab 仍具有较好的耐受性。共有 10% 的患者因为不良事件终止了治疗，其中大部分都是 1 级或 2 级不良反应。无白血病生存（LFS）在 lirilumab 间歇性治疗组和安慰剂组类似，即 lirilumab 间歇性治疗组 vs. 安慰剂组：17.6 个月（11.2～25 个月）vs. 13.9 个月（7.9～27.9 个月），HR=0.96（95% CI，0.61～1.56）[34]。

类似的，在另一项Ⅱ期临床研究中，lirilumab 与 AZA 联用治疗既往经过多次化疗的难治 AML 患者，也显示出良好的安全性。共入组 35 例复发 AML 患者，其中 12 例为继发性 AML，7 例为异基因移植后复发，这些患者既往接受的中位治疗线数为 3（范围 1~8），入组后接受 AZA（$75mg/m^2 \times 7$ 天）和 lirilumab（剂量分两组，分别是 1mg/kg 和 3mg/kg，4 周 1 次，每组 6 例患者）治疗。后来 3mg/kg 的 lirilumab 剂量被推荐为Ⅱ期试验的剂量。共有 4 例患者（11%）达到 CR/CRi，1 例（3%）达到血液学改善，整体缓解率为 14%。另有 3 例（9%）原始细胞数下降≥50%。4 周和 8 周的死亡率分别为 7% 和 15%。中位随访 3.6 个月（1.1~15.1 个月），所有患者的中位 OS 为 4.2 个月（0.4~5.1 个月）。3 级以上不良事件发生率与基于 AZA 的挽救治疗方案相似。在 3 例患者中观察到与免疫相关的≥3 级不良事件（肺炎 1 例，结肠炎 2 例）；但激素治疗所有患者均起效迅速。另外，该方案治疗的 7 例移植后患者均未出现≥3 级的免疫相关不良事件[35]。

T 淋巴细胞结合抗体

在 AML 基于抗体的免疫疗法中，有一类新药由两种具有各自特异性和生物学功能的抗体组合而成，其中一种为抗体靶向肿瘤相关抗原，而另一种为靶向效应 T 淋巴细胞，通过这两种抗体拉近 T 淋巴细胞和肿瘤细胞，从而增强 T 淋巴细胞活性和抗肿瘤活性[36]。近期的研究数据提示，这种抗体不仅可通过 T 淋巴细胞介导的细胞毒效应，也可通过靶向髓样抑制细胞避免肿瘤细胞的免疫逃逸来增加免疫反应的质和量，其中后者与免疫性抗肿瘤活性受损相关[37,38]。

双向特异性 T 淋巴细胞结合子（BiTE）包含 4 个轻链重链可变区，由一个多肽连接子连接，是 T 淋巴细胞结合单克隆抗体中的第一种。在获得不错的临床前数据后，三种药物进入了治疗复发或难治 AML 的Ⅰ期临床研究，目前正在招募患者。这三种药物分别是抗 CD3/CD33，AMG-330；抗 CD123/CD3，JNJ-63709178；以及抗 CD3/CD123，XmAb（表 4.1）。

为了改善 BiTE 的稳定性、安全性和疗效，关于各种 T 淋巴细胞结合单克隆抗体的研发正处于不同的临床前和临床研究阶段，如靶向 NK 细胞表面 CD16 的双向特异性和三向特异性杀伤细胞结合子（BiKE/TriKE）[39]，或者是二价双向亲和重复靶向双特异性抗体（DART），该抗体由两个抗原结合特异性连接在两条独立多肽链上，并具有 2 种抗原结合特性的抗体组成[40]。

最近 CD123/CD3 DART flotetuzumab（MGD006）相关的临床试验表明，DART 的安全性与 BiTE 相比可能有轻度的改善。

在获得了不错的临床前数据之后[41]，flotetuzumab 在复发或难治 AML 和中危2/高危MDS患者中进行了首项人类临床试验。近期报道了Ⅰ期剂量爬坡结果。共入组45例患者（89%为AML患者），患者中位年龄为64岁。整体看来，flotetuzumab毒性可控，44%的患者出现药物相关≥3级不良事件，最常见的不良事件为输注相关反应和细胞因子释放综合征（CRS，总发生率为76%，≥3级不良事件占13%）。17例患者中有8例患者出现药物抗白血病效应（47%），其中包括3例CR患者。目前该研究正在美国和欧洲为500ng/（kg·d）组扩大样本量[42]。后续的数据表明，在治疗第一周分步导入治疗剂量，并使用塔西单抗(tocilizumab)早期干预，可降低CRS的严重程度，平均降低0.54级。初步的数据也显示基线循环T淋巴细胞数与患者早期CRS严重程度上限呈正相关[43]。研究者们证实，初发AML标本中，原始细胞表面PD-L1高表达者，在体外对flotetuzumab介导的杀伤作用更不敏感。另外，经过flotetuzumab治疗后，早期复发的患者AML细胞表面PD-L1基线水平更高。体外实验也证实，flotetuzumab和抗-PD-L1抗体对AML细胞系具有协同杀伤作用[44]。

过继T淋巴细胞疗法

过继T淋巴细胞疗法（ACT）是高度个体化的治疗方法，其过程是将患者体内的T淋巴细胞在体外扩增，然后回输至肿瘤患者体内。这些经肿瘤激活的T淋巴细胞经过遗传学修饰，可表达特异性抗体的结合位点（嵌合抗原受体，CAR-T），因此可靶向杀伤肿瘤细胞[45]。CAR由以下元件组成：细胞外单链免疫球蛋白可变片段（scFvs）、一个跨膜短肽连接子、细胞内T淋巴细胞信号区，通常是TCR受体的CD3-ζ，以及各种共刺激分子，如CD28、OX40、4-1BB等（二代及三代CAR）或包含额外的细胞因子（IL-2、IL-15、IL-12、IL-21，为四代复合物组成部分）[46]。

目前CAR-T在AML患者中的应用还处于早期研发阶段。第一个相关的临床试验评估的是抗-LeY CAR-T在复发或难治AML患者中的安全性和可行性。在该研究的5例受试者中，2例达到疾病稳定状态，其中较长的1例疗效维持时间为23个月。更重要的是，没有发现≥3级的不良事件或CRS[47]。

近来，另一个直接针对CD123的CAR-T复合物在复发或难治AML和BPDCN患者中显示出良好的安全性和疗效。6例在异基因造血干细胞移植后出现疾病复发或难治的AML患者，中位既往治疗线数为4线，在接受了1次或2次CD123 CAR-T细胞后，2例次达CR，成功桥接至再次异基因造血干细胞移植。另有2例患者出现原始细胞数降低，但达不到CR标准。所有观察到的毒性均为可逆、可控，仅有1例出现3级不良事件（皮疹），未出现治疗限制性不良事件[48]。

近期有一项新的有趣的过继 T 淋巴细胞疗法，利用 CAR 将 $CD56^+$ NK 细胞介导至 AML 原始细胞上的特异性抗原（CD33、CD23、CD7 等）。NK 细胞是一种非常有趣的细胞，可在没有抗原提呈的前提下，依靠其本身的自然杀伤功能来攻击恶性细胞，这一特点也让它们能够从异体供者获取（而不仅仅局限于患者自身来源）[49]。另一种分离 NK 细胞的方法是从外周血单核细胞中，通过特定的细胞因子来培养它们（亦即细胞因子诱导的杀伤细胞，CIK）[50]。

最近，Zhang 等报道了他们单中心应用 CIK 和 NK 细胞治疗低中危 AML 患者 11 年的经验。共入组 152 例患者，接受联合化疗（氟达拉滨、环磷酰胺和阿糖胞苷）和免疫治疗（53 例接受 CIK，67 例轮流接受 CIK 和 NK 细胞治疗）。患者在 80 个月的 OS 率分别为 92%和 72%。轮流使用 CIK 和 NK 细胞治疗的患者组生存率较仅用 CIK 患者组更好（OS 95.5% vs.71.4%，$P<0.001$），（DFS 85% vs.63.5%，$P=0.001$）。不良反应较轻，为发热、寒战和疲乏[51]。

免疫检查点抑制剂

通过检查点抑制剂，利用免疫系统来对抗肿瘤是实体瘤和霍奇金淋巴瘤治疗的重大突破。检查点抑制剂，包括 CTLA-4 抑制剂和 PD-1 抑制剂，均为可阻断 T 淋巴细胞抑制信号的相关抗体，可松开抗肿瘤细胞毒性 T 淋巴细胞的"刹车"。免疫检查点在免疫内环境稳定和自体耐受中发挥着关键作用，也是肿瘤细胞逃脱免疫检测的重要机制[52]。

研究已经证实，AML 原始细胞表面 PD-1 和 CTLA-4 的高表达与白血病的高侵袭性相关，可能是因为降低了抗肿瘤 T 淋巴细胞的功能[53,54]。在哺乳动物模型中，阻断 CTLA-4 和 PD-1/PD-L1 通路可增强（治疗的）抗白血病效应并延长模型的存活时间[55,56]。近期有研究表明，与健康供者（$n=8$）相比，AML 患者（$n=107$）骨髓中 $PD1^+$ T 淋巴细胞数量明显增多，包括 $PD-1^+CD8^+$ 细胞、$PD-1^+$ 效应 T 细胞和 $PD-1^+$ 调节性 T 细胞等。调节性 T 细胞出现的频率，从健康供者到初发 AML 患者再到复发或难治 AML 患者依次递增（1.6% vs.2.8%vs.4.5%，$P<0.01$）。另外，Treg 浸润增加，也与表达 PD-1 的 $CD8^+T$ 淋巴细胞比例升高和表达 PD-L1/L2 的 AML 原始细胞增多密切相关[57]。以上发现表明，AML 患者中存在 T 淋巴细胞免疫耗竭的情况，也为检查点抑制剂的治疗提供了可能的依据。

近期的临床研究显示，PD-1/PD-L1 抑制剂纳武利尤单抗（Opdivo，BMS-936558）（Bristol-Myers Squibb，美国）或帕博利珠单抗（Keytruda，MK-3475/former lambrolizumab，Merck，美国）或 CTLA-4 抑制剂伊匹木单抗（Yervoy，BMS-734016），这些药物单药或与其他治疗 AML/MDS 的药物联用，对

复发 AML 患者具有很好的缓解率和缓解持续时间。检查点抑制剂单药使用对 AML 患者疗效有限，需要与其他标准抗白血病药物联用，以改善缓解率和缓解持续时间。HMA（AZA 和 DAC）为 FDA 批准的治疗 MDS 的表观遗传学药物，已被证实可上调抑制性免疫检测点蛋白，如 PD-1、PD-L1、PD-L2 等，因此这一类药物可能会增敏 T 淋巴细胞对抗 PD-1/PD-L1 抗体的反应。HMA 这类药物对免疫系统的作用比较广泛，因为它们既有免疫激活作用，也有免疫抑制作用。HMA 可通过放大抗原性（上调肿瘤细胞表面抗原表达，MHC-Ⅰ类分子的提呈）、过表达共刺激分子（包括 PD-1、PD-L1 和 PD-L2）、诱导 T 淋巴细胞启动和效应功能[58]。相反的，PD-1 上调可导致细胞对 AZA 耐药，通过抑制 PD-1/PD-L1 轴可能可以克服这种耐药[59]。

免疫检查点抑制剂单药在白血病的治疗中，让人印象最深刻的结果来源于 CTLA4 抑制剂伊匹木单抗对异基因造血干细胞移植后复发 AML 患者的疗效。该项研究共纳入 14 例移植后复发或难治 AML/MDS 患者（中位 3 种既往挽救治疗），接受 10mg/kg 的伊匹木单抗治疗后有 5 例获得 CR/Cri[60]。该项研究最近有更新，公布了中位随访 15 个月的结果。在伊匹木单抗 10mg/kg 组 5 例缓解的 AML/MDS 患者中，3 例皮肤白血病的患者中有 2 例持续缓解，另有 1 例骨髓 AML 持续缓解，以上 3 例持续缓解时间分别为 30 个月、32 个月和 34 个月。疗效数据没有报道扩展组单药伊匹木单抗 5mg/kg 的疗效（入组 6 例 AML，1 例 MDS）和单药纳武利尤单抗 0.5~1mg/kg 组的疗效（入组 4 例 AML，1 例 MDS）。报道中治疗毒性反应与免疫相关的≥4 级的不良事件，包括致死性心肌炎（1 例）、肺炎（1 例）和败血症（2 例），还有 4 级发热（1 例）和 4 级 AIHA（1 例）。另外，鉴于 1mg/kg 纳武利尤单抗组的毒性，目前仅有 0.5mg/kg 组还在继续，该剂量组目前没有观察到明显的毒性（$n=2$）[61]。

单药伊匹木单抗（3mg/kg）在 HMA 治疗失败的难治性 MDS 中也证实有效，整体有效率为 22%（2/9），毒性可耐受（≥3 级不良事件发生率为 33%）。在该项研究中，单药纳武利尤单抗（3mg/kg）对 15 例难治患者无效。

在该项研究中，最好的疗效来源于第三组——纳武利尤单抗（3mg/kg）与 AZA（75mg/m^2×5 天）联合用药组，两药联合在一线高危 MDS 患者（9/11；2 例 CR，5 例 mCR/HI，2 例 HI）中的缓解率为 80%，≥3 级不良事件发生率 27%，在可接受范围内[62]。

Daver 等最近报道了 AZA（75mg/m^2，1~7 天）联合纳武利尤单抗（3mg/kg，每 2 周 1 次）/伊匹木单抗（3mg/kg，每月 1 次），或者上述 3 药联合治疗 AML 的效果，结果令人鼓舞。该研究第一组评估的是 AZA 联合纳武利尤单抗治疗复发或难治 AML 的疗效，共纳入 70 例患者。接下来的两组目前正在招募患者中：AZA 联合纳武利尤单抗在年龄≥65 岁不适合诱导治疗的初发 AML 患者（第二组）和

AZA联合纳武利尤单抗+伊匹木单抗治疗复发或难治AML组（第三组）。第一组的结果显示，70例复发或难治AML患者（其中34%具有不良预后的细胞遗传学指标），中位年龄为70岁（22～90岁），整体的CR/CRi率为22%（4例CR，11例CRi），10%的患者达到了血液学改善，24%患者骨髓原始细胞数减少≥50%。具有二倍体核型、既往无HMA用药史和ASXL1突变的患者具有更高的缓解率。8周死亡率为7%。CR/CRi患者的中位OS为15.3个月（范围2.29～17.25个月余），该数据比同一单位使用包含AZA进行挽救治疗患者的历史数据要好（$P=0.004$）。在8例患者（12%）中观察到免疫相关的3/4级不良事件，主要包括肺炎、结肠炎、肾炎和皮疹。免疫相关不良事件出现的中位时间是治疗开始6周（4天～14周）。第二组患者目前的初步数据显示，入组9例患者，有5例出现CR/CRp（包括2例CR），1例PR。CR/CRi的患者，治疗前骨髓中的$CD3^+T$淋巴细胞和$CD8^+T$淋巴细胞比例更高，且在治疗过程中，骨髓中$CD8^+T$淋巴细胞和$CD4^+T$淋巴细胞浸润逐渐增加[63]。

Ravandi等展示了纳武利尤单抗联合大剂量化疗治疗AML患者的可行性。共入组32例初发AML（$n=30$）或高危MDS（原始细胞≥10%，$n=2$）患者，接受伊达比星（$12mg/m^2\times3$天）加阿糖胞苷（$1.5g/m^2$，24小时输注×4天），后续在第(24 ± 2)天开始用纳武利尤单抗 3mg/kg，一直治疗2年。整体的有效率（CR/CRi）为72%（23例）。早期死亡率（8周）为6%，16%的患者出现≥3级的不良事件。中位随访8.3个月，中位OS尚未达到。与之前的研究结果一致，CR/CRi与治疗前的$CD3^+T$淋巴细胞浸润水平呈正相关。而治疗无反应率则与治疗前高比例的$CD4^+PD-1^+/TIM3^+$效应T淋巴细胞水平相关[64]。

另有一项Ⅱ期、多中心评估帕博利珠单抗（200mg）联合大剂量阿糖胞苷（1.5～$2g/m^2\times5$天）治疗复发或难治AML（$n=13$）的研究结果较好。患者中位年龄为54岁，约50%的患者有欧洲白血网（ELN）分级标准的不良预后或为继发性AML。在10例可评估患者中，整体缓解率（CR/CRi）为50%，其中4例为CR。该方案毒性可控，观察到2例3级免疫相关不良事件（肝酶升高和皮疹）。CR患者中2例进行了异基因干细胞移植，移植后未见明显严重不良事件。4周和8周的死亡率分别为0和10%[65]。

讨论

在过去数十年中，我们对AML生物学的理解逐渐进步，促进了AML治疗领域——特别是靶向治疗领域突飞猛进的发展。多种靶向治疗药物（FLT3抑制剂、IDH抑制剂、Bcl-2抑制剂等）或是与一线化疗联用，或是与去甲基化药物联用作为挽救性治疗，或是在移植后使用，都显著改善了 AML 患者的预后。单克隆抗体、T 淋巴细胞结合药物和免疫检查点抑制剂是这一类免疫治疗药物中具有良好临床数据的代表。未来这类药物研究中关键的一步是鉴别出相关生物标志物（biomarker），并加以应用，使得我们能够将可以从这些治疗中获益的 AML/MDS 患者筛选出来。另外，给药时机、剂量、最佳药物组合和治疗的前后顺序，都是需要积极研究的内容，并希望这些研究能让我们将以上治疗手段安全、有效地提供给患者。

经费来源 本文部分资助来源于 MD Anderson 癌症中心经费（CCSG）CA16672。

声明 L.M. 和 G.G.M——无。N.D.——接受来自以下单位的研究经费：BMS，Pfzer，Immunogen，AbbVie，Astellas，Servier，Daiichi-Sankyo，Nohla，Genentech。同时为以下单位指导/顾问：Novartis，BMS，Daiichi-Sankyo，Astellas，AbbVie，Pfzer，Jazz，Agios，and Celgene。H.K.——接受来自以下单位的研究经费：AbbVie，Agios，Amgen，Ariad，Astex，BMS，Cyclacel，Daiichi-Sankyo，Immunogen，Jazz Pharma，Novartis，Pfzer。honoraria：AbbVie，Actinium（advisory board），Agios，Amgen，Immunogen，Orsinex，Pfzer，Takeda。F.R.——接受以下公司的研究经费和酬金：BMS。P.S.——拥有以下单位的股票：Jounce，Neon，Constellation，Oncolytics，BioAtla，Forty-Seven，Apricity，Polaris，Marker Therapeutics，Codiak。同时为以下单位的顾问委员会成员：Constellation，Jounce，Kite Pharma，Neon，BioAtla，Pieris Pharmaceuticals，Oncolytics Biotech，Merck，BioMx，Forty-Seven，Polaris，Apricity，Marker Therapeutics，Codiak。

参考文献

1. Yates JW, Wallace HJ Jr, Ellison RR, Holland JF. Cytosine arabinoside (NSC-63878) and daunorubicin (NSC-83142) therapy in acute nonlymphocytic leukemia. Cancer Chemother Rep. 1973;57:485–8.
2. Kantarjian HM. Therapy for elderly patients with acute myeloid leukemia: a problem in search of solutions. Cancer. 2007;109:1007–10. https://doi.org/10.1002/cncr.22502.
3. Saito Y, et al. Identification of therapeutic targets for quiescent, chemotherapy-resistant human leukemia stem cells. Sci Transl Med. 2010;2:17ra19. https://doi.org/10.1126/scitranslmed.3000349.
4. Hauswirth AW, et al. Expression of the target receptor CD33 in CD34+/CD38-/CD123+ AML stem cells. Eur J Clin Invest. 2007;37:73–82. https://doi.org/10.1111/j.1365-2362.2007.01746.x.
5. Larson RA, et al. Final report of the efficacy and safety of gemtuzumab ozogamicin (Mylotarg) in patients with CD33-positive acute myeloid leukemia in first recurrence. Cancer. 2005;104:1442–52. https://doi.org/10.1002/cncr.21726.
6. Sievers EL, et al. Efficacy and safety of gemtuzumab ozogamicin in patients with CD33-positive acute myeloid leukemia in first relapse. J Clin Oncol. 2001;19:3244–54.
7. Petersdorf SH, et al. A phase 3 study of gemtuzumab ozogamicin during induction and postconsolidation therapy in younger patients with acute myeloid leukemia. Blood. 2013;121:4854–

60. https://doi.org/10.1182/blood-2013-01-466706.
8. Burnett AK, et al. Identification of patients with acute myeloblastic leukemia who benefit from the addition of gemtuzumab ozogamicin: results of the MRC AML15 trial. J Clin Oncol. 2011;29:369–77. https://doi.org/10.1200/jco.2010.31.4310.
9. Burnett AK, et al. Addition of gemtuzumab ozogamicin to induction chemotherapy improves survival in older patients with acute myeloid leukemia. J Clin Oncol. 2012;30:392431. https://doi.org/10.1200/jco.2012.42.2964.
10. Castaigne S, et al. Effect of gemtuzumab ozogamicin on survival of adult patients with de-novo acute myeloid leukaemia (ALFA-0701): a randomised, open-label, phase 3 study. Lancet. 2012;379:1508–16. https://doi.org/10.1016/s0140-6736(12)60485-1.
11. Amadori S, et al. Gemtuzumab ozogamicin versus best supportive care in older patients with newly diagnosed acute myeloid leukemia unsuitable for intensive chemotherapy: results of the randomized phase III EORTC-GIMEMA AML-19. J Clin Oncol. 2016;34:972–9. https://doi.org/10.1200/jco.2015.64.0060.
12. Taksin AL, et al. High efficacy and safety profile of fractionated doses of Mylotarg as induction therapy in patients with relapsed acute myeloblastic leukemia: a prospective study of the alfa group. Leukemia. 2007;21:66–71. https://doi.org/10.1038/sj.leu.2404434.
13. Kung Sutherland MS, et al. SGN-CD33A: a novel CD33-targeting antibody-drug conjugate using a pyrrolobenzodiazepine dimer is active in models of drug-resistant AML. Blood. 2013;122:1455–63. https://doi.org/10.1182/blood-2013-03-491506.
14. Sutherland MK, et al. 5-azacytidine enhances the anti-leukemic activity of lintuzumab (SGN-33) in preclinical models of acute myeloid leukemia. MAbs. 2010;2:440–8.
15. Stein EM, et al. A phase 1 trial of vadastuximab talirine as monotherapy in patients with CD33-positive acute myeloid leukemia. Blood. 2018;131:387–96. https://doi.org/10.1182/blood-2017-06-789800.
16. Erba HP, Levy MY, Vasu S, et al. A phase 1b study of vadastuximab talirine in combination with 7+3 induction therapy for patients with newly diagnosed acute myeloid leukemia (AML). Blood. 2016;128:211. Abstract 906
17. Fathi AT, Erba HP, Lancet JE, et al. Vadastuximab talirine plus hypomethylating agents: a well-tolerated regimen with high remission rate in frontline older patients with acute myeloid leukemia. Leukemia. 2016;128(22):591.
18. Bothell W. Seattle genetics. 2017. 4 Immunotherapy in AML114.
19. Watkins K, Walker R Fishkin N, Audette C, Kovtun Y, Romanelli A. IMGN779, a CD33-targeted antibody-drug conjugate (ADC) with a novel DNA-alkylating effector molecule, induces DNA damage, cell cycle arrest, and apoptosis in AML cells. Blood. 2015;126. Abstract No 1366.
20. Whiteman KR, Noordhuis P Walker R, Watkins K, Kovtun Y, Harvey L, Wilhelm A, et al. The antibody-drug conjugate (ADC) IMGN779 is highly active in vitro and in vivo against acute myeloid leukemia (AML) with FLT3-ITD mutations. Blood. 2014. Abstract No 2321.
21. Adams S, Watkins K, McCarthy R, Wilhelm A, et al. IMGN779, a next generation CD33-targeting ADC, combines effectively with cytarabine in acute myeloid leukemia (AML) pre-clinical models, resulting in increased DNA damage response, cell cycle arrest and apoptosis in vitro and prolonged survival in vivo. Blood. 2017;130:1357.
22. Cortes J, Traer E, Wang E, Erba HP, et al. IMGN779, a next-generation CD33-targeting antibody-drug conjugate (ADC) demonstrates initial antileukemia activity in patients with relapsed or refractory acute myeloid leukemia. Blood. 2017;130:1312.
23. Bagley CJ, Woodcock JM, Stomski FC, Lopez AF. The structural and functional basis of cytokine receptor activation: lessons from the common beta subunit of the granulocyte-macrophage colony-stimulating factor, interleukin-3 (IL-3), and IL-5 receptors. Blood. 1997;89:1471–82.
24. Testa U, et al. Elevated expression of IL-3Ralpha in acute myelogenous leukemia is associated with enhanced blast proliferation, increased cellularity, and poor prognosis. Blood. 2002;100:2980–8. https://doi.org/10.1182/blood-2002-03-0852.
25. Smith BD, Roboz GJ, Walter RB, et al. First-in man, phase 1 study of CSL362 (anti-IL3Rα/anti-CD123 monoclonal antibody) in patients with CD123+ acute myeloid leukemia (AML) in CR at high risk for early relapse. Blood. 2014. Abstract 616.

26. Frankel AE, Ramage J, Kiser M, Alexander R, Kucera G, Miller MS. Characterization of diphtheria fusion proteins targeted to the human interleukin-3 receptor. Protein Eng. 2000;13:575–81.
27. Pemmaraju N, Sweet KL, Lane AA, Stein AS, et al. Results of pivotal phase 2 trial of SL-401 in patients with blastic plasmacytoid dendritic cell neoplasm (BPDCN). Blood. 2017;130:1298.
28. Frankel AE, et al. Activity of SL-401, a targeted therapy directed to interleukin-3 receptor, in blastic plasmacytoid dendritic cell neoplasm patients. Blood. 2014;124:385–92. https://doi.org/10.1182/blood-2014-04-566737.
29. Konopleva M, Hogge DE, Rizzieri D, Cirrito T, Liu JS, Kornblau S, Grable M, Hwang IL, Borthakur G, et al. Phase I trial results for SL-401, a novel cancer stem cell (CSC) targeting agent, demonstrate clinical efficacy at tolerable doses in patients with heavily pre-treated AML, poor risk elderly AML, and high risk MDS. In: 53th ASH Annual Meeting and Exposition Abstract No 3298; 2010.
30. Sweet K, Pemmaraju N, Lane A, Stein A, Vasu S, Blum W, Rizzieri DA, et al. Lead-in stage results of a pivotal trial of SL-401, an interleukin-3 receptor (IL-3R) targeting biologic, in patients with blastic plasmacytoid dendritic cell neoplasm (BPDCN) or acute myeloid leukemia (AML). Blood. 2015;126. Abstract No 3795.
31. Lane AA, Sweet KL, Wang ES, et al. Results from ongoing phase 2 trial of SL-401 as consolidation therapy in patients with acute myeloid leukemia (AML) in remission with high relapse risk including minimal residual disease (MRD). Blood. 2016;128:215.
32. Stephansky J, Togami K, Ghandi M, Montero J, et al. Resistance to SL-401 in AML and BPDCN is associated with loss of the diphthamide synthesis pathway enzyme DPH1 and is reversible by azacitidine. Blood. 2017;130:797.
33. Romagne F, Andre P, Spee P et al. Preclinical characterization of 1-7F9, a novel human anti-KIR receptor therapeutic antibody that augments natural killer-mediated killing of tumor cells. Blood 2009;114:2667–2677.
34. Vey N, Dumas P-Y, Recher C, Gastaud L, et al. Randomized phase 2 trial of lirilumab (anti-KIR monoclonal antibody, mAb) as maintenance treatment in elderly patients (pts) with acute mveloid leukemia(AML): Results of the Effikir Trial. Blood. 2017;130:889.L.Masarova et al.115
35. Daver N, Boddu P, Garcia-Manero G, Ravandi F, et al. Phase IB/II study of lirilumab with azacytidine (AZA) in relapsed AML. Blood. 2017;130:2634.
36. Baeuerle PA, Reinhardt C. Bispecific T-cell engaging antibodies for cancer therapy. Cancer Res. 2009;69:4941–4. https://doi.org/10.1158/0008-5472.can-09-0547.
37. Cheng P, Eksioglu E, Chen X, et al. Immunodepletion of MDSC By AMV564, a novel tetravalent bispecific CD33/CD3 T cell engager restores immune homeostasis in MDS in vitro. Blood. 2017;130:51.
38. Mougiakakos D, Saul D, Braun M, et al. CD33/CD3-bispecific T-cell engaging (BiTE®) antibody constructs efficiently target monocytic CD14+ hla-DRlow IDO+ aml-MDSCs. Blood. 2017;130:1363.
39. Vallera DA, et al. IL15 trispecific killer engagers (TriKE) make natural killer cells specific to CD33+ targets while also inducing persistence, in vivo expansion, and enhanced function. Clin Cancer Res. 2016;22:3440–50. https://doi.org/10.1158/1078-0432.ccr-15-2710.
40. Rader C. DARTs take aim at BiTEs. Blood. 2011;117:4403–4. https://doi.org/10.1182/blood-2011-02-337691.
41. Chichili GR, et al. A CD3xCD123 bispecific DART for redirecting host T cells to myelogenous leukemia: preclinical activity and safety in nonhuman primates. Sci Transl Med. 2015;7:289ra282. https://doi.org/10.1126/scitranslmed.aaa5693.
42. Uy GL, Godwin J, Rettig PM, et al. Preliminary results of a phase 1 study of flotetuzumab, a CD123 × CD3 Bispecific Dart® protein, in patients with relapsed/refractory acute myeloid leukemia and myelodysplastic syndrome. Blood. 2017;130:637.
43. Jacobs K, Godwin J, Foster M, Vey N, et al. Lead-in dose optimization to mitigate cytokine release syndrome in AML and MDS patients treated with flotetuzumab, a CD123 × CD3 Dart® molecule for T-cell redirected therapy. Blood. 2017;130:3856.
44. Rettig M, Godwin J, Vey N, Fox B, et al. Preliminary translational results from an ongoing phase 1 study of flotetuzumab, a CD123 × CD3 Dart®, in AML/MDS: rationale for combining flotetuzumab and anti-PD-1/PD-L1 immunotherapies. Blood. 2017;130:1365.

45. Rosenberg SA, Restifo NP. Adoptive cell transfer as personalized immunotherapy for human cancer. Science. 2015;348:62–8. https://doi.org/10.1126/science.aaa4967.
46. Pegram HJ, Park JH, Brentjens RJ. CD28z CARs and armored CARs. Cancer J. 2014;20:127–33. https://doi.org/10.1097/ppo.0000000000000034.
47. Ritchie DS, et al. Persistence and efficacy of second generation CAR T cell against the LeY antigen in acute myeloid leukemia. Mol Ther. 2013;21:2122–9. https://doi.org/10.1038/mt.2013.154.
48. Budde L, Song JY, Blanhcard S, Wagner J, et al. Remissions of acute myeloid leukemia and blastic plasmacytoid dendritic cell neoplasm following treatment with CD123-specific CAR T cells: a first-in-human clinical trial. Blood. 2017;130:811.
49. Hermanson DL, Kaufman DS. Utilizing chimeric antigen receptors to direct natural killer cell activity. Front Immunol. 2015;6:195. https://doi.org/10.3389/fimmu.2015.00195.
50. Yang XY, Zeng H, Chen FP. Cytokine-induced killer cells: a novel immunotherapy strategy for leukemia. Oncol Lett. 2015;9:535–41. https://doi.org/10.3892/ol.2014.2780.
51. Zhang X, Yang J, Zhang G, Lu P. A 11-year clinical summary of DC—CIK/NK cell immunotherapy for 152 patients with acute myeloid leukemia. Blood. 2017;130:1369.
52. Pardoll DM. The blockade of immune checkpoints in cancer immunotherapy. Nat Rev Cancer. 2012;12:252–64. https://doi.org/10.1038/nrc3239.
53. Fevery S, et al. CTLA-4 blockade in murine bone marrow chimeras induces a host-derived antileukemic effect without graft-versus-host disease. Leukemia. 2007;21:1451–9. https://doi.org/10.1038/sj.leu.2404720.
54. Mumprec t S, Schurch C, Schwaller J, Solenthaler M, Ochsenbein AF. Programmed death 1 signaling on chronic myeloid leukemia-specific T cells results in T-cell exhaustion and disease progression. Blood. 2009;114:1528–36. https://doi.org/10.1182/blood-2008-09-179697. 4 Immunotherapy in AML116.
55. Zhang L, Gajewski TF, Kline J. PD-1/PD-L1 interactions inhibit antitumor immune responses in a murine acute myeloid leukemia model. Blood. 2009;114:1545–52. https://doi.org/10.1182/blood-2009-03-206672.
56. Zhou Q, et al. Coexpression of Tim-3 and PD-1 identifies a CD8+ T-cell exhaustion phenotype in mice with disseminated acute myelogenous leukemia. Blood. 2011;117:4501–10. https://doi.org/10.1182/blood-2010-10-310425.
57. Williams P, Basu S, Garcia-Manero G, Cortes J, et al. Checkpoint expression by acute myeloid leukemia (AML) and the immune microenvironment suppresses adaptive immunity. Blood. 2017;130:185.
58. Heninger E, Krueger TE, Lang JM. Augmenting antitumor immune responses with epigenetic modifying agents. Front Immunol. 2015;6:29. https://doi.org/10.3389/fimmu.2015.00029.
59. Yang H, et al. Expression of PD-L1, PD-L2, PD-1 and CTLA4 in myelodysplastic syndromes is enhanced by treatment with hypomethylating agents. Leukemia. 2014;28(6):1280–8. https://doi.org/10.1038/leu.2013.355.
60. Davids MS, et al. Ipilimumab for patients with relapse after allogeneic transplantation. N Engl J Med. 2016;375:143–53. https://doi.org/10.1056/NEJMoa1601202.
61. Davids MS, Kim HT, Costello C, Herrera AF, et al. Optimizing checkpoint blockade as a treatment for relapsed hematologic malignancies after allogeneic hematopoietic cell transplantation. Blood. 2017;130:275.
62. Garcia-Manero G, Daver NG, Montalban-Bravo G, Jabbour EJ, et al. A phase II study evaluating the combination of nivolumab (Nivo) or ipilimumab (Ipi) with azacitidine in Pts with previously treated or untreated myelodysplastic syndromes (MDS). Blood. 2016;128:344.
63. Daver N, Basu S, Garcia-Manero G, Cortes EJ, et al. Phase IB/II study of nivolumab with azacytidine (AZA) in patients (pts) with relapsed AML. J Clin Oncol. 2017;35:7026–702.
64. Ravandi F, Daver N, Garcia-Manero G, Benton CB, et al. Phase 2 study of combination of cytarabine, idarubicin, and nivolumab for initial therapy of patients with newly diagnosed acute myeloid leukemia. Blood. 2017;130:815.
65. Zeidner FJ, Vincent BG, Ivanova A, Foster M, et al. Phase II study of high dose cytarabine followed by pembrolizumab in relapsed/refractory acute myeloid leukemia (AML). Blood. 2017;130:1349.

第 5 章

免疫检查点抑制剂的皮肤不良事件

Anisha B. Patel, Omar Pacha

译者：储香玲　蔡修宇

摘要 近期研究发现，免疫检查点抑制剂可导致皮肤不良事件，很多临床医生不熟悉这种皮肤病变的诊断和治疗，常因皮肤问题的频繁发生而停止免疫检查点抑制剂治疗。在临床过程中，常出现的前 5 种皮肤病变中，主要是瘙痒和皮疹。在 FDA 批准的三种药物中，皮肤不良事件发病率为 35%～50%，在伊匹木单抗临床试验中，虽然报道的 3 级和 4 级皮肤不良事件仅占 2%，但严重影响患者的生活质量。研究发现，43.5%的伊匹木单抗治疗患者合并有皮肤不良事件，其中 20%的患者需减少伊匹木单抗治疗剂量，这就意味着，有 9%的伊匹木单抗治疗人群因为皮肤病变而需调整剂量。接下来，将讨论免疫检查点抑制剂的种类，皮肤病变的临床表现、分级、治疗选择。

关键词 免疫检查点抑制剂　皮炎　伊匹木单抗　纳武利尤单抗　抗 PD-1 抗体　抗 CTLA-4 抗体　皮疹　免疫治疗　瘙痒

近期研究发现，免疫检查点抑制剂可导致皮肤不良事件，很多临床医生不熟悉这种皮肤病变的诊断和治疗，常因皮肤问题的频繁发生而停止免疫检查点抑制剂治疗。在临床过程中，常出现的前 5 种皮肤病变中，主要是瘙痒和皮疹。在 FDA 批准的三种药物中，皮肤不良事件发病率为 35%～50%，在伊匹木单抗 临床试验中，虽然报道的 3 级和 4 级皮肤不良事件仅占 2%，但严重影响患者的生活质量。研究发现，43.5%的伊匹木单抗治疗的患者合并有皮肤不良事件，其中 20%的患者需减少伊匹木单抗治疗剂量，这就意味着，有 9%的伊匹木单抗治疗人群因为皮肤病变而需调整剂量[1]。接下来，我们讨论免疫检查点抑制剂的种类，皮肤病变的临床表现、分级、治疗选择。

A. B. Patel (✉) · O. Pacha
Department of Dermatology, The University of Texas MD Anderson Cancer Center, Houston, TX, USA
e-mail: APatel11@mdanderson.org; opacha@mdanderson.org

© Springer Nature Switzerland AG 2018
A. Naing, J. Hajjar (eds.), *Immunotherapy*, Advances in Experimental Medicine and Biology 995, https://doi.org/10.1007/978-3-030-02505-2_5

通常情况下，细胞毒性T淋巴细胞相关蛋白4（CTLA-4）抑制剂和程序性死亡受体-1（PD-1）的抑制剂具有类似的不良反应。有报道称PD-1抑制剂通常比CTLA-4抑制剂耐受性更好，皮肤不良事件更少（分别为18%和43.5%）[1]。此外，这两种不良反应的出现似乎都有延迟的趋势，CTLA-4抑制剂大约在治疗后1个月出现皮疹，而PD-1抑制剂稍晚[1]。PD-L1抑制剂和第二代CTLA-4抑制剂目前正在进行临床试验，还没有大量的皮肤不良事件相关数据。然而，这两种药物似乎与第一代药物结构类似，也可导致皮肤不良事件，皮肤病变的严重程度可能较低。有趣的是，皮肤毒性与病情改善呈正相关，如果皮肤不良反应处理得当，可以作为预后良好的一个指标[2-4]。

免疫检查点抑制剂的皮肤不良事件

这类药物引起的皮肤病变与其他药物导致的典型皮疹不同，免疫反应并不明显。组织学上，表现为轻度的麻疹样改变，严重的有Stevens-Johnson综合征（SJS）/中毒性表皮坏死溶解症（TEN）[5]。

麻疹样药疹（通常称为"斑丘疹"），临床表现为红斑和薄而无鳞屑的丘疹，融合成泛白的斑块或薄斑块，从躯干向四肢末端扩散。组织学表现为浅表血管周围大小不一的空泡样改变、角化不良和嗜酸性粒细胞浸润。患者通常无症状，偶有瘙痒，如果伴有疼痛或进展为水疱，应考虑早期多形性红斑（EM）或SJS/TEN。多形性红斑表现为成靶形分布的红色斑丘疹，常累及肢端和皮肤黏膜，丘疹中央呈深色并伴有水疱。当弥漫性皮疹和黏膜受累范围低于体表面积（BSA）10%时，称为SJS；当皮疹大于体表面积30%时，称为TEN，从SJS到TEN这个过程非常迅速。对于麻疹样皮疹，局部类固醇使用和停用免疫检查点抑制剂通常有效。对于多形性红斑，视严重程度而定，口服或静脉注射类固醇或停药。对于SJS和TEN，停药和支持治疗至关重要，可能需要静脉注射类固醇或免疫球蛋白。

荨麻疹也是一种常见的Ⅰ型变态反应，在免疫检查点抑制剂皮肤不良事件中十分常见。组织学表现为轻度的水肿性乳头状表皮改变，表浅网状真皮层中淋巴细胞、嗜酸性粒细胞和中性粒细胞浸润。发病时间迅速，数天内即可出现，这种红色斑疹样瘙痒性荨麻疹通常经口服抗组胺药或停药可得到控制。

CTLA-4抑制剂和PD-1的抑制剂共有的皮肤不良事件

"皮疹"是最常见的药物不良反应之一，仅次于瘙痒，在帕博利珠单抗和纳武利尤单抗的临床试验中，发病率为 11%，在伊匹木单抗的临床试验中，发病率为 19%。这一非特异性描述包含多种炎性皮肤病变，包括牛皮癣样皮疹、湿疹、苔藓样皮疹和麻疹样药疹。与抗 CTLA -4 抗体抑制剂相比，抗 PD-1 抗体治疗中皮疹发生率略低。然而，严重的皮肤不良事件（3 级和 4 级）的发生率却是类似的（分别为 2.4%和 2.6%）。湿疹、瘙痒和白癜风样改变在两类药物中均可见[6-12]。

明确炎性皮肤病变的严重程度十分必要，其相应的治疗方式也不同。轻度病变可以用局部类固醇治疗，弥漫性病变需要系统性综合治疗，其中一些特殊类型的病变需要针对性治疗（图 5.1，图 5.2）。

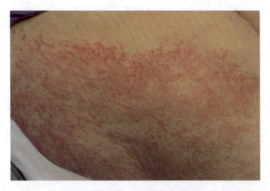

图 5.1　湿疹-红斑样丘疹融合成粗糙的块状，伴随少量的脱屑

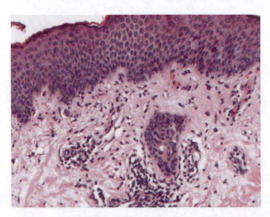

图 5.2　伴真皮层嗜酸性粒细胞浸润的湿疹样皮肤棘细胞层水肿性皮炎

湿疹可出现各种程度的瘙痒、水肿和红色丘疹，这种红色丘疹可融合成块，偶尔在严重情况下可伴有水疱，随着病情进展，斑块变得粗糙，颜色变红，可见脱屑。异位性皮炎的典型特征是皮疹呈弥漫性分布，多累及躯干和四肢的屈侧，而面部较少累及，头皮和生殖器区域常出现弥漫性表现。斑块通常表现为瘙痒及小裂隙或浅表感染区域的疼痛，组织学表现为明显的海绵层水肿和各种程度的嗜

酸性粒细胞浸润[13]。其治疗包括外用类固醇，通常是中等强度的乳膏如 0.1% 的曲安奈德乳膏，然后逐渐过渡到强力多效的氯倍他索乳膏，如 0.05% 的氯倍他索乳膏。面部、腋窝和腹股沟通常使用温和低效的类固醇，如 2.5% 的氢化可的松或 0.05% 的地奈德乳膏。一天 2 次局部类固醇外用可有效控制皮疹的复发，然后一周 2 次维持治疗。同时口服第一代抗组胺药物如二苯氢胺或羟嗪，这点非常重要。

根据作者的经验，晨服第二代非镇静抗组胺药，如西替利嗪或氯雷他定，也是有益的。对于不良事件 3 级、累及体表面积大于 30%，而且对局部治疗无效的患者，口服类固醇如泼尼松 1mg/kg 通常是有效的，剂量可逐渐减少，缓慢减量直至局部外用类固醇维持治疗。

初步文献筛查，并未发现关于口服类固醇治疗效果减弱方面的报道，因此在局部类固醇耐药的患者中，口服类固醇成为首选的全身治疗策略[14,15]。

重度的皮肤病变治疗疗程较长，可能停药后还可持续数月，因此需要类固醇替代品。针对白细胞介素 4 受体-亚单位（IL-4Ra）拮抗来治疗特异性皮炎的这种生物治疗，也是长期类固醇维持治疗的严重难治性湿疹患者的一种潜在治疗选择。

对于没有皮疹的瘙痒，临床表现各不相同，即使出现药物性皮肤病变，大多数情况下，患者的皮肤看起来仍无异常。瘙痒可导致各种程度的糜烂、溃疡、瘙痒性结节和线性糜烂。瘙痒性结节表现不一，呈离散性、红色高色素沉着的棘皮丘疹，常伴有中心部位糜烂。组织学表现为纤维化，浅表真皮垂直方向的血管上方覆盖棘状表皮。治疗的第一步是清除原发性炎症。对于原发性瘙痒，最好是根据严重程度采取相应措施。对于病情较轻的患者，第一代抗组胺药通常就足够了，它还具有镇静的额外益处，睡前服用可以帮助患者在瘙痒最严重的时候入睡。随着病情加重，睡前高剂量的三环抗抑郁药多塞平和 GABA 激动剂如加巴喷丁治疗可控制疾病（图 5.3，图 5.4）。

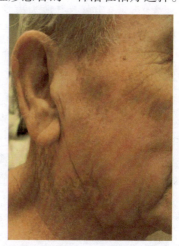

图 5.3　白癜风样病变-头颈部白斑

白癜风样皮肤病变表现为色素缺失，分界清晰的斑点融合成斑块，偶有红斑和瘙痒。白癜风样皮肤病变仅在黑色素瘤患者中有报道，抗 CTLA-4 和抗 PD-1 治疗人群中患病率大约 2%。组织学显示真皮-表皮交界处黑色素细胞的缺失。患者常无症状，但可能有过瘙痒。白癜风的治疗包括局部类固醇和紫外线联合治疗。然而，在黑色素瘤患者出现这种皮肤损害时，由于紫外线照射可增加患皮肤癌的风险，因此紫外线不能频繁使用。

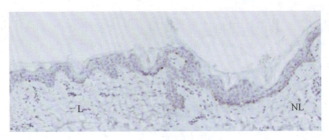

图 5.4 与非病变（NL）皮肤的 MART1 免疫印迹相比，白癜风样病变皮肤（L）表皮和真皮交界处黑色素细胞减少

抗 CTLA-4 抗体类药物常见的皮肤不良事件

在接受伊匹木单抗治疗的患者中，最常见的不良事件是"皮疹"，占 25%~50%，1/4~1/3 的患者出现瘙痒[16]。皮疹表现从轻度湿疹到中毒性表皮坏死松解性皮疹[17]，其中大多数为更常见的麻疹样药疹或湿疹样特应性皮炎样疹[16]。据报道，皮疹多在用药 3 周后出现，通常 2.5 个月左右消退[16]。通过复习本中心未发表的研究数据，大多数患者需要停止用药后才能获得完全缓解。上面讨论的这类药物最常见的皮肤不良事件中，痤疮样皮疹[12]和肉芽肿性皮炎[18]较少见。

抗 CTLA-4 抗体类药物是通过干扰 T 淋巴细胞 CTLA-4 而激活 T 淋巴细胞，从而导致机体免疫系统上调而达到抗肿瘤活性（具体见本文其他部分所述）。分别使用抗 CTLA-4 抗体 10mg/kg 与 3mg/kg 的患者，可出现相似的皮肤发病率，由此可见，皮肤不良事件的发生率与使用剂量无关，然而，按照常见的皮肤病标准定义分类≥3 级的皮疹发生率低于 2.4%[19]。

抗 PD-1 抗体类药物的皮肤不良事件

除了前面讨论的皮肤炎症外，抗 PD-1 抗体还可诱发银屑病[20,21]和大疱性类天疱疮[22,23]。近期发现，在接受抗 PD-1 抗体治疗的患者中出现了暴发性角化棘皮瘤[24]（图 5.5，图 5.6）。

银屑病样皮炎的临床表现为典型的寻常型银屑病，界线清晰的红色略硬斑块，轻度鳞屑粘连，呈局灶或弥漫性分布，肢体病变通常较躯干严重，头皮为好发部位，可能呈逆向分布，尤其是三叉神经区域[21]，或呈脓疱样改变，可有瘙痒或疼痛，皮肤微裂隙，并导致四肢水肿。组织学表现为海绵状银屑病样皮炎，伴有角膜下脓疱，嗜酸性粒细胞浸润。作者发现，银屑病比湿疹更难治疗，这使其成为了皮疹预后判断的参考指标。这种皮肤病变需要局部类固醇与口服抗组胺药联合治疗，升级治疗包括口服维 A 酸、阿普斯特片、紫外-B（UV-B）治疗或口服类固醇。生物制剂如 IL-17 抑制剂，是治疗难治性病例的一种潜在疗法，并已有治疗成功的报道。

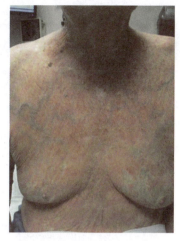

图 5.5　牛皮癣样皮炎——黏附着屑样物的红色分界清楚的斑块

大疱性类天疱疮是由抗体介导的高张力大疱性疾病，呈大小不一、充满浆液的水疱，剧痒。组织学表现为表皮下水疱性皮炎，真皮浅表层和大疱内可见丰富的嗜酸性粒细胞；真皮-表皮交界处裂开，表皮顶部完整，没有角化不良。直接免疫荧光可见高强度 IgG 沉积于真皮-表皮交界处。局部和口服类固醇，以及利妥昔单抗已经成功用于治疗这种缓慢出现的皮肤病变[25]。

暴发性角化棘皮瘤相对较易诊断，属于低级别鳞状细胞癌。本章中的此类皮肤病变患者均采取保守治疗，并未中断抗 PD-1 治疗[24]。

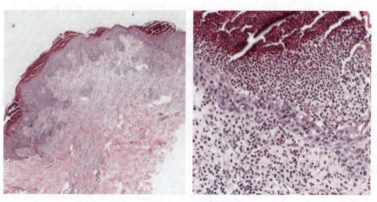

图 5.6　伴角层下脓疱、不规则棘皮和大量嗜酸性粒细胞浸润的海绵状银屑病性皮炎

分级

临床广泛使用通用术语标准对不良事件进行分级，近期美国临床肿瘤学会（American Society of Clinical Oncology）修订后的版本将其作为"实践指南"，这种分级标准侧重于症状和生活质量的描述，而不是病变皮疹的面积，即使高分级皮疹累及较少的体表面积，也可能需要调整药物剂量（表 5.1，图 5.7）。

表 5.1　不良事件的通用术语分级标准[26]

分级	1	2	3	4	5
皮疹	黄斑或丘疹占体表面积<10%,有或无症状（如瘙痒、烧灼感、紧绷感）	黄斑或丘疹占体表面积10%～30%,有或无症状（如瘙痒、烧灼感、紧绷感），并且限制工具性日常生活能力	黄斑或丘疹占体表面积>30%,有或无症状（如瘙痒、烧灼感、紧绷感），并且限制工具性日常生活能力	广泛表皮剥脱，溃疡性或大疱性皮炎	死亡
脱发	通常情况下不明显,通过仔细检查才能发现的50%以下的脱发,需要改变发型以掩盖脱发,但并不需要假发	很容易发现的超过50%以上的脱发,如果想不被人发现或者脱发已经导致心理问题,需要假发来遮掩脱发			
色素减退	皮肤色素减退面积低于体表面积的10%,而且色素减退没有导致心理疾病	皮肤色素减退面积大于体表面积10%,或色素减退导致了心理疾病			
瘙痒	轻度或局部瘙痒,可自发缓解或局部治疗可以控制	广泛的剧烈瘙痒,可自发缓解或系统治疗可以控制	广泛的剧烈瘙痒,治疗后无缓解		

表 5.2　免疫检查点抑制剂相关不良事件中皮肤毒性的管理

1.0 皮肤毒性
1.1 皮疹/炎症性皮炎
定义：多形性红斑（皮肤和黏膜上的靶形损害，通常由感染如单纯疱疹病毒引起，但也可能与免疫相关的药疹有关，如果进展为多形性红斑，则可能预示着 SCAR 的发生，例如 SJS），苔藓样变（扁平状，多边形，有时是鳞状或肥大性的扁平苔藓病变），湿疹（炎症性皮炎，特征是皮肤瘙痒，出现红斑，鳞状或结痂的丘疹或斑块，易反复感染），牛皮癣（边界清楚，呈红斑状、鳞屑状丘疹和银屑病斑块），麻疹[非脓疱性，非大疱状麻疹样皮疹，常被称为斑丘疹且无全身症状或实验室检查异常，不包括偶发的周围性嗜酸性粒细胞增多症），感觉丧失性红斑（手足综合征；泛红，麻木，烧灼感，瘙痒和浅表脱屑），嗜中性皮肤病（如 SWEET 综合征）等。
诊断检查：
患者病史及体格检查；
排除其他致病因素，如感染、另一种药物的作用，或与另一种全身性疾病相关的皮肤损害或原发性皮肤疾病；
必要时进行实验室检验，包括血常规和肝、肾功能；
若怀疑自身免疫性疾病，如狼疮或皮肌炎，则进行直接血清学检验：抗核抗体筛选试验，SS-A/抗 Ro、SS-B/抗 La（如果主要是光分布/光敏性），抗组蛋白、双链 DNA 和其他相关血清学。若考虑为其他自身免疫性疾病，则考虑增加血清学检查或诊断性检查。
皮肤活检；
使用连续拍照的方式密切监测病情；
检查患者用药记录，排除其他药物引起的光敏反应。

续表

分级	管理建议
根据常见不良反应事件评价标准（CTCAE）对皮肤毒性进行分级具有挑战性。皮肤毒性的严重程度可能取决于体表面积（BSA）、耐受性、发病率及持续时间。	
1级：症状不影响生活质量或经局部治疗和（或）口服止痒剂可以控制。	继续 ICPi 治疗； 使用局部润肤剂和（或）使用中到高强度的糖皮质激素（局部外用）； 避免皮肤刺激和阳光暴露。
2级：炎症反应影响生活质量且需要诊断性治疗。	暂缓 ICPi 治疗且每周监测病情，若未改善，则暂停 ICPi 治疗，直至皮肤不良反应降至1级； 使用泼尼松龙（或等效）全身治疗，起始剂量1mg/kg，至少4周内逐渐减量； 此外，可局部使用润肤剂、口服抗组胺药和使用中到高强度的糖皮质激素（局部外用）。
3级：2级反应，但对2级治疗措施无效者。	暂停 ICPi 治疗并请皮肤科会诊； 局部使用润肤剂、口服抗组胺药物和使用高强度的糖皮质激素（局部外用）； 使用（甲基）泼尼松龙（或等效）全身治疗，起始剂量1～2mg/kg，至少4周内逐渐减量。
4级：所有严重难治的皮疹，之前的治疗措施无效或无法耐受。	立即停药，当泼尼松龙（或等效）减少至≤10mg 时请皮肤科会诊以确定是否恢复 ICPi 治疗； 静脉使用（甲基）泼尼松龙（或等效）1～2mg/kg，完全恢复正常后缓慢减量； 密切监测严重皮肤不良反应的进展； 立即住院治疗并请皮肤科紧急会诊； 若皮肤不良反应不能降至1级及以下，则考虑更换抗肿瘤治疗方案；若 ICPi 为患者仅有的选择，则考虑在皮肤不良反应降至1级时重新开始 ICPi 治疗。

1.2 大疱皮肤病

定义：包括大疱性类天疱疮或其他自身免疫性大疱性皮肤病，大疱性药物反应。

诊断检查：

体格检查；

排除其他致病因素，如感染、另一种药物的作用，或与另一种全身性疾病相关的皮肤损害；

必要时可进行实验室检验，包括血常规和肝、肾功能；

考虑通过血清抗体检测来排除大疱性类天疱疮或者在皮肤科的指导下，送患者血清进行间接免疫荧光检测来排除其他自身免疫性病；

非传染性或暂时性的其他原因（如单纯疱疹、带状疱疹、大疱性脓疱、虫咬性大疱、摩擦或压力性水疱）转诊至皮肤科治疗；

考虑进行皮肤活检（苏木素-伊红法染色评估病变皮肤，直接免疫荧光法评估病变周围皮肤）

续表

分级	管理建议
1级：无症状，水疱区域低于10%的BSA，无相关红斑。	如果水疱区域低于10%的BSA，无症状且无炎症（例如摩擦性水疱或压力性水疱），则无须停止ICPi，仅需观察和（或）局部伤口护理； 当在皮肤或黏膜表面观察到有症状的大疱或糜烂（脱皮的小疱或大疱）时，根据定义至少将其视为2级，见2级管理建议。
2级：根据诊断未达到2级，但影响生活质量并需要进行干预； 或水疱覆盖10%~30%的体表面积。	暂停ICPi治疗，并请皮肤科会诊决定是否继续治疗； 注意局部伤口护理，如用凡士林油和绷带包扎由水疱破裂或顶部脱落形成的开放性糜烂； 避免皮肤刺激和阳光暴露，穿防晒衣，使用防晒霜； 排查自身免疫性大疱性疾病； 局部外用1类高效皮质类固醇（例如氯倍他索、倍他米松或同类药物），每3天重新评估其进展或改善情况； 使用泼尼松（或同等药物）全身治疗，起始剂量为0.5~1mg/kg，至少4周内逐渐减量； 密切监测是否累及更多的BSA或黏膜； 使用连续拍照的方式密切监测病情； 监测复杂皮肤不良药物反应的基础检查： ·系统回顾：皮肤疼痛（如晒伤）、发热、乏力、肌痛、关节痛、腹痛、眼部不适或畏光、鼻腔疼痛或不适、口腔疼痛或不适、咽痛、声音嘶哑、排尿困难、女性阴道区疼痛或不适、男性阴茎口疼痛、肛周疼痛或排便疼痛 ·体格检查：包括生命体征和全身皮肤检查。具体包括：评估所有皮肤表面和黏膜（眼睛、鼻孔、口咽、生殖器和肛周区域）；评估淋巴结病、面部或远端肢体肿胀（可能是DIHS/DRESS的征象）；评估脓疱、水疱或糜烂，以及"暗色红斑"区域（触诊时可感疼痛）。若要检测尼氏征，可将戴手套的手指在与红斑性皮肤相切方向，平行于皮肤表面施加摩擦，若出现表皮脱落，则尼氏征为阳性，表明表皮与真皮的附着不良，在自身免疫性疾病（如天疱疮）和SJS/TEN中可见。
3级：皮肤脱落超过30%的BSA并伴有疼痛和日常生活自理能力受限。	暂停ICPi治疗，并请皮肤科会诊决定是否继续治疗； 静脉使用（甲基）泼尼松龙（或等效）1~2mg/kg，至少4周内逐渐减量； 如果诊断为大疱性类天疱疮，有可能需要避免长期使用全身性皮质类固醇激素并用利妥昔单抗替代治疗； 如果患者可能患有继发性蜂窝织炎或存在其他感染的危险因素，例如中性粒细胞减少症等，应请传染科会诊。
4级：水疱覆盖超过30%的BSA，并伴有液体或电解质异常。	永久停止ICPi治疗； 立即住院治疗，请皮肤科紧急会诊； 静脉使用（甲基）泼尼松龙（或等效）1~2mg/kg，完全恢复正常后，至少4周内逐渐减量。 如果诊断为大疱性类天疱疮，有可能需要避免长期使用全身性皮质类固醇激素并用利妥昔单抗替代治疗； 如果患者可能患有继发性蜂窝织炎或存在其他感染的危险因素，例如中性粒细胞减少症等，应请传染科会诊。

续表

1.3 严重皮肤不良反应（SCARS），包括 Stevens-Johnson 综合征（SJS）、中毒性表皮坏死松解症（TEN）、急性全身发疹性脓疱病和伴嗜酸性粒细胞增多和系统症状的药疹（DRESS）或药物超敏反应综合征（DIHS）。

定义：由于药物引起的皮肤、附属物或黏膜的结构或功能的严重变化。

诊断检查：

全身皮肤检查，注意检查所有的黏膜及所有的系统。排除其他致病因素，感染、另一种药物的作用，或与另一种全身性疾病相关的皮肤损害。

实验室检验包括血常规、肝肾功能的检查、尿常规，如果病人发热，还应考虑血培养。

皮肤活检可用于评估全层表皮坏死，可见于 SJS/TEN，以及其他可能的病因，如副肿瘤性天疱疮或其他自身免疫性疱病或其他药物反应，如急性全身发疹性脓疱病。

使用连续拍照的方式密切监测病情。

如果在皮肤上发现黏膜受损或起水疱，考虑尽早到烧伤中心进行进一步的监测和处理。

监测复杂皮肤不良药物反应的基础检查：

系统回顾：皮肤疼痛（如晒伤）、发热、乏力、肌痛、关节痛、腹痛、眼部不适或畏光、鼻腔疼痛或不适、口腔疼痛或不适、咽痛、声音嘶哑、排尿困难、女性阴道区疼痛或不适、男性阴茎口疼痛、肛周疼痛或排便疼痛。

体格检查：包括生命体征和全身皮肤检查。具体包括：评估所有皮肤表面和黏膜（眼睛、鼻孔、口咽、生殖器和肛周区域）；评估淋巴结病、面部或远端肢体肿胀（可能是 DIHS/DRESS 的征象）；评估脓疱、水疱或糜烂，以及"暗色红斑"区域（触诊时可感疼痛）。若要检测尼氏征，可将戴手套的手指在与红斑性皮肤相切方向，平行于皮肤表面施加摩擦，若出现表皮脱落，则尼氏征为阳性，表明表皮与真皮的附着不良，在自身免疫性疾病（如天疱疮）和 SJS/TEN 中可见。

分级	管理建议
所有级别	如怀疑有 SJS 或黏膜受累者，无论其程度如何，应停止 ICPi 治疗并密切监测病情。
1 级：无症状。	对于 SCARS，没有 1 级；大疱或糜烂累及的体表面积（BSA）较少时就应引起高度重视，以防发展到 3 级或 4 级。
2 级：麻疹样皮疹（斑丘疹）区域占 10%～30% 的 BSA，伴有全身症状、淋巴结病或面部肿胀。	暂停 ICPi，密切监测，每 3 天评估一次，以防疾病进展，累及更多的 BSA 或黏膜，可使用连续拍照的方式密切监测病情；局部使用润肤剂、口服抗组胺药和使用中到高强度的糖皮质激素（局部外用）；使用（甲基）泼尼松龙（或等效）0.5～1mg/kg，至少 4 周内逐渐减量。
3 级：皮肤脱落区域<10% 的 BSA，伴有黏膜受累（红斑、紫癜、表皮剥离、黏膜剥离）	暂停 ICPi，请皮肤科会诊，局部使用润肤剂比如凡士林油、二甲硅油，口服抗组胺剂和使用高强度的糖皮质激素（局部外用）；静脉使用（甲基）泼尼松龙（或等效）0.5～1 mg/kg，好转后改为口服，至少 4 周内逐渐减量；请烧伤科会诊，注意支持性护理，包括液体和电解质平衡，尽量减少隐性水分流失，并防止感染；鉴于这些药物的免疫作用机制，使用免疫抑制性药物是必要的；对于黏膜受累的 SJS 或 TEN，应进行多学科会诊指导毒性管理，以预防后遗症（如眼科、耳鼻喉科、泌尿外科、妇科等）。

续表

分级	管理建议
4级：皮肤红斑、水泡、脱落区域超过10%的BSA，伴有相关症状（如红斑、紫癜、表皮剥离、黏膜剥离），伴或不伴有全身症状和相关血液学异常（如DRESS或DIHS患者会出现肝功能指标升高）。	永久停止ICPi，立即将病人送往烧伤病房或ICU，请皮肤科紧急会诊； 基于黏膜表面管理的多学科会诊（如眼科、泌尿外科、妇科、耳鼻喉科等）。 静脉使用（甲基）泼尼松龙（或等效）1~2mg/kg，完全恢复至正常时缓慢减量。 静脉注射免疫球蛋白或环孢素也可用于严重或皮质类固醇无效的病例。 考虑疼痛科或姑息性治疗科会诊，临床表现为DRESS综合征的病人需住院治疗。
注意：对于SJS患者，常规的禁止使用皮质激素不再适用，因为免疫相关的SJS的潜在机制是T细胞免疫介导的毒性，糖皮质激素或其他药物的充分抑制是必要的，并且在DRESS或DIHS患者中可延长免疫抑制时间。	
所有的建议都是基于专家的共识，利大于弊，推荐力度为中等推荐。	
英文缩写：ADL, activities of daily living; BSA, body surface area; CTCAE, Common Terminology Criteria for Adverse Events; DIHS, drug-induced hypersensitivity syndrome; DRESS, drug reaction with eosinophilia and systemic symptoms; G, grade; ICPi, immune checkpoint inhibitor; ICU, intensive care unit; irAE, immune-related adverse event; IV, intravenous; IVIG, intravenous immunoglobulin; NA, not applicable; SCAR, severe cutaneous adverse reactions; SJS, Stevens-Johnson syndrome; TENS, toxic epidermal necrolysis.	

作为预后因子的皮肤不良事件

白癜风大多情况下是无症状的，而且不需要治疗，是一种相对较轻的皮肤不良事件。然而，当使用免疫检查点抑制剂的患者出现白癜风时，反而提示患者有较高的无疾病进展生存率和肿瘤缓解率。人们普遍认为白癜风是一种被低估的不良事件，如果不进行全身皮肤检查，很容易遗漏。此外，白癜风仅在黑色素瘤患者中有报道[2,3,28,29]，且皮疹的发生率与存活率和肿瘤缓解率相关[2]。

参考文献

1. Villadolid J, Amin A. Immune checkpoint inhibitors in clinical practice: update on management of immune-related toxicities. Transl Lung Cancer Res. 2015;4(5):560–75.
2. Sanlorenzo M, Vujic I, Daud A, et al. Pembrolizumab cutaneous adverse events and their association with disease progression. JAMA Dermatol. 2015;151(11):1206–12.
3. Teulings HE, Limpens J, Jansen SN, et al. Vitiligo-like depigmentation in patients with stage III-IV melanoma receiving immunotherapy and its association with survival: a systematic review and meta-analysis. J Clin Oncol. 2015;33(7):773–81.
4. Attia P, Phan GQ, Maker AV, et al. Autoimmunity correlates with tumor regression in patients

with metastatic melanoma treated with anti-cytotoxic T-lymphocyte antigen-4. J Clin Oncol. 2005;23(25):6043–53.
5. Sundaresan S, Nguyen KT, Nelson KC, Ivan D, Patel AB. Erythema multiforme major in a patient with metastatic melanoma treated with nivolumab. Dermatol Online J. 2017;23(9).
6. Hodi FS, O'Day SJ, McDermott DF, et al. Improved survival with ipilimumab in patients with metastatic melanoma. N Engl J Med. 2010;363:711–23.5.
7. Robert C, Thomas L, Bondarenko I, et al. Ipilimumab plus dacarbazine for previously untreated metastatic melanoma. N Engl J Med. 2011;364:2517–26.
8. Robert C, Ribas A, Wolchok JD, et al. Anti-programmed-death-receptor-1 treatment with pembrolizumab in ipilimumab-refractory advanced melanoma: a randomised dose-comparison cohort of a phase 1 trial. Lancet. 2014;384:1109–7.7.
9. Robert C, Long GV, Brady B, et al. Nivolumab in previously untreated melanoma without BRAF mutation. N Engl J Med. 2015;372:320–30.
10. Weber JS, D'Angelo SP, Minor D, et al. Nivolumab versus chemotherapy in patients with advanced melanoma who progressed after anti-CTLA-4 treatment (CheckMate037): a randomised, controlled, open-label, phase 3 trial. Lancet Oncol. 2015;16:375–84.
11. Rizvi NA, Mazières J, Planchard D, et al. Activity and safety of nivolumab, an anti-PD-1 immune checkpoint inhibitor, for patients with advanced, refractory squamous non-small-cell lung cancer (CheckMate 063): a phase 2, single-arm trial. Lancet Oncol. 2015;16:257–65.
12. Garon EB, Rizvi NA, Hui R, et al. Pembrolizumab for the treatment of non-small-cell lung cancer. N Engl J Med. 2015;372:2018–28.
13. Di Giacomo AM, Biagioli M, Maio M. The emerging toxicity profiles of anti-CTLA-4 antibodies across clinical indications. Semin Oncol. 2010;37(5):499–507.
14. Fujii T, Colen RR, Bilen MA, et al. Incidence of immune-related adverse events and its association with treatment outcomes: the MD Anderson Cancer Center experience. Invest New Drugs. 2018;36(4):638–46.
15. Horvat TZ, Adel NG, Dang TO, et al. Immune-related adverse events, need for systemic immunosuppression, and effects on survival and time to treatment failure in patients with melanoma treated with ipilimumab at Memorial Sloan Kettering Cancer Center. J Clin Oncol. 2015;33(28):3193–8.
16. Lacouture ME, Wolchok JD, Yosipovitch G, Kähler KC, Busam KJ, Hauschild A. Ipilimumab in patients with cancer and the management of dermatologic adverse events. J Am Acad Dermatol. 2014;71(1):161–9.
17. Nayar N, Briscoe K, Fernandez Penas P. Toxic epidermal necrolysis-like reaction with severe satellite cell necrosis associated with nivolumab in a patient with ipilimumab refractory metastatic melanoma. J Immunother. 2016;39(3):149–52.
18. Kubicki SL, Welborn ME, Garg N, Aung PP, Patel AB. Granulomatous dermatitis associated with ipilimumab therapy (Ipilimumab associated granulomatous dermatitis). J Cutan Pathol. 2018;45(8):636–8.
19. Minkis K, et al. The risk of rash associated with ipilimumab in patients with cancer: a systematic review of the literature and meta-analysis. J Am Acad Dermatol. 2013;69(3):e121–8.
20. Ohtsuka M, Miura T, Mori T, Ishikawa M, Yamamoto T. Occurrence of psoriasiform eruption during nivolumab therapy for primary oral mucosal melanoma. JAMA Dermatol. 2015;151(7):797–9.
21. Totonchy MB, Ezaldein HH, Ko CJ, Choi JN. Inverse psoriasiform eruption during pembrolizumab therapy for metastatic melanoma. JAMA Dermatol. 2016;152(5):590–2.
22. Jour G, Glitza IC, Ellis RM, et al. Autoimmune dermatologic toxicities from immune checkpoint blockade with anti-PD-1 antibody therapy: a reporton bullous skin eruptions. J Cutan Pathol. 2016;43(8):688–96.
23. Naidoo J, Schindler K, Querfeld C, et al. Autoimmune bullous skin disorders with immune checkpoint inhibitors targeting PD-1 and PD-L1. Cancer Immunol Res. 2016;4(5):383–9.
24. Freites-martinez A, Kwong BY, Rieger KE, Coit DG, Colevas AD, Lacouture ME. Eruptive keratoacanthomas associated with pembrolizumab therapy. JAMA Dermatol. 2017;153(7):694–7.
25. Sowerby L, Dewan AK, Granter S, Gandhi L, Leboeuf NR. Rituximab treatment of nivolumab-induced bullous pemphigoid. JAMA Dermatol. 2017;153(6):603–5.

26. Common Terminology Criteria for Adverse Events (CTCAE) v4.0. 2008. http://ctep.cancer.gov/protocolDevelopment/electronic_applications/ctc.htm. Accessed 26 Jul 2016.
27. Brahmer JR, Lacchetti C, Schneider BJ, Atkins MB, Brassil KJ, Caterino JM, et al. Management of immune-related adverse events in patients treated with immune checkpoint inhibitor therapy: American Society of Clinical Oncology Clinical Practice Guideline. J Clin Oncol. 2018;36(17):1714–68. https://doi.org/10.1200/JCO.2017.77.6385.
28. Hua C, Boussemart L, Mateus C, et al. Association of vitiligo with tumor response in patients with metastatic melanoma treated with pembrolizumab. JAMA Dermatol. 2016;152(1):45–51.
29. Freeman-Keller M, Kim Y, Cronin H, Richards A, Gibney G, Weber JS. Nivolumab in resected and unresectable metastatic melanoma: characteristics of immune-related adverse events and association with outcomes. Clin Cancer Res. 2016;22(4):886–94.

第6章

免疫相关不良事件之肺炎

Akash Jain，Vickie R. Shannon，Ajay Sheshadri

译者：周　娟　苏春霞

摘要　免疫检查点抑制剂是免疫治疗家族的一部分，并越来越多地用于治疗各种癌症。免疫相关的不良事件是癌症患者面临的重大挑战。肺炎是一种少见的免疫相关不良事件，临床上有不同的表现形式。本章的目的是指导读者了解肺炎的发生率和临床表现，并为肺炎患者的评估和治疗提供指导。

关键词　免疫检查点抑制剂　免疫相关不良事件　肺炎　胸部影像学　机化性肺炎　非特异性间质性肺炎　过敏性肺炎　弥漫性肺泡损伤

引言

随着人类预期寿命的增加[1]，癌症患病率也逐年上升，复发、难治性癌症的治疗给临床医生带来了巨大挑战，需要新的治疗策略来延缓癌症的进展[2]。免疫治疗就是这样一种新的治疗方式，它通过激活免疫系统来对抗癌症，从而持续降低肿瘤负荷[3-5]。免疫治疗药物的常见治疗靶点包括程序性细胞死亡蛋白 1（PD-1）通路和细胞毒性 T 淋巴细胞相关蛋白 4（CTLA-4）通路，将在下述内容详细讨论[6]。肿瘤细胞通过 PD-L1（PD-1 的配体）和 CTLA-4[7]的表达等多种机制抑制 T 淋巴细胞的天然抗肿瘤活性，PD-1 通路和 CTLA-4 通路的抑制剂通过阻止 T 淋巴细胞活性的稳态下调（通常发生在慢性感染期间）来提高抗肿瘤免疫反应，从而防止过度的组织损伤[8,9]。然而，激活的免疫系统可能破坏正常的免疫平衡，从而可能诱导许多靶外器官免疫相关不良事件（irAE）的发生。本章中，将重点讨论免疫治疗药物引起的肺部免疫相关不良事件。

经 PD-1 通路和 CTLA-4 通路抑制 T 淋巴细胞功能

PD-1 是免疫球蛋白超家族中的单分子跨膜蛋白，存在于巨噬细胞、T 淋巴细胞和 B 淋巴细胞表面[10-12]。PD-1 主要在成熟的 T 淋巴细胞中表达，并在 T 淋巴细胞活化后 24 小时内出现，用以调节 T 淋巴细胞的活性，防止损伤健康组织[13]。PD-1 主要与两个配体结合，PD-L1 和 PD-L2。PD-L1 广泛表达于造血细胞系、各种上皮细胞和内皮细胞，而 PD-L2 主要表达于树突状细胞和 B 淋巴细胞[10]。多种炎症因子可诱导淋巴细胞和非免疫细胞[11]PD-L1 的表达。PD-1 与其配体结合可促进磷酸酶 Src 同源蛋白 2（SHP2）的募集，进而导致 PI3K/AKT 信号通路失活[14,15]。在 T 淋巴细胞中，PD-1 通路的激活可以阻止其增殖，减弱炎性反应，降低存活率[16]。PD-1 与 PD-L2 结合，可降低 T 淋巴细胞细胞因子的产生，但不抑制其增殖[17]。

此外，PD-1 通路的激活诱导幼稚 T 淋巴细胞向调节性 T 淋巴细胞分化，并诱导免疫耐受[18,19]。癌细胞通过表达 PD-L1 和 PD-L2 来抑制 PD-1 的活化，从而抑制肿瘤免疫反应[20]。PD-1 也可表达于肿瘤组织巨噬细胞上，这可能与利于肿瘤进展的肿瘤微环境有关[21]。

T 淋巴细胞的激活，需要将 T 淋巴细胞表面表达的 CD28 等共刺激分子与其抗原提呈细胞上表达的受体 B7-1（CD80）和 B7-2（CD86）结合[22,23]。CTLA-4 是一种 CD28 同源物，它与 B7 的亲和力高于 CD28，但不产生刺激信号。CTLA-4 有一个缺乏酶活性的 36-氨基酸细胞质尾，也有一个具有抑制功能的基于酪氨酸免疫受体的抑制基团[24,25]。CTLA-4 的激活可诱导 T 淋巴细胞功能的抑制[23,26-29]，从而降低 T 淋巴细胞增殖，减少 IL-2 的分泌[22,23,26,27,30]。在健康人群中，CTLA-4 主要由调节性 T 淋巴细胞表达，激活 CTLA-4 是促进免疫耐受的重要机制[31]。小鼠 CTLA-4 功能的丧失可产生致命的自身免疫病[32,33]。同样，肿瘤患者肿瘤细胞表面表达的 CTLA-4 可致 T 淋巴细胞功能减弱，而使瘤细胞得以存活[34,35]。

通过免疫检查点的抑制来治疗肿瘤

癌细胞通过 PD-1 和 CTLA-4 途径来诱导抗肿瘤的淋巴细胞活性丧失，相反，抑制免疫检查点可导致肿瘤消退。在本章中，将简要讨论 CTLA-4 抑制剂伊匹木单抗、PD-1 抑制剂纳武利尤单抗和帕博利珠单抗、PD-L1 抑制剂阿特珠单抗、阿维鲁单抗和度伐鲁单抗。这些药物已经被美国 FDA（Federal Drug Administration）批准用于治疗数种癌症，更多的 ICPI 疗法的临床试验正在进行中。

伊匹木单抗是 FDA 唯一批准的 CTLA-4 抑制剂，伊匹木单抗结合 CTLA-4 的前 β-片段从而阻止 CTLA-4：B7 复合物的形成[36]。2011 年，FDA 批准了伊匹木单抗上市，此前一项关键研究显示，伊匹木单抗可以提高转移性黑色素瘤患者的生存率[37]。另一种 CTLA-4 抑制剂曲美木单抗正在研发中，尚未获得 FDA 的批准，本章暂不讨论。

PD-1 通路的抑制剂大致可分为两类：PD-1 功能抑制剂和 PD-L1 功能抑制剂。纳武利尤单抗和帕博利珠单抗与 PD-1 竞争性结合，形成 PD-1：单克隆抗体复合物[38]。然而，这两种药物结合 PD-1 的部位略有不同。纳武利尤单抗在 2014 年被 FDA 批准用于治疗黑色素瘤，2015 年被批准用于治疗鳞状细胞肺癌和晚期肾细胞癌，2016 年被批准用于治疗非霍奇金淋巴瘤和经典霍奇金淋巴瘤，2018 年被批准与伊匹木单抗联合用于晚期肾细胞癌的治疗。2014 年帕博利珠单抗被 FDA 批准用于治疗黑色素瘤，2015 年被批准用于治疗转移性非小细胞肺癌，2016 年被批准用于治疗晚期头颈部癌症，2017 年被批准用于治疗错配修复缺陷或微卫星不稳定的实体肿瘤。

阿维鲁单抗和度伐鲁单抗与 PD-L1 竞争性结合的部位略微不同[39]。2017 年，阿维鲁单抗被 FDA 批准用于治疗尿路上皮细胞癌和 Merkel 细胞癌。2016 年，FDA 批准阿特珠单抗用于治疗尿路上皮细胞癌和非小细胞肺癌。度伐鲁单抗于 2017 年被 FDA 批准用于治疗转移性尿路上皮细胞癌，2018 年被批准用于治疗非小细胞肺癌。其他一些 PD-1 和 PD-L1 抑制剂正在开发中，但超出了本章的范围。

肺炎的临床表现和影像学表现

接下来，将讨论免疫检查点抑制剂（ICI）相关性肺炎的临床表现。肺炎是 ICI 治疗后出现的一种少见的免疫相关不良事件，通常表现为间质性肺疾病[40]。ICI 治疗后肺炎表现为四种类型：机化性肺炎（OP）、非特异性间质性肺炎（NSIP）、过敏性肺炎（HP）、弥漫性肺泡损伤（DAD）。本章中，将把 NSIP 和 HP 合并到一个类别中，因为两者在临床表现和治疗上有相似之处。表 6.1 总结了各种类型肺炎的临床特征、影像学特征和病理学特征，图 6.1 显示了胸部 CT 扫描的特征图像。关于各种间质性肺炎的临床特征和病理生理学的更详尽的讨论参见其他相关章节和文献[41,42]。

表 6.1　常见肺炎的临床、放射学和组织病理学特点

类型	临床特点	放射学特点	组织病理学特点	特点
隐源性机化性肺炎（COP）	通常 2 个月内出现干咳、呼吸困难、体重下降	肺外周通常可见斑片状实变或毛玻璃样模糊影，多发肺泡、单叶或浸润性模糊影	远端支气管和肺泡肉芽组织增生伴轻度至中度浆细胞和淋巴细胞浸润	无肺功能损害的轻度 COP，可自发缓解，但需要对呼吸道症状、影像学检查和（或）肺功能密切监测。进展性和（或）症状持续伴有肺功能下降者，开始应用泼尼松 0.5～1mg/（kg·d）或等量的其他激素 3～6 个月
非特异性间质性肺炎（NSIP）	数周至数月后出现干咳、呼吸困难。大多数患者可闻及双肺底湿啰音	肺底多可见网状纹理、牵拉性支气管扩张和毛玻璃样混浊	纤维化伴弥漫性炎性细胞浸润和肺泡壁的弥漫性增厚，但是无肺泡结构完整性的丧失	对轻微症状与肺功能无影响的患者，观察即可；中度症状或肺功能下降的患者，给予泼尼松 0.5～1mg/（kg·d）或等量的其他激素治疗 8～12 周；激素难治的疾病，静脉使用泼尼松或细胞毒性药物
弥漫性肺泡损伤（DAD）	数天至数周内迅速出现进展性呼吸困难和咳嗽	肺的病变区域广泛的气腔模糊影	肺泡增厚伴透明膜沉积和炎性细胞浸润	对呼吸衰竭患者的支持治疗及静脉使用大剂量糖皮质激素

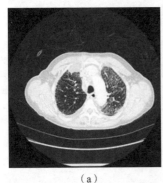 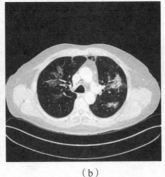 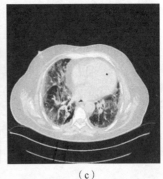

(a) (b) (c)

图 6.1　肿瘤患者接受免疫检查点抑制剂治疗后出现的肺部不良事件的典型图像
（a）非特异性间质性肺炎；（b）机化性肺炎；（c）弥漫性肺泡损伤

OP：是 ICI 治疗相关性肺炎的常见表现之一[43]。OP 主要影响远端细支气管、呼吸性细支气管、肺泡导管和肺泡壁[44]。OP 的症状可能包括低热、不适和咳嗽，症状通常是亚急性的[45-48]。呼吸道感染常与 OP 的发生和发展有关，但其机制尚不清楚[49]。OP 患者胸部 CT 主要表现为毛玻璃样或实变得模糊影，多见于肺周围胸膜下区域[50]，以反光晕征和毛玻璃样模糊影为特征，周围有较致密的浸润影，

但并非特征性[51]，影像学表现因病例而不同。OP 组织学特征为远端气道中肉芽组织栓的过度增殖（图 6.2），伴随淋巴细胞和浆细胞浸润[50]。这些栓子由松散的胶原、成纤维细胞和肌成纤维细胞组成。尽管支气管肺泡灌洗术（BAL）中发现的炎症性病变不足以诊断 OP[50]，仍推荐对疑似 OP 的患者进行 BAL 检查，用以排除感染。OP 的治疗取决于疾病的严重程度，建议使用不良事件的通用术语标准（CTCAE，表 6.2）来对肺炎的严重程度进行分级[52]。轻度（1 级）OP 可能会自行消退，但密切监测肺部情况是必要的[53]，2 级以上患者应给予皮质类固醇治疗。皮质类固醇在 OP 中疗效明显，治疗剂量通常从泼尼松 0.5～1mg/（kg·d）开始，治疗 3～6 个月。皮质类固醇治疗中断可能导致 OP 复发[54]。非皮质类固醇治疗，如环磷酰胺、环孢霉素、利妥昔单抗和大环内酯，在少部分类固醇难治性患者中偶有治疗成功的报道，但无广泛应用经验[55-58]。有报道称英夫利昔单抗对严重肺炎有效，需要在前瞻性研究中进一步验证[43]。通常情况下，建议至少暂时停止 ICI 治疗直至肺炎吸收。

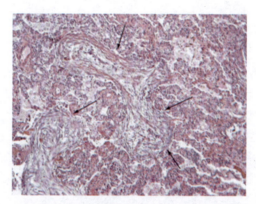

图 6.2　肺泡腔内的肉芽组织（箭头）

经允许引自 Clinical Respiratory Medicine. Cottin V.and Cordier J，2012，Elsevier Publishing

表 6.2　不良事件通用术语标准 5.0 肺炎的分级

分级	1 级	2 级	3 级	4 级	5 级
症状	无症状	有症状，工具性日常生活能力受限	严重症状，日常生活自理能力下降	威胁生命的呼吸衰竭	死亡
需要干预	仅需要临床或诊断性观察，无须干预	需要医学干预	需要医学干预和吸氧	需要紧急医学干预（如器官切开或插管）	

　　NSIP：是一种少见的间质性肺病，常与自身免疫性疾病或人类免疫缺陷病毒感染有关，NSIP 与 OP 均为 ICI 治疗相关性肺炎的常见表现[59]。NSIP 通常表现为咳嗽和呼吸困难等非特异性症状，尽管症状的持续时间可能因人而异。典型的 NSIP 胸部 CT 表现为毛玻璃模糊影、网状浸润和牵拉性支气管扩张[60-62]。肺部浸

润导致胸膜下分离的情况有助于区分 NSIP 与特发性肺纤维化[63]。ICI 治疗相关性 HP，以胸部 CT 呼气相空气滞留为特征[64]，与普通人群发生的 HP 不同，它与肺部暴露于雾化霉菌[65]或有毒化学物质[66]没有相关性。组织学上 NSIP 表现为致密纤维化，弥漫性炎性细胞浸润，肺泡壁均匀弥漫性增厚，与特发性肺纤维化不同，特发性肺纤维化的肺泡完整性并未丧失[67]，成纤维细胞灶可能存在，而在 NSIP 病例中这种表现较少见[68]。HP 的特征可能是少泡沫的非干酪性肉芽肿[64]。通常情况下，ICI 治疗后出现 NSIP 的患者需要进行 8～12 周的皮质类固醇治疗[泼尼松龙 0.5～1mg/（kg·d）或同等剂量]。类固醇难治性 NSIP 较 OP 更为常见，可能需要静脉注射皮质类固醇和（或）细胞毒性药物治疗[53]。对于 NSIP，常规推荐中断 ICI 治疗[69]。

DAD：是一种由弥漫肺泡损伤引起的严重肺炎；可导致严重的毛细血管渗漏和非心源性肺水肿[69,70]。临床表现与急性呼吸窘迫综合征相似，以呼吸急促、严重低氧血症和广泛的肺泡浸润为特征。通常，DAD 比 OP 和 NSIP 进展更快，症状在数天内迅速出现。DAD 的病理组织学表现为肺泡膜增厚、透明膜沉积、炎性细胞浸润（图 6.3）[71,72]。DAD 的急性期以炎症反应和肺泡结构水肿为特征，组织期以成纤维细胞胶原沉积为特征[73]。胸部 CT 图像显示广泛的空气征，这可能在病变累及区域更为明显[74-76]。其他类似药物相关性 DAD 的疾病应予以排除。肺部感染和嗜酸性肺炎可通过 BAL 排除，而充血性心力衰竭应通过彻底的临床检查、超声心动图和右心导管检查排除。支持性治疗包括无创或有创机械通气，通常是治疗 DAD 合并呼吸衰竭的必要措施，关于全身大剂量皮质类固醇应用方面的资料虽然非常有限，仍常规推荐尽早开始系统性使用大剂量皮质类固醇治疗，即使经过这些积极的治疗措施，死亡率仍然很高[77]。

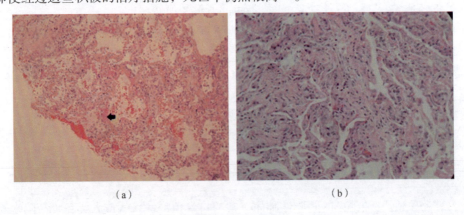

图 6.3 弥漫性肺泡损伤的病理学表现

（a）急性期的弥漫性肺泡损伤，表现为间质水肿、肺泡管上透明膜形成（箭头）（苏木精伊红染色，×100）；
（b）机化期的弥漫性肺泡损伤，表现为间质增厚、机化性结缔组织形成、典型的 2 型肺泡上皮细胞增生（苏木精伊红染色，×200）[73]

评估 ICI 相关性肺炎的方法

因为 ICI 相关性肺炎的症状可能是轻微的，可能被潜在的肿瘤相关症状所掩盖（如大块肺癌或广泛肺转移），因此，建议临床医生，对轻微 ICI 相关性肺炎，尽早进行全面的评估和治疗。患者出现呼吸困难、咳嗽、发热和胸痛等症状时，应考虑肺炎的可能[78,79]。我们推荐胸片和肺功能测试，胸片检查对肺炎的细微表现不够敏感，对于有症状的患者应推荐行胸部 CT 检查[80]。目前的胸部 CT 检查放射剂量较低，使得胸部 CT 成为评估肺炎进展或缓解的一种安全有效的方法[81]。评估时应进行肺功能检测，因为肺功能早期受损可能预示着肺炎的发生[82]。此外，对于肺炎确诊的患者，应连续监测肺功能，以评估肺炎的进展或缓解，疑似有 ICI 相关肺炎的患者，建议早期咨询肺部专家，尽早行支气管镜支气管肺泡灌洗术检查，以排除其他疾病如感染性肺炎，部分患者需要对病变累及的肺实质进行手术活检，以评估肺炎的组织病理学特征，一般不推荐经支气管活组织检查，因为对间质性肺病诊断的敏感度较低[83]。

ICI 相关性肺炎的发病率和临床特点

ICI 相关性肺炎的发生率因使用的药物不同而不同。在伊匹木单抗治疗的患者中，约 1% 的患者会发生肺炎，而 PD-1 和 PD-L1 抑制剂单药治疗的发生率为 3%~5%，与 CTLA-4 抑制剂联合治疗的发生率高达 10%[84-88]。通常情况下，肺炎的中位发病时间约为 3 个月[43,89-91]。ICI 治疗相关性肺炎通常表现为 OP 或 NSIP，偶可表现为暴发性 DAD。在本章中，我们将讨论每一种 FDA 批准的 ICI 治疗药物发生肺炎的发生率和表现形式。

CTLA-4 抑制剂

伊匹木单抗是在撰写本文时 FDA 批准的唯一一种 CTLA-4 抑制剂。使用伊匹木单抗治疗时肺炎发生率较低，所有级别的肺炎发生率共 1.3%，而高级别（3 级或 4 级）肺炎发生率为 0.3%[92]。据报道，从治疗开始到肺炎发作的中位时间约为 2.3 个月，最常见的肺炎类型为 OP[93]。虽然与 PD-1 或 PD-L1 抑制剂相比，免疫相关性不良事件在 CTLA-4 抑制剂更常见[94,95]，但肺炎并不常见，其机制尚不清楚[96]。接受伊匹木单抗治疗的患者中，黑色素瘤患者发生肺炎的比例约为肾细胞癌或小细胞肺癌患者的 1/3[96]，吸烟可能也是引起的肺部疾病的原因之一，这一点在其他 ILD 有所描述[97]。

PD-1 和 PD-L1 抑制剂

在本章中，将讨论 PD-1 抑制剂纳武利尤单抗和帕博利珠单抗，以及 PD-L1 抑制剂阿特珠单抗、阿维鲁单抗和度伐鲁单抗。在数种类型的癌症中，PD-1 抑制剂治疗后发生肺炎的频率是常规化疗方案的三倍[98]。最近对纳武利尤单抗和帕博利珠单抗临床试验的荟萃分析发现,抗 PD-1 治疗引起的肺炎总体发生率约为 3%，而高级别肺炎的发生率为 1.5%[98]。然而，在数个临床试验中，黑色素瘤人群肺炎的发病率在 0.5%左右[94]，非小细胞肺癌肺炎的发病率在 5%左右[99]。与伊匹木单抗相似，在吸烟导致的癌症患者中，PD-1 抑制剂治疗相关性肺炎的发病率更高一些。任何级别肺炎和高级别肺炎（CTCAE 标准为 3 级或更高）的发生率，在肾细胞癌患者中（分别是 4.4%和 1.7%）和非小细胞肺癌患者中（分别为 4.3%和 2.0%），均高于黑色素瘤患者（分别是 1.4%和 0.9%）[98]。同样，在 PD-1 抑制剂治疗后发生肺炎的病例对照研究中，吸烟状况与肺炎的患病风险无关，但慢性阻塞性肺部疾病（COPD）或肺部放疗史是肺炎的预测因子[100]。然而，PD-1 抑制剂的剂量对肺炎的发生率似乎没有任何影响，这表明 irAE 并没有以剂量依赖的方式与这些治疗直接相关[98]。这与我们的观察一致，即检查点抑制剂治疗相关性肺炎似乎是一个特殊的现象。PD-L1 抑制剂相关的肺炎发生率可能低于 PD-1 抑制剂，在非小细胞肺癌中，与 PD-L1 抑制剂相比，PD-1 抑制剂治疗的患者中所有级别和高级别肺炎的总发生率更高（PD-1 vs.PD-L1：所有级别为 3.6% vs.1.3%；高级别为 1.1% vs.0.4%）。

一个关键的补充说明是，由于这些临床试验多是单臂、开放性研究，结果可能容易产生偏差。事实上，在两个大型机构的临床试验中，PD-1 抑制剂和 PD-L1 抑制剂治疗的患者中,肺炎发生率在黑色素瘤患者和非小细胞肺癌患者中相似（分别是 5%和 4%）[86]，在该研究中，从治疗开始到肺炎发生的中位时间为 2.8 个月，这种方法已被批准用于新的癌症治疗，但仍需要进一步研究肺炎的发生率，在一个小的亚组群中，Naidoo 等[86]发现血液系统肿瘤患者肺炎发生率为 11%，明显高于黑色素瘤患者或非小细胞肺癌患者。

PD-1/PD-L1 抑制剂和 CTLA-4 抑制剂联合治疗

同时抑制 CTLA-4 通路和 PD-1 通路，有可能获得更强的免疫激活，增强抗癌效果[101]，却增加了免疫相关不良反应的发生风险，其中包括肺炎。与单药治疗相比，联合治疗时肺炎的发生率可能高达10%，且发病时间通常较早[86]。Naidoo等发现，接受ICI联合治疗的患者发生肺炎的平均时间为2.7个月，而接受ICI单药治疗的为4.6个月[86]。Wu等发现，联合ICI治疗的肺炎发生率约7%，高级别肺炎发生率约2%，与单药治疗的肺炎发生率相仿[98]，这表明，与单药治疗相比，ICI联合治疗引起任何级别和高级别肺炎的患病风险更高，发病时间更早。ICI疗法通常由于诱导免疫记忆而具有持久的疗效[102]，因此，先后使用PD-1/PD-L1抑制剂、CTLA-4抑制剂治疗导致肺炎的患病风险可能与同时使用ICI药物相同。Bowyer等对40名接受纳武利尤单抗或帕博利珠单抗联合伊匹木单抗治疗的患者进行了一项小型研究，发现8%的患者出现了严重的肺炎[103]。这一现象还需要在更大的研究队列中予以证实，但这表明，当依次进行ICI疗法时，肺炎的患病风险与联合治疗相似。

ICI 治疗相关性肺炎的放射学表现

ICI治疗相关性肺炎通常表现为NSIP或COP。在一项接受ICI单药治疗或联合治疗的915例患者的临床研究中发现，最常见的肺炎类型是NSIP（分别为18例和27例），其次是COP（分别为5例和27例）。也有研究表明，PD-1[43]抑制剂或CTLA-4抑制剂治疗后，COP更为常见[93]，DAD较少见。典型的DAD临床表现通常更为严重，但仍可通过早期免疫抑制治疗得以控制。

关于免疫相关性肺炎的其他表现在文献中也有所描述。1例接受纳武利尤单抗治疗的非小细胞肺癌患者，可见气道炎症伴毛细支气管炎[104]。有2例患者在开始纳武利尤单抗治疗8周内，出现了快速复发的胸腔积液和心包积液[105]。非小细胞肺癌患者的纳武利尤单抗治疗的临床试验早期，也发现胸腔积液的发生率增加。尽管这些积液归因于疾病进展而不是药物纳武利尤单抗治疗[106]，但与ICI相关的胸腔积液和心包积液仍可能是免疫相关不良事件的一种表现形式，也有可能是一种假性疾病进展。停用ICI药物和胸膜/心包引流术是主要的治疗方式，尽管类固醇激素在这种情况下的作用效果尚未明确，但对顽固性积液启动免疫抑制治疗也是合理的。

伊匹木单抗[93,107,108]和PD-1抑制剂[109,110]治疗时观察到有类肉瘤样反应。类肉瘤样反应是少见的免疫相关不良事件之一，其临床表现因人而异，可能为纵隔淋巴结病、肺浸润、皮疹或肾脏疾病。虽然这种表现类似于结节病，但其免疫反应过程与普通人群中的结节病并不完全一致[107,111]。抑制免疫检查点通路可能增加Th17细胞的数量，这些细胞可能参与了非ICI相关的结节病的发病过程[112,113]，因此，有理由认为，在使用ICI抑制剂治疗的患者中，可能发生类似于结节病样反应的生物学过程。类肉瘤样反应的治疗包括停止 ICI 治疗和全身使用类固醇激素，但还需要进一步明确 ICI 治疗相关的类肉瘤样反应的发病率。

盲区

ICI 相关性肺炎停药后再用药

免疫相关不良事件如肺炎等疾病的发生是否预示着更好的药物疗效，是 ICI 治疗的一个关键问题。研究发现，合并免疫相关不良事件的患者显示出更好的治疗效果[91,114]，反之亦然[115]，因此，在 ICI 相关性肺炎治愈后，再次使用 ICI 治疗也是有效的。有几项研究已经报道，在免疫相关性不良事件治愈后，恢复 ICI 治疗是安全的[116,117]。然而，再次接受免疫检查点抑制剂药物治疗时，患者的免疫相关性不良事件的总体发病率更高，约有一半患者出现各个级别的不良事件，此外，约 20%的患者出现了与初始治疗不同的不良事件[117]，换句话说，ICI 治疗后出现肺炎的患者，再次接受药物治疗后，可能会出现肺炎以外的其他不良事件。通常情况下，这些不良事件是可以用糖皮质激素治愈的，并不致命[91]，但也有罕见的死亡报告[117]。然而，ICI 在治疗导致免疫相关不良事件的高发病率与临床获益方面，风险利弊关系尚不清楚[35]。在 2 级和 3 级肺炎完全缓解后，评估 ICI 疗法的益处大于不良事件复发的前提下，可再次启动免疫治疗[118]，4 级肺炎患者不应再次启用 ICI 治疗，但还需要更多的研究来指导治疗。

明确肺炎患病的危险因素

如本章前面所述，某些患者可能是肺炎高风险人群，尤其是有吸烟史或辐射造成的肺损伤患者，ICI 相关性肺炎的患病风险更高。近些年来，影像学技术的进步使得胸部 CT 图像能够在像素水平上进行分析，以检测与疾病或健康相关的纹理特征[119]，类似的方法促使了放射学的发展。接受 ICI 治疗的患者治疗前胸部 CT 可预测肺炎的发病可能[120]，当然这需要进一步研究验证，但这强调了影像学作为疾病风险的生物学标志物的地位。

IL-17 是一种炎性细胞因子，在包括炎症性肠病在内的许多自身免疫性疾病中均表达上调[121]。血清 IL-17 水平升高可预测使用伊匹木单抗治疗黑色素瘤患者结肠炎的发病可能[122]。同样，与没有接受 ICI 治疗的白血病合并肺炎患者相比，在接受 ICI 治疗的白血病合并肺炎患者中，肺泡灌洗液中 Th1/Th17 细胞明显增多[123]。进一步研究血液和支气管肺泡灌洗液中的炎症指标，可以帮助预测 ICI

治疗后肺炎的发病可能。

结论

肺炎是一种少见但严重的发生在 PD-1 抑制剂、PD-L1 抑制剂和 CTLA-4 抑制剂治疗后的免疫相关不良事件，如果患者出现新的肺部症状，如咳嗽或呼吸短促，应尽早明确是否是免疫相关性肺炎。疑似肺炎患者的检查应包括肺功能测试、胸部 CT 和支气管镜 BAL 检查，以排除感染可能。使用皮质类固醇治疗通常是有效的，并能迅速缓解症状，然而，未进行治疗的肺炎可能是致命的。临床还需要进一步研究，来明确 ICI 治疗相关性肺炎的高发人群。

参考文献

1. Ahmad AS, Ormiston-Smith N, Sasieni PD. Trends in the lifetime risk of developing cancer in Great Britain: comparison of risk for those born from 1930 to 1960. Br J Cancer. 2015;112(5):943–7.
2. Miller KD, Siegel RL, Lin CC, Mariotto AB, Kramer JL, Rowland JH, et al. Cancer treatment and survivorship statistics, 2016. CA Cancer J Clin. 2016;66(4):271–89.
3. Baxevanis CN, Perez SA, Papamichail M. Cancer immunotherapy. Crit Rev Clin Lab Sci. 2009;46(4):167–89.
4. Farkona S, Diamandis EP, Blasutig IM. Cancer immunotherapy: the beginning of the end of cancer? BMC Med. 2016;14:73.
5. Dillman RO. Cancer immunotherapy. Cancer Biother Radiopharm. 2011;26(1):1–64.
6. Oiseth SJ, Aziz MS. Cancer immunotherapy: a brief review of the history, possibilities, and challenges ahead. J Cancer Metastasis Treat. 2017;3(10):250–61.
7. Finn OJ. Immuno-oncology: understanding the function and dysfunction of the immune system in cancer. Ann Oncol. 2012;23(Suppl 8):viii6–9.
8. Sharma P, Allison JP. Immune checkpoint targeting in cancer therapy: toward combination strategies with curative potential. Cell. 2015;161(2):205–14.
9. Barber DL, Wherry EJ, Masopust D, Zhu B, Allison JP, Sharpe AH, et al. Restoring function in exhausted CD8 T cells during chronic viral infection. Nature. 2006;439(7077):682–7.
10. Francisco LM, Sage PT, Sharpe AH. The PD-1 pathway in tolerance and autoimmunity. Immunol Rev. 2010;236:219–42.
11. Keir ME, Butte MJ, Freeman GJ, Sharpe AH. PD-1 and its ligands in tolerance and immunity. Annu Rev Immunol. 2008;26:677–704.
12. Fife BT, Pauken KE. The role of the PD-1 pathway in autoimmunity and peripheral tolerance. Ann N Y Acad Sci. 2011;1217:45–59.
13. Ishida Y, Agata Y, Shibahara K, Honjo T. Induced expression of PD-1, a novel member of the immunoglobulin gene superfamily, upon programmed cell death. EMBO J. 1992;11(11):3887–95.
14. Parry RV, Chemnitz JM, Frauwirth KA, Lanfranco AR, Braunstein I, Kobayashi SV, et al. CTLA-4 and PD-1 receptors inhibit T-cell activation by distinct mechanisms. Mol Cell Biol. 2005;25(21):9543–53.
15. Freeman GJ, Long AJ, Iwai Y, Bourque K, Chernova T, Nishimura H, et al. Engagement of the PD-1 immunoinhibitory receptor by a novel B7 family member leads to negative regula-

tion of lymphocyte activation. J Exp Med. 2000;192(7):1027–34.
16. Riley JL. PD-1 signaling in primary T cells. Immunol Rev. 2009;229(1):114–25.
17. Latchman Y, Wood CR, Chernova T, Chaudhary D, Borde M, Chernova I, et al. PD-L2 is a second ligand for PD-1 and inhibits T cell activation. Nat Immunol. 2001;2(3):261–8.
18. Francisco LM, Salinas VH, Brown KE, Vanguri VK, Freeman GJ, Kuchroo VK, et al. PD-L1 regulates the development, maintenance, and function of induced regulatory T cells. J Exp Med. 2009;206(13):3015–29.
19. Amarnath S, Mangus CW, Wang JC, Wei F, He A, Kapoor V, et al. The PDL1-PD1 axis converts human TH1 cells into regulatory T cells. Sci Transl Med. 2011;3(111):111ra20.
20. Wang X, Teng F, Kong L, Yu J. PD-L1 expression in human cancers and its association with clinical outcomes. Onco Targets Ther. 2016;9:5023–39.
21. Gordon SR, Maute RL, Dulken BW, Hutter G, George BM, McCracken MN, et al. PD-1 expression by tumour-associated macrophages inhibits phagocytosis and tumour immunity. Nature. 2017;545(7655):495–9.
22. Buchbinder EI, Desai A. CTLA-4 and PD-1 pathways: similarities, differences, and implications of their inhibition. Am J Clin Oncol. 2016;39(1):98–106.
23. Sharpe AH, Abbas AK. T-cell costimulation—biology, therapeutic potential, and challenges. N Engl J Med. 2006;355(10):973–5.
24. Egen JG, Kuhns MS, Allison JP. CTLA-4: new insights into its biological function and use in tumor immunotherapy. Nat Immunol. 2002;3(7):611–8.
25. Teft WA, Kirchhof MG, Madrenas J. A molecular perspective of CTLA-4 function. Annu Rev Immunol. 2006;24:65–97.
26. Krummel MF, Allison JP. CD28 and CTLA-4 have opposing effects on the response of T cells to stimulation. J Exp Med. 1995;182(2):459–65.
27. Walunas TL, Bakker CY, Bluestone JA. CTLA-4 ligation blocks CD28-dependent T cell activation. J Exp Med. 1996;183(6):2541–50.
28. Tivol EA, Borriello F, Schweitzer AN, Lynch WP, Bluestone JA, Sharpe AH. Loss of CTLA-4 leads to massive lymphoproliferation and fatal multiorgan tissue destruction, revealing a critical negative regulatory role of CTLA-4. Immunity. 1995;3(5):541–7.
29. Waterhouse P, Penninger JM, Timms E, Wakeham A, Shahinian A, Lee KP, et al. Lymphoproliferative disorders with early lethality in mice deficient in Ctla-4. Science. 1995;270(5238):985–8.
30. Walunas TL, Lenschow DJ, Bakker CY, Linsley PS, Freeman GJ, Green JM, et al. CTLA-4 can function as a negative regulator of T cell activation. Immunity. 1994;1(5):405–13.
31. Darrasse-Jèze G, Deroubaix S, Mouquet H, Victora GD, Eisenreich T, Yao K-H, et al. Feedback control of regulatory T cell homeostasis by dendritic cells in vivo. J Exp Med. 2009;206(9):1853.
32. Mandelbrot DA, McAdam AJ, Sharpe AH. B7-1 or B7-2 is required to produce the lymphoproliferative phenotype in mice lacking cytotoxic T lymphocyte-associated antigen 4 (CTLA-4). J Exp Med. 1999;189(2):435–40.
33. Piccirillo CA, Shevach EM. Naturally-occurring $CD4^+$ $CD25^+$ immunoregulatory T cells: central players in the arena of peripheral tolerance. Semin Immunol. 2004;16(2):81–8.
34. Syn NL, Teng MWL, Mok TSK, Soo RA. De-novo and acquired resistance to immune checkpoint targeting. Lancet Oncol. 2017;18(12):e731–e41.
35. Schadendorf D, Hodi FS, Robert C, Weber JS, Margolin K, Hamid O, et al. Pooled analysis of long-term survival data from phase II and phase III trials of ipilimumab in unresectable or metastatic melanoma. J Clin Oncol. 2015;33(17):1889–94.
36. Ramagopal UA, Liu W, Garrett-Thomson SC, Bonanno JB, Yan Q, Srinivasan M, et al. Structural basis for cancer immunotherapy by the first-in-class checkpoint inhibitor ipilimumab. Proc Natl Acad Sci U S A. 2017;114(21):E4223–E32.
37. Hodi FS, O'Day SJ, McDermott DF, Weber RW, Sosman JA, Haanen JB, et al. Improved survival with ipilimumab in patients with metastatic melanoma. N Engl J Med. 2010;363(8):711–23.
38. Tan S, Zhang H, Chai Y, Song H, Tong Z, Wang Q, et al. An unexpected N-terminal loop in PD-1 dominates binding by nivolumab. Nat Commun. 2017;8:14369.
39. Tan S, Chen D, Liu K, He M, Song H, Shi Y, et al. Crystal clear: visualizing the intervention

mechanism of the PD-1/PD-L1 interaction by two cancer therapeutic monoclonal antibodies. Protein Cell. 2016;7(12):866–77.
40. Antoniou KM, Margaritopoulos GA, Tomassetti S, Bonella F, Costabel U, Poletti V. Interstitial lung disease. Eur Respir Rev. 2014;23(131):40–54.
41. Lim G, Lee KH, Jeong SW, Uh S, Jin SY, Lee DH, et al. Clinical features of interstitial lung diseases. Korean J Intern Med. 1996;11(2):113–21.
42. Glasser SW, Hardie WD, Hagood JS. Pathogenesis of interstitial lung disease in children and adults. Pediatr Allergy Immunol Pulmonol. 2010;23(1):9–14.
43. Nishino M, Ramaiya NH, Awad MM, Sholl LM, Maattala JA, Taibi M, et al. PD-1 inhibitor-related pneumonitis in advanced Cancer patients: radiographic patterns and clinical course. Clin Cancer Res. 2016;22(24):6051–60.
44. Epler GR. Bronchiolitis obliterans organizing pneumonia: definition and clinical features. Chest. 1992;102(1 Suppl):2S–6S.
45. Epler GR, Colby TV, McLoud TC, Carrington CB, Gaensler EA. Bronchiolitis obliterans organizing pneumonia. N Engl J Med. 1985;312(3):152–8.
46. Cordier JF, Loire R, Brune J. Idiopathic bronchiolitis obliterans organizing pneumonia. Definition of characteristic clinical profiles in a series of 16 patients. Chest. 1989;96(5):999–1004.
47. Guerry-Force ML, Muller NL, Wright JL, Wiggs B, Coppin C, Pare PD, et al. A comparison of bronchiolitis obliterans with organizing pneumonia, usual interstitial pneumonia, and small airways disease. Am Rev Respir Dis. 1987;135(3):705–12.
48. King T Jr. Organizing pneumonia. In: Schwarz M, King T, editors. Interstitial lung disease. Shelton, CT: People's Medical Publishing House; 2011.
49. Cordier JF. Organising pneumonia. Thorax. 2000;55(4):318–28.
50. Cordier JF. Cryptogenic organising pneumonia. Eur Respir J. 2006;28(2):422–46.
51. Godoy MCB, Viswanathan C, Marchiori E, Truong MT, Benveniste MF, Rossi S, et al. The reversed halo sign: update and differential diagnosis. Br J Radiol. 2012;85(1017):1226–35.
52. Friedman CF, Proverbs-Singh TA, Postow MA. Treatment of the immune-related adverse effects of immune checkpoint inhibitors: a review. JAMA Oncol. 2016;2(10):1346–53.
53. Wells AU, Hirani N. Interstitial lung disease guideline. Thorax. 2008;63(Suppl 5):v1–v58.
54. Bradley B, Branley HM, Egan JJ, Greaves MS, Hansell DM, Harrison NK, et al. Interstitial lung disease guideline: the British Thoracic Society in collaboration with the Thoracic Society of Australia and New Zealand and the Irish Thoracic Society. Thorax. 2008;63(Suppl 5):v1–58.
55. Pathak V, Kuhn JM, Durham C, Funkhouser WK, Henke DC. Macrolide use leads to clinical and radiological improvement in patients with cryptogenic organizing pneumonia. Ann Am Thorac Soc. 2014;11(1):87–91.
56. Ding QL, Lv D, Wang BJ, Zhang QL, Yu YM, Sun SF, et al. Macrolide therapy in cryptogenic organizing pneumonia: a case report and literature review. Exp Ther Med. 2015;9(3):829–34.
57. Purcell IF, Bourke SJ, Marshall SM. Cyclophosphamide in severe steroid-resistant bronchiolitis obliterans organizing pneumonia. Respir Med. 1997;91(3):175–7.
58. Koinuma D, Miki M, Ebina M, Tahara M, Hagiwara K, Kondo T, et al. Successful treatment of a case with rapidly progressive Bronchiolitis obliterans organizing pneumonia (BOOP) using cyclosporin A and corticosteroid. Intern Med. 2002;41(1):26–9.
59. Romagnoli M, Nannini C, Piciucchi S, Girelli F, Gurioli C, Casoni G, et al. Idiopathic non-specific interstitial pneumonia: an interstitial lung disease associated with autoimmune disorders? Eur Respir J. 2011;38(2):384–91.
60. Park IN, Jegal Y, Kim DS, Do KH, Yoo B, Shim TS, et al. Clinical course and lung function change of idiopathic nonspecific interstitial pneumonia. Eur Respir J. 2009;33(1):68–76.
61. Silva CI, Muller NL, Lynch DA, Curran-Everett D, Brown KK, Lee KS, et al. Chronic hypersensitivity pneumonitis: differentiation from idiopathic pulmonary fibrosis and nonspecific interstitial pneumonia by using thin-section CT. Radiology. 2008;246(1):288–97.
62. Travis WD, Hunninghake G, King TE Jr, Lynch DA, Colby TV, Galvin JR, et al. Idiopathic nonspecific interstitial pneumonia: report of an American Thoracic Society project. Am J Respir Crit Care Med. 2008;177(12):1338–47.

63. Akira M, Inoue Y, Kitaichi M, Yamamoto S, Arai T, Toyokawa K. Usual interstitial pneumonia and nonspecific interstitial pneumonia with and without concurrent emphysema: thin-section CT findings. Radiology. 2009;251(1):271–9.
64. American Thoracic Society/European Respiratory Society International Multidisciplinary Consensus Classification of the Idiopathic Interstitial Pneumonias. This joint statement of the American Thoracic Society (ATS), and the European Respiratory Society (ERS) was adopted by the ATS board of directors, June 2001 and by the ERS Executive Committee, June 2001. Am J Respir Crit Care Med. 2002;165(2):277–304.
65. Malmberg P, Rask-Andersen A, Rosenhall L. Exposure to microorganisms associated with allergic alveolitis and febrile reactions to mold dust in farmers. Chest. 1993;103(4):1202–9.
66. Zeiss CR, Kanellakes TM, Bellone JD, Levitz D, Pruzansky JJ, Patterson R. Immunoglobulin E-mediated asthma and hypersensitivity pneumonitis with precipitating anti-hapten antibodies due to diphenylmethane diisocyanate (MDI) exposure. J Allergy Clin Immunol. 1980;65(5):347–52.
67. Hashisako M, Fukuoka J. Pathology of idiopathic interstitial pneumonias. Clin Med Insights Circ Respir Pulm Med. 2015;9(Suppl 1):123–33.
68. Flaherty KR, Martinez FJ, Travis W, Lynch JP 3rd. Nonspecific interstitial pneumonia (NSIP). Semin Respir Crit Care Med. 2001;22(4):423–34.
69. Schwaiblmair M. Drug induced interstitial lung disease. Open Respir Med J. 2012;6:63–74.
70. Kaarteenaho R, Kinnula VL. Diffuse alveolar damage: a common phenomenon in progressive interstitial lung disorders. Pulm Med. 2011;2011:1.
71. Matthay MA, Zemans RL. The acute respiratory distress syndrome: pathogenesis and treatment. Annu Rev Pathol. 2011;6:147–63.
72. Spira D, Wirths S, Skowronski F, Pintoffl J, Kaufmann S, Brodoefel H, et al. Diffuse alveolar hemorrhage in patients with hematological malignancies: HRCT patterns of pulmonary involvement and disease course. Clin Imaging. 2013;37(4):680–6.
73. Kao KC, Hu HC, Chang CH, Hung CY, Chiu LC, Li SH, et al. Diffuse alveolar damage associated mortality in selected acute respiratory distress syndrome patients with open lung biopsy. Crit Care. 2015;19:228.
74. Goodman LR. Congestive heart failure and adult respiratory distress syndrome. New insights using computed tomography. Radiol Clin N Am. 1996;34(1):33–46.
75. Gattinoni L, Presenti A, Torresin A, Baglioni S, Rivolta M, Rossi F, et al. Adult respiratory distress syndrome profiles by computed tomography. J Thorac Imaging. 1986;1(3):25–30.
76. Pelosi P, Crotti S, Brazzi L, Gattinoni L. Computed tomography in adult respiratory distress syndrome: what has it taught us? Eur Respir J. 1996;9(5):1055–62.
77. Rogers S. Spencer's pathology of the lung. Histopathology. 1999;34(5):470.
78. Naidoo J, Page DB, Li BT, Connell LC, Schindler K, Lacouture ME, et al. Toxicities of the anti-PD-1 and anti-PD-L1 immune checkpoint antibodies. Ann Oncol. 2015;26(12):2375–91.
79. Michot JM, Bigenwald C, Champiat S, Collins M, Carbonnel F, Postel-Vinay S, et al. Immune-related adverse events with immune checkpoint blockade: a comprehensive review. Eur J Cancer. 2016;54:139–48.
80. Claessens YE, Debray MP, Tubach F, Brun AL, Rammaert B, Hausfater P, et al. Early chest computed tomography scan to assist diagnosis and guide treatment decision for suspected community-acquired pneumonia. Am J Respir Crit Care Med. 2015;192(8):974–82.
81. Hammond E, Sloan C, Newell JD Jr, Sieren JP, Saylor M, Vidal C, et al. Comparison of low- and ultralow-dose computed tomography protocols for quantitative lung and airway assessment. Med Phys. 2017;44(9):4747–57.
82. Franzen D, Schad K, Kowalski B, Clarenbach CF, Stupp R, Dummer R, et al. Ipilimumab and early signs of pulmonary toxicity in patients with metastastic melanoma: a prospective observational study. Cancer Immunol Immunother. 2018;67(1):127–34.
83. Raghu G, Mageto YN, Lockhart D, Schmidt RA, Wood DE, Godwin JD. The accuracy of the clinical diagnosis of new-onset idiopathic pulmonary fibrosis and other interstitial lung disease: a prospective study. Chest. 1999;116(5):1168–74.
84. Nishino M, Giobbie-Hurder A, Hatabu H, Ramaiya NH, Hodi FS. Incidence of programmed cell death 1 inhibitor-related pneumonitis in patients with advanced cancer: a systematic review and meta-analysis. JAMA Oncol. 2016;2(12):1607–16.

85. Khunger M, Rakshit S, Pasupuleti V, Hernandez AV, Mazzone P, Stevenson J, et al. Incidence of pneumonitis with use of programmed death 1 and programmed death-ligand 1 inhibitors in non-small cell lung Cancer: a systematic review and meta-analysis of trials. Chest. 2017;152(2):271–81.
86. Naidoo J, Wang X, Woo KM, Iyriboz T, Halpenny D, Cunningham J, et al. Pneumonitis in patients treated with anti–programmed death-1/programmed death ligand 1 therapy. J Clin Oncol. 2017;35(7):709–17.
87. Robert C, Long GV, Brady B, Dutriaux C, Maio M, Mortier L, et al. Nivolumab in previously untreated melanoma without BRAF mutation. N Engl J Med. 2015;372(4):320–30.
88. Reck M, Rodríguez-Abreu D, Robinson AG, Hui R, Csőszi T, Fülöp A, et al. Pembrolizumab versus chemotherapy for PD-L1–positive non–small-cell lung Cancer. N Engl J Med. 2016;375(19):1823–33.
89. Nishino M, Hatabu H, Hodi FS, Ramaiya NH. Drug-related pneumonitis in the era of precision Cancer therapy. JCO Precision Oncol. 2017;1:1–12.
90. Shohdy KS, Abdel-Rahman O. Risk of pneumonitis with different immune checkpoint inhibitors in NSCLC. Ann Transl Med. 2017;5(17):365.
91. Fujii T, Colen RR, Bilen MA, Hess KR, Hajjar J, Suarez-Almazor ME, et al. Incidence of immune-related adverse events and its association with treatment outcomes: the MD Anderson Cancer Center experience. Investig New Drugs. 2018;36(4):638–46.
92. Kwon ED, Drake CG, Scher HI, Fizazi K, Bossi A, van den Eertwegh AJ, et al. Ipilimumab versus placebo after radiotherapy in patients with metastatic castration-resistant prostate cancer that had progressed after docetaxel chemotherapy (CA184-043): a multicentre, randomised, double-blind, phase 3 trial. Lancet Oncol. 2014;15(7):700–12.
93. Tirumani SH, Ramaiya NH, Keraliya A, Bailey ND, Ott PA, Hodi FS, et al. Radiographic profiling of immune-related adverse events in advanced melanoma patients treated with ipilimumab. Cancer Immunol Res. 2015;3(10):1185–92.
94. Robert C, Schachter J, Long GV, Arance A, Grob JJ, Mortier L, et al. Pembrolizumab versus Ipilimumab in advanced melanoma. N Engl J Med. 2015;372(26):2521–32.
95. Larkin J, Chiarion-Sileni V, Gonzalez R, Grob JJ, Cowey CL, Lao CD, et al. Combined nivolumab and ipilimumab or monotherapy in untreated melanoma. N Engl J Med. 2015;373(1):23–34.
96. Khoja L, Day D, Wei-Wu Chen T, Siu LL, Hansen AR. Tumour- and class-specific patterns of immune-related adverse events of immune checkpoint inhibitors: a systematic review. Ann Oncol. 2017;28(10):2377–85.
97. Ryu JH, Colby TV, Hartman TE, Vassallo R. Smoking-related interstitial lung diseases: a concise review. Eur Respir J. 2001;17(1):122–32.
98. Wu J, Hong D, Zhang X, Lu X, Miao J. PD-1 inhibitors increase the incidence and risk of pneumonitis in cancer patients in a dose-independent manner: a meta-analysis. Sci Rep. 2017;7:44173.
99. Herbst RS, Baas P, Kim DW, Felip E, Perez-Gracia JL, Han JY, et al. Pembrolizumab versus docetaxel for previously treated, PD-L1-positive, advanced non-small-cell lung cancer (KEYNOTE-010): a randomised controlled trial. Lancet. 2016;387(10027):1540–50.
100. Cui P, Liu Z, Wang G, Ma J, Qian Y, Zhang F, et al. Risk factors for pneumonitis in patients treated with anti-programmed death-1 therapy: a case-control study. Cancer Med. 2018;7:4115.
101. Wolchok JD, Chiarion-Sileni V, Gonzalez R, Rutkowski P, Grob JJ, Cowey CL, et al. Overall survival with combined nivolumab and ipilimumab in advanced melanoma. N Engl J Med. 2017;377(14):1345–56.
102. Ribas A, Shin DS, Zaretsky J, Frederiksen J, Cornish A, Avramis E, et al. PD-1 blockade expands intratumoral memory T cells. Cancer Immunol Res. 2016;4(3):194–203.
103. Bowyer S, Prithviraj P, Lorigan P, Larkin J, McArthur G, Atkinson V, et al. Efficacy and toxicity of treatment with the anti-CTLA-4 antibody ipilimumab in patients with metastatic melanoma after prior anti-PD-1 therapy. Br J Cancer. 2016;114(10):1084–9.
104. Balagani A, Arain M, Sheshadri A. Bronchiolitis obliterans after combination immunotherapy with pembrolizumab and ipilimumab. J Immunother Precision Oncol. 2018;1(1):49–52.

105. Kolla BC, Patel MR. Recurrent pleural effusions and cardiac tamponade as possible manifestations of pseudoprogression associated with nivolumab therapy—a report of two cases. J Immunother Cancer. 2016;4:80.
106. Borghaei H, Paz-Ares L, Horn L, Spigel DR, Steins M, Ready NE, et al. Nivolumab versus docetaxel in advanced nonsquamous non-small-cell lung cancer. N Engl J Med. 2015;373(17):1627–39.
107. Berthod G, Lazor R, Letovanec I, Romano E, Noirez L, Mazza Stalder J, et al. Pulmonary sarcoid-like granulomatosis induced by ipilimumab. J Clin Oncol. 2012;30(17):e156–9.
108. Bronstein Y, Ng CS, Hwu P, Hwu WJ. Radiologic manifestations of immune-related adverse events in patients with metastatic melanoma undergoing anti-CTLA-4 antibody therapy. AJR Am J Roentgenol. 2011;197(6):W992–w1000.
109. Reuss JE, Kunk PR, Stowman AM, Gru AA, Slingluff CL Jr, Gaughan EM. Sarcoidosis in the setting of combination ipilimumab and nivolumab immunotherapy: a case report & review of the literature. J Immunother Cancer. 2016;4:94.
110. Tetzlaff MT, Nelson KC, Diab A, Staerkel GA, Nagarajan P, Torres-Cabala CA, et al. Granulomatous/sarcoid-like lesions associated with checkpoint inhibitors: a marker of therapy response in a subset of melanoma patients. J Immunother Cancer. 2018;6(1):14.
111. Ramstein J, Broos CE, Simpson LJ, Ansel KM, Sun SA, Ho ME, et al. IFN-gamma-producing T-helper 17.1 cells are increased in sarcoidosis and are more prevalent than T-helper type 1 cells. Am J Respir Crit Care Med. 2016;193(11):1281–91.
112. Facco M, Cabrelle A, Teramo A, Olivieri V, Gnoato M, Teolato S, et al. Sarcoidosis is a Th1/Th17 multisystem disorder. Thorax. 2011;66(2):144–50.
113. von Euw E, Chodon T, Attar N, Jalil J, Koya RC, Comin-Anduix B, et al. CTLA4 blockade increases Th17 cells in patients with metastatic melanoma. J Transl Med. 2009;7:35.
114. Attia P, Phan GQ, Maker AV, Robinson MR, Quezado MM, Yang JC, et al. Autoimmunity correlates with tumor regression in patients with metastatic melanoma treated with anti-cytotoxic T-lymphocyte antigen-4. J Clin Oncol. 2005;23(25):6043–53.
115. Horvat TZ, Adel NG, Dang TO, Momtaz P, Postow MA, Callahan MK, et al. Immune-related adverse events, need for systemic immunosuppression, and effects on survival and time to treatment failure in patients with melanoma treated with ipilimumab at Memorial Sloan Kettering Cancer Center. J Clin Oncol. 2015;33(28):3193–8.
116. Santini FC, Rizvi H, Wilkins O, van Voorthuysen M, Panora E, Halpenny D, et al. Safety of retreatment with immunotherapy after immune-related toxicity in patients with lung cancers treated with anti-PD(L)-1 therapy. J Clin Oncol. 2017;35:9012.
117. Pollack MH, Betof A, Dearden H, Rapazzo K, Valentine I, Brohl AS, et al. Safety of resuming anti-PD-1 in patients with immune-related adverse events (irAEs) during combined anti-CTLA-4 and anti-PD1 in metastatic melanoma. Ann Oncol. 2018;29(1):250–5.
118. Puzanov I, Diab A, Abdallah K, Bingham CO 3rd, Brogdon C, Dadu R, et al. Managing toxicities associated with immune checkpoint inhibitors: consensus recommendations from the Society for Immunotherapy of Cancer (SITC) Toxicity Management Working Group. J Immunother Cancer. 2017;5(1):95.
119. Cunliffe A, Armato SG 3rd, Castillo R, Pham N, Guerrero T, Al-Hallaq HA. Lung texture in serial thoracic computed tomography scans: correlation of radiomics-based features with radiation therapy dose and radiation pneumonitis development. Int J Radiat Oncol Biol Phys. 2015;91(5):1048–56.
120. Colen RR, Fujii T, Bilen MA, Kotrotsou A, Abrol S, Hess KR, et al. Radiomics to predict immunotherapy-induced pneumonitis: proof of concept. Invest New Drugs. 2018;36(4):601–7.
121. Abraham C, Cho J. Interleukin-23/Th17 pathways and inflammatory bowel disease. Inflamm Bowel Dis. 2009;15(7):1090–100.
122. Tarhini AA, Zahoor H, Lin Y, Malhotra U, Sander C, Butterfield LH, et al. Baseline circulating IL-17 predicts toxicity while TGF-beta1 and IL-10 are prognostic of relapse in ipilimumab neoadjuvant therapy of melanoma. J Immunother Cancer. 2015;3:39.
123. Kim S, Shannon V, Sheshadri A, Kantarjian HM, Garcia-Manero G, Im J, et al. Th1/Th17 hybrid CD4+ cells in bronchial alveolar lavage fluid from leukemia patients with checkpoint inhibitor-induced pneumonitis. J Clin Oncol. 2017;36(5 suppl):204.

第7章

免疫检查点抑制剂诱发的结肠炎

Yun Tian，Hamzah Abu-Sbeih，Yinghong Wang

译者：乔　梦　宫晓梅

摘要　免疫检查点抑制剂（ICI）在癌症患者中效果明显，但会导致免疫相关的不良事件（irAE），也可累及胃肠道，表现为腹泻和结肠炎，从轻微的自限性腹泻至致死性结肠炎均可发生，这也使 ICI 药物不能在临床中广泛使用。ICI 相关性结肠炎的诊断主要基于临床表现、体格检查、大便测试、肠镜评估和（或）肠道显像。目前针对结肠炎的治疗策略主要是对轻微症状患者使用止泻剂治疗，对较严重的病例使用免疫抑制剂（如皮质类固醇、英夫利昔单抗或维多利单抗）治疗。

关键词　免疫检查点抑制剂　结肠炎　腹泻　糖皮质激素　英夫利昔单抗　类固醇　免疫治疗

ICI 诱发的结肠炎发病率

在接受抗 CTLA-4 药物治疗的患者中，有 25%～30%的患者出现了与炎症性肠病（IBD）相似的 ICI 诱发的结肠炎[1-3]。抗 PD-1 抗体产生的胃肠道（GI）不良事件发生率较低，约 10%[4]。然而，CTLA-4 与 PD-1 抑制剂联合治疗可升高胃肠道毒性，达 45%，远远高于单药治疗[5]。据报道，ICI 抑制剂治疗中，3 级或 4 级腹泻是最常见的严重不良事件，发生率为 10%[3,6]。

Y. Tian
Department of Oncology, Shanghai Dermatology Hospital, Tongji University, Shanghai, China
Tongji University Cancer Center, The Shanghai Tenth People's Hospital, Tongji University, Shanghai, China

H. Abu-Sbeih · Y. Wang (✉)
Department of Gastroenterology, Hepatology and Nutrition, Division of Internal Medicine, The University of Texas MD Anderson Cancer Center, Houston, TX, USA
e-mail: YWang59@mdanderson.org

© Springer Nature Switzerland AG 2018
A. Naing, J. Hajjar (eds.), *Immunotherapy*, Advances in Experimental Medicine and Biology 995, https://doi.org/10.1007/978-3-030-02505-2_7

ICI 诱发的结肠炎的临床表现

在 ICI 诱发的胃肠道毒性中,最常见的是水样腹泻,其次是腹痛、便血、恶心/呕吐和发热[1,2,7],也有患者表现为体重减轻[1],许多患者通常仅有非血性自限性腹泻而无其他相关症状[8,9],而严重的结肠炎可能导致结肠穿孔和死亡[10-12]。腹泻和结肠炎的严重程度根据不良事件的通用术语标准进行分级(4.03 版),CTCAE 分类标准详见表 7.1[13]。

表 7.1 不良事件通用术语标准腹泻和结肠炎的分级

不良事件	胃肠道功能紊乱 分级				
	1	2	3	4	5
腹泻	与基线相比,每天增加的大便次数少于 4 次,肠造瘘排泄物轻度增加	与基线相比,每天增加的大便次数 4~6 次,肠造瘘排泄物中度增加	与基线相比,每天增加的大便次数 ≥7 次,大便失禁,需要住院,肠造瘘排泄物明显增加,生活自理能力受限	威胁生命的后果,需要紧急医学干预	死亡
结肠炎	无症状,仅临床或诊断性观察即可,无须医学干预	腹痛,伴黏液或血便	严重腹痛,大便习性改变,需要医学干预,有腹膜炎征象	威胁生命的后果,需要紧急医学干预	死亡

腹泻一般发生在 ICI 治疗结束后 6~7 周[11,14],然而,也可以从第一次服药后迅速起病到最后一次服药后 4 个月,期间均有可能[7,15,16]。

评估 ICI 诱发的结肠炎的诊断学工具

ICI 治疗的患者发生急性腹泻时应首先明确是否由感染诱发[12],粪便测试需排除细菌、艰难梭菌、病毒、寄生虫或真菌感染,才能确诊为 ICI 相关性腹泻或结肠炎[17,18]。值得注意的是,在某些情况下,ICI 引起的结肠炎和胃肠道感染可能同时存在[19]。

目前,还没有可用的特定血清学或粪便标志物来确诊 ICI 诱发的结肠炎[20]。粪便钙保护素是一种广泛应用于炎症性肠病患者的炎症性标志物,它被报道可以作为 ICI 诱发性肠炎的诊断或预测工具[2]。然而,粪便钙保护素水平的升高与 ICI 诱发的结肠炎之间的关系还需要进一步验证[20]。

对于≥2级的腹泻和结肠炎患者,强烈建议采用内镜活检进一步评估ICI诱发的胃肠道毒性的严重程度[21,22]。内镜下常表现为红斑、水肿、糜烂、溃疡、渗出物、颗粒状、血管形态丧失和出血[23]。大约43%的患者会出现回肠和结肠炎症,而34%的患者仅限于左半结肠,其余肠段无异常表现[24]。病理可表现为环形弥漫浸润、斑片状、节段性、孤立性和局灶病变。对于肠镜检查正常的患者,需要常规活检来排除亚型结肠炎,这种亚型结肠炎类似于显微镜下结肠炎[7,25]。内镜下表现为明显结肠炎的患者仅占79%,仍有21%的患者内镜检查未见异常。

ICI相关性结肠炎的肠镜下表现可分为三类:急性炎症、慢性炎症和显微镜下炎症[22,25]。急性炎症以中性粒细胞和(或)嗜酸性粒细胞浸润、上皮细胞凋亡、隐窝炎和隐窝微脓肿为特征,23%的结肠炎患者有此表现。慢性炎症表现以隐窝结构变形、基底部淋巴细胞胞质增多、肉芽肿、盘状细胞化生为特征,60%的结肠炎有此表现。显微镜下结肠炎表现为上皮细胞浸润和(或)上皮下胶原带沉积,占结肠炎的8%。慢性炎症的组织学特征与克罗恩病和溃疡性结肠炎相似。此外,在结肠组织的组织病理学检查中应明确有无巨细胞病毒感染。

放射学尤其是CT,对于评估严重的ICI相关性肠炎的肠穿孔、肠梗阻和毒性巨结肠是非常重要的。结肠炎症在影像学上表现为弥漫性肠壁增厚、肠系膜血管充血、结肠周围脂肪淤滞、黏膜CT值增强等特征[2,26],腹腔内游离气体提示存在肠穿孔[27]。然而,如果以内镜作为诊断结肠炎的金标准,影像学诊断结肠炎的敏感度仅为50%[24]。对于某些高度怀疑毒性巨结肠或肠穿孔的患者,应进行腹部影像学检查,尽早为后续治疗提供依据。

ICI 相关性结肠炎的临床管理和预后

现阶段,对ICI诱发的腹泻和结肠炎的治疗仍取决于症状的严重程度[28]。对于1级腹泻患者,通常建议保守使用非处方药进行止泻治疗,适当口服补液、饮食调整和密切的随访监测,也有报道称,5-氨基水杨酸(5-ASA)可能对轻度腹泻有效[29]。通常情况下,ICI治疗可导致1级腹泻持续存在,如果保守治疗失败或症状进展到更高级别,则需要更积极的管理。

对于2级及以上的腹泻和结肠炎患者,强烈建议采用免疫治疗[30,31]。ICI诱发的高级别腹泻或结肠炎的主要治疗药物是免疫抑制剂,以减弱ICI的作用,从而抑制炎症反应。这些药物包括糖皮质激素和其他非甾体免疫抑制剂,如英夫利昔单抗和(或)vedolizumab [3,32,33]。据报道,用于治疗的糖皮质激素包括氢化可的松灌肠、口服布地奈德和全身使用糖皮质激素(静脉注射类固醇和口服泼尼松)。静脉注射糖皮质激素用于有严重症状需要住院治疗的患者,尤其是

3级及以上的患者，建议在4～6周内缓慢减量然后停用，以减少反弹现象。初始糖皮质激素治疗的标准剂量为1mg/（kg·d），但如果在2～3天内无效，则可增加到2mg/kg。使用类固醇灌肠和布地奈德口服仅在病例研究中有所报道[14,17,29,34]。对于糖皮质激素难治的病例，抗TNF药物如英夫利昔单抗和黏附分子阻滞剂如vedolizumab在病例研究中报道是成功的[3,32,35]。的确，早期使用英夫利昔单抗可缩短免疫抑制的时间，改善临床预后[32,33,36]。生物制剂治疗的禁忌证包括肠穿孔和感染，尤其是脓毒症[11]。英夫利昔单抗的治疗通常在1～3天可见疗效[7]，而一些患者可能需要多次治疗[29]。英夫利昔单抗治疗反应率高达83%～100%[2]。

在类固醇激素治疗后结肠炎症状缓解或改善到1级或以下时，可以考虑恢复免疫检查点抑制剂的治疗，尤其是非CTLA-4药物治疗[11]。初次发作后的胃肠道症状如果在成功治疗数月后复发，可能需要对相同的病因进行全面的评估[17]。

有病例研究报道，其他免疫抑制剂如他克莫司或霉酚酸酯也可用于治疗ICI诱发的结肠炎[33]。值得注意的是，对于高度怀疑肠穿孔或毒性巨结肠的患者，应停用类固醇激素，并进行外科会诊。有严重胃肠道并发症的患者如结肠穿孔，需进行结肠切除手术[33,37,38]。有病例报道不推荐使用非甾体抗炎药（NSAID），以防止胃肠道症状的进一步加重[1,39]。

结论

近年来，随着ICI药物的广泛应用，对ICI相关性结肠炎的认识不断提高，它与IBD有一些共同的特点，但比IBD的临床表现更为复杂，需要通过多种方式来进行诊断，以及对其严重程度进行全面评估。严重病例中早期使用免疫抑制剂，如糖皮质激素、英夫利昔单抗和（或）vedolizumab，可迅速改善症状。最终目标是使结肠炎处于长期缓解状态，而同时让ICI治疗效果好的患者继续接受ICI治疗，从而使患者获益最大化。当然还需要进一步研究以优化ICI相关性结肠炎的诊治。

声明

作者无相关利益。

参考文献

1. Marthey L, Mateus C, Mussini C, et al. Cancer immunotherapy with Anti-CTLA-4 monoclonal antibodies induces an inflammatory bowel disease. J Crohns Colitis. 2016;10:395–401.
2. Gupta A, De Felice KM, Loftus EV Jr, Khanna S. Systematic review: colitis associated with anti-CTLA-4 therapy. Aliment Pharmacol Ther. 2015;42:406–17.
3. Michot JM, Bigenwald C, Champiat S, et al. Immune-related adverse events with immune checkpoint blockade: a comprehensive review. Eur J Cancer. 2016;54:139–48.
4. Kumar V, Chaudhary N, Garg M, Floudas CS, Soni P, Chandra AB. Current diagnosis and management of immune related adverse events (irAEs) induced by immune checkpoint inhibitor therapy. Front Pharmacol. 2017;8:49.
5. Larkin J, Chiarion-Sileni V, Gonzalez R, et al. Combined nivolumab and ipilimumab or monotherapy in untreated melanoma. N Engl J Med. 2015;373:23–34.
6. Wang Y, Abu-Sbeih H, Mao E, Ali N, Ali FS, Qiao W, et al. Immune-checkpoint inhibitor-induced diarrhea and colitis in patients with advanced malignancies: retrospective review at MD Anderson. J Immunother Cancer. 2018;6(1):37.
7. Beck KE, Blansfield JA, Tran KQ, et al. Enterocolitis in patients with cancer after antibody blockade of cytotoxic T-lymphocyte-associated antigen 4. J Clin Oncol. 2006;24:2283–9.
8. Johnston RL, Lutzky J, Chodhry A, Barkin JS. Cytotoxic T-lymphocyte-associated antigen 4 antibody-induced colitis and its management with infliximab. Dig Dis Sci. 2009;54:2538–40.
9. de Guillebon E, Roussille P, Frouin E, Tougeron D. Anti program death-1/anti program death-ligand 1 in digestive cancers. World J Gastrointest Oncol. 2015;7:95–101.
10. Garon EB, Rizvi NA, Hui R, et al. Pembrolizumab for the treatment of non-small-cell lung cancer. N Engl J Med. 2015;372:2018–28.
11. Howell M, Lee R, Bowyer S, Fusi A, Lorigan P. Optimal management of immune-related toxicities associated with checkpoint inhibitors in lung cancer. Lung Cancer. 2015;88:117–23.
12. Ledezma B, Binder S, Hamid O. Atypical clinical response patterns to ipilimumab. Clin J Oncol Nurs. 2011;15:393–403.
13. Common terminology criteria for adverse events (CTCAE) version 4.0. US Department of Health and Human Services.
14. Weber JS, Kahler KC, Hauschild A. Management of immune-related adverse events and kinetics of response with ipilimumab. J Clin Oncol. 2012;30:2691–7.
15. Weber J. Review: anti-CTLA-4 antibody ipilimumab: case studies of clinical response and immune-related adverse events. Oncologist. 2007;12:864–72.
16. Lord JD, Hackman RC, Moklebust A, et al. Refractory colitis following anti-CTLA4 antibody therapy: analysis of mucosal FOXP3+ T cells. Dig Dis Sci. 2010;55:1396–405.
17. Pernot S, Ramtohul T, Taieb J. Checkpoint inhibitors and gastrointestinal immune-related adverse events. Curr Opin Oncol. 2016;28:264–8.
18. Eggermont AM, Chiarion-Sileni V, Grob JJ. Correction to Lancet Oncol 2015; 16: 522-30. Adjuvant ipilimumab versus placebo after complete resection of high-risk stage III melanoma (EORTC 18071): a randomised, double-blind, phase 3 trial. Lancet Oncol. 2015;16:e262.
19. McCutcheon JL, McClain CM, Puzanov I, Smith TA. Infectious colitis associated with ipilimumab therapy. Gastroenterol Res. 2014;7:28–31.
20. Berman D, Parker SM, Siegel J, et al. Blockade of cytotoxic T-lymphocyte antigen-4 by ipilimumab results in dysregulation of gastrointestinal immunity in patients with advanced melanoma. Cancer Immun. 2010;10:11.
21. Abu-Sbeih H, Ali FS, Luo W, Qiao W, Raju GS, Wang Y. Importance of endoscopic and histological evaluation in the management of immune checkpoint inhibitor-induced colitis. J Immunother Cancer. 2018;6(1):95.
22. Wang Y, Abu-Sbeih H, Mao E, Ali N, Qiao W, Trinh VA, et al. Endoscopic and histologic features of immune checkpoint inhibitor-related colitis. Inflamm Bowel Dis. 2018;24(8):1695–705.
23. Di Giacomo AM, Biagioli M, Maio M. The emerging toxicity profiles of anti-CTLA-4 anti-

bodies across clinical indications. Semin Oncol. 2010;37:499–507.
24. Wang Y, Abu-Sbeih H, Mao E, et al. Endoscopic and histologic features of immune checkpoint inhibitor-related colitis. Inflamm Bowel Dis. 2018;24(8):1695–705.
25. Choi K, Abu-Sbeih H, Samdani R, Nogueras Gonzalez G, Raju GS, Richards DM, et al. Can immune checkpoint inhibitors induce microscopic colitis or a brand new entity? Inflamm Bowel Dis. 2018.
26. Kim KW, Ramaiya NH, Krajewski KM, et al. Ipilimumab-associated colitis: CT findings. Am J Roentgenol. 2013;200:W468–74.
27. Mitchell KA, Kluger H, Sznol M, Hartman DJ. Ipilimumab-induced perforating colitis. J Clin Gastroenterol. 2013;47:781–5.
28. Singal AK, Jampana SC, Singal V, Kuo YF. Hepatocellular carcinoma predicts in-hospital mortality from acute variceal hemorrhage among patients with cirrhosis. J Clin Gastroenterol. 2012;46:613–9.
29. Tarhini A, Lo E, Minor DR. Releasing the brake on the immune system: ipilimumab in melanoma and other tumors. Cancer Biother Radiopharm. 2010;25:601–13.
30. Puzanov I, Diab A, Abdallah K, et al. Managing toxicities associated with immune checkpoint inhibitors: consensus recommendations from the Society for Immunotherapy of Cancer (SITC) Toxicity Management Working Group. J Immunother Cancer. 2017;5:95.
31. Hwang JH, Shergill AK, Acosta RD, et al. The role of endoscopy in the management of variceal hemorrhage. Gastrointest Endosc. 2014;80:221–7.
32. Dadu R, Zobniw C, Diab A. Managing adverse events with immune checkpoint agents. Cancer J. 2016;22:121–9.
33. Spain L, Diem S, Larkin J. Management of toxicities of immune checkpoint inhibitors. Cancer Treat Rev. 2016;44:51–60.
34. Collins M, Michot JM, Danlos FX, et al. Inflammatory gastrointestinal diseases associated with PD-1 blockade antibodies. Ann Oncol. 2017;28:2860–5.
35. Minor DR, Chin K, Kashani-Sabet M. Infliximab in the treatment of anti-CTLA4 antibody (ipilimumab) induced immune-related colitis. Cancer Biother Radiopharm. 2009;24:321–5.
36. Johnson DH, Zobniw CM, Trinh VA, Ma J, Bassett RL Jr, Abdel-Wahab N, et al. Infliximab associated with faster symptom resolution compared with corticosteroids alone for the management of immune-related enterocolitis. J Immunother Cancer. 2018;6(1):103.
37. Yang JC, Hughes M, Kammula U, et al. Ipilimumab (anti-CTLA4 antibody) causes regression of metastatic renal cell cancer associated with enteritis and hypophysitis. J Immunother. 2007;30:825–30.
38. Burdine L, Lai K, Laryea JA. Ipilimumab-induced colonic perforation. J Surg Case Rep. 2014;2014:rju010.
39. Ananthakrishnan AN, Higuchi LM, Huang ES, et al. Aspirin, nonsteroidal anti-inflammatory drug use, and risk for Crohn disease and ulcerative colitis: a cohort study. Ann Intern Med. 2012;156:350–9.

第 8 章

免疫检查点抑制剂诱发的肝炎

Yun Tian，Hamzah Abu-Sbeih，Yinghong Wang

译者：石　琴　苏春霞

摘要　免疫检查点抑制剂（ICI）、CTLA-4 抑制剂（如伊匹木单抗）、PD-1 和 PD-L1 抑制剂（如纳武利尤单抗和帕博利珠单抗），在过去的十年中被越来越多地用于治疗多种癌症。ICI 相关性肝毒性并不少见。在 ICI 治疗后 8～12 周，可出现天冬氨酸转氨酶（AST）和丙氨酸转氨酶（ALT）升高。由 ICI 诱发的肝炎通常无症状，但也有出现发热、不适甚至死亡的报道。ICI 相关性肝毒性是根据病史、实验室检查、影像学和组织学检测排除其他病因后的排他性诊断。ICI 诱发的肝炎可能需要停用 ICI 药物和（或）免疫抑制剂治疗。

关键词　免疫检查点抑制剂　肝炎　抗 CTLA-4　抗 PD-1/抗 PD-L1　糖皮质激素　转氨酶升高　肝损伤

ICI 诱发的肝炎的发病率

免疫检查点抑制剂（ICI）诱发的肝损伤发生率为 5%～30%[1,2]，与抗 PD-1/PD-L1 治疗的患者相比，抗 CTL-4 治疗的患者肝毒性风险较高，可高达 15%[3,4]，而抗 PD-1/PD-L1 药物相关的肝损伤发生率为 5%～10%，然而，接受抗 CTLA-4 与抗 PD-1/PD-L1 联合治疗的患者，肝毒性高达 30%[3-5]。

Y. Tian
Department of Oncology, Shanghai Dermatology Hospital, Tongji University, Shanghai, China
Tongji University Cancer Center, The Shanghai Tenth People's Hospital, Tongji University, Shanghai, China
H. Abu-Sbeih · Y. Wang (✉)
Department of Gastroenterology, Hepatology and Nutrition, Division of Internal Medicine, The University of Texas MD Anderson Cancer Center, Houston, TX, USA
e-mail: YWang59@mdanderson.org

© Springer Nature Switzerland AG 2018
A. Naing, J. Hajjar (eds.), *Immunotherapy*, Advances in Experimental Medicine and Biology 995, https://doi.org/10.1007/978-3-030-02505-2_8

ICI 最常见的肝细胞损伤病理表现为全小叶性肝炎[5-12]。据报道,接受 ICI 单药治疗的患者出现 3 级或 4 级肝炎占 1%～3%,接受抗 PD-1 和抗 CTLA-4 联合治疗的患者出现 3 级或 4 级肝炎占 8%～14%[5,7-10,13-16]。

ICI 诱发的肝炎的临床表现

ICI 诱发的肝炎是通过免疫介导的,表现为肝细胞破坏或胆汁淤积[14,17-19]。ICI 诱发的肝炎表现为高度异质性,从完全无症状的氨基转移酶轻度升高到致死性的肝衰竭均有报道[6,20,21]。部分 ICI 诱发的肝炎患者可表现为发热、不适、黄疸、大便颜色改变等[17,22]。所有 ICI 药物均可导致天冬氨酸转移酶(AST)、丙氨酸转氨酶(ALT)和胆红素水平的升高[13,17,20,23]。

ICI 诱发的肝炎可在任何时刻发生,但大多数在 ICI 治疗开始后 8～12 周出现[16,20,24],迟发性肝炎通常病情较轻[14,25]。值得注意的是,尽管患者能耐受 ICI 长期治疗,仍有可能部分患者出现暴发性重症肝炎[26]。

评估 ICI 诱发的肝炎的诊断工具

肝炎、肝衰竭生化指标的 CTCAE 分级系统见表 8.1[27]。

表 8.1 肝胆疾病

不良事件	等级				
	1	2	3	4	5
肝炎					
1. ALT 和 AST	(1～3)×ULN	(3～5)×ULN	(5～20)×ULN	>20×ULN	-
2. 总胆红素	(1～1.5)×ULN	(1.5～3)×ULN	(3～10)×ULN	>10×ULN	
肝衰竭	-	-	震颤;轻度脑病;自理性日常生活活动受限(ADL)	中度至重度脑病;昏迷;危及生命	死亡

疑似 ICI 诱发的肝炎,除了密切监测肝功能外,还需通过实验室和影像学检查排除其他可能诱发肝损伤的原因,如药物、自身免疫病、病毒感染或酒精性肝损伤[13,28]。对标准免疫抑制治疗失败的 ICI 肝炎,肝脏活检是必要的[29]。

生物化学检查可以帮助排除病毒性肝炎或其他自身免疫性肝病。对 ICI 诱发的肝炎,CT、MRI 和超声(US)的成像结果通常呈非特异性表现[30],但是,这些检测对其他导致肝酶异常的原因,如肝转移、血栓栓塞事件等,都具有一定的价值[17,31]。ICI 诱发的重型肝炎，在 CT 和 MRI 上的影像学特征包括门静脉周围水肿、肝大、门静脉周围 MRI T_2 强化、肝实质密度弱化、门静脉周围淋巴结肿大[17,25,32]。轻度肝炎在影像学上无异常表现[17,33]。有报道称，ICI 相关性肝炎在治疗后，影像学上可见的肝大和门静脉周围淋巴结肿大得以改善[17]。

ICI 诱发性肝炎的组织学检查呈非特异性表现，表现为小叶性肝炎和胆管损伤，包括纤维蛋白环样肉芽肿[34]、中央静脉内皮炎[20,35]、明显的窦性淋巴组织细胞浸润、中央静脉内皮炎[20]在内的小叶性肝炎和胆管损伤[22]。抗 PD-1/PD-L1 药物诱发的肝炎组织学表现与抗 CTLA-4 药有所不同。PD-1/PD-L1 抗体诱发的肝炎可导致小叶性非肉芽肿性肝炎[16]，而 CTLA4 抗体诱发的肝炎可导致肉芽肿性肝炎伴有纤维蛋白沉积[16]。此外，与自身免疫性肝炎和药物性肝损伤相比，ICI 诱发的肝炎中，$CD3^+$ 和 $CD8^+$ 淋巴细胞较多，$CD20^+B$ 淋巴细胞和 $CD4^+T$ 淋巴细胞较少[35]。

ICI 相关性肝炎的管理和预后

对于轻微病例，如 1 级肝炎，建议进行严密的实验室监测[36]，ICI 可以继续使用；对于 2 级及以上肝炎，在排除其他病因后，可予免疫抑制剂如糖皮质激素治疗，并停用 ICI。糖皮质激素的剂量为 0.5~2mg/（kg·d），建议治疗 4 周以上，并逐渐减量[11,13]。当糖皮质激素剂量逐渐减少到 10mg/d 时（毒性等级≤1），可以恢复 ICI 治疗。对于 3 级和 4 级肝炎，建议永久停止 ICI，并予糖皮质激素治疗[36]。通常情况下，糖皮质激素可使大多数患者肝酶恢复正常或部分改善[20,26,35]。一些患者可能需要多个周期的糖皮质激素治疗[17]。糖皮质激素治疗的平均周期约为 8 周[37]。在临床实践中，停用 ICI 后而不使用糖皮质激素情况下，也有少部分患者肝功能指标可自行改善[16]。

在一些病例研究中发现，对于高剂量糖皮质激素无效的 ICI 相关性肝炎患者，可能需要霉酚酸酯来治疗[6,21]。由于英夫利昔单抗有潜在的肝毒性作用（非常罕见），因此不推荐用于治疗 ICI 诱发的肝炎[22,24]。也有报道显示，抗胸腺细胞球蛋白治疗为糖皮质激素不耐受情况下的另一种替代治疗方法[21]。

对于 ICI 诱发的肝炎，氨基转移酶下降至 1 级或以下，可恢复 ICI 治疗。如果是持续性 3 级或 4 级肝炎，肝损伤的恢复可能需要 1 个月以上的时间，这可能导致 ICI 永久停药。部分患者即使在糖皮质激素治疗使肝炎达到临床缓解后，仍可能出现 AST 和 ALT 再次反弹，因此应严密监测肝功能[20]。

结论

近年来,由于 ICI 的广泛应用,文献报道 ICI 诱发的肝炎发病率也明显上升。ICI 相关性肝炎通常发生在 ICI 治疗开始后 8~12 周,通常无症状,与病毒性肝炎有一些共同特征,表现为 AST、ALT 和总胆红素水平升高,但也可能伴有发热、不适,甚至在极少数病例中导致死亡。通常情况下,在排除其他导致肝炎的病因后,才能诊断为 ICI 相关性肝炎。对于 ICI 诱发的肝炎的治疗,停用 ICI 和早期使用免疫抑制剂如糖皮质激素,可迅速改善重型肝炎。最终的目标是维持正常的肝功能,同时继续 ICI 治疗,以使 ICI 治疗效果明显的患者获得最大限度的效益,但还需要进一步研究对 ICI 相关性肝炎的管理。

声明

作者无相关利益。

参考文献

1. Foller S, Oppel-Heuchel H, Fetter I, Winkler Y, Grimm MO. [Adverse events of immune checkpoint inhibitors]. Der Urologe Ausg A. 2017;56:486–91.
2. Ali AK, Watson DE. Pharmacovigilance assessment of immune-mediated reactions reported for checkpoint inhibitor cancer immunotherapies. Pharmacotherapy. 2017;37:1383–90.
3. Topalian SL, Sznol M, McDermott DF, et al. Survival, durable tumor remission, and long-term safety in patients with advanced melanoma receiving nivolumab. J Clin Oncol. 2014;32:1020–30.
4. Bernardo SG, Moskalenko M, Pan M, et al. Elevated rates of transaminitis during ipilimumab therapy for metastatic melanoma. Melanoma Res. 2013;23:47–54.
5. Larkin J, Chiarion-Sileni V, Gonzalez R, et al. Combined Nivolumab and Ipilimumab or monotherapy in untreated melanoma. N Engl J Med. 2015;373:23–34.
6. O'Day SJ, Maio M, Chiarion-Sileni V, et al. Efficacy and safety of ipilimumab monotherapy in patients with pretreated advanced melanoma: a multicenter single-arm phase II study. Ann Oncol. 2010;21:1712–7.
7. Schachter J, Ribas A, Long GV, et al. Pembrolizumab versus ipilimumab for advanced melanoma: final overall survival results of a multicentre, randomised, open-label phase 3 study (KEYNOTE-006). Lancet. 2017;390:1853–62.
8. Robert C, Long GV, Brady B, et al. Nivolumab in previously untreated melanoma without BRAF mutation. N Engl J Med. 2015;372:320–30.
9. Weber JS, D'Angelo SP, Minor D, et al. Nivolumab versus chemotherapy in patients with advanced melanoma who progressed after anti-CTLA-4 treatment (CheckMate 037): a randomised, controlled, open-label, phase 3 trial. Lancet Oncol. 2015;16:375–84.
10. Garon EB, Rizvi NA, Hui R, et al. Pembrolizumab for the treatment of non-small-cell lung cancer. N Engl J Med. 2015;372:2018–28.

11. Hofmann L, Forschner A, Loquai C, et al. Cutaneous, gastrointestinal, hepatic, endocrine, and renal side-effects of anti-PD-1 therapy. Eur J Cancer. 2016;60:190–209.
12. van den Eertwegh AJ, Versluis J, van den Berg HP, et al. Combined immunotherapy with granulocyte-macrophage colony-stimulating factor-transduced allogeneic prostate cancer cells and ipilimumab in patients with metastatic castration-resistant prostate cancer: a phase 1 dose-escalation trial. Lancet Oncol. 2012;13:509–17.
13. Spain L, Diem S, Larkin J. Management of toxicities of immune checkpoint inhibitors. Cancer Treat Rev. 2016;44:51–60.
14. Boutros C, Tarhini A, Routier E, et al. Safety profiles of anti-CTLA-4 and anti-PD-1 antibodies alone and in combination. Nat Rev Clin Oncol. 2016;13:473–86.
15. Sznol M, Ferrucci PF, Hogg D, et al. Pooled analysis safety profile of nivolumab and ipilimumab combination therapy in patients with advanced melanoma. J Clin Oncol. 2017;35:3815–22.
16. De Martin E, Michot JM, Papouin B, et al. Liver injury from cancer immunotherapy using monoclonal immune checkpoint inhibitors. J Hepatol. 2018 Oct 5. pii: S0168-8278(18)32379-1. doi: 10.1016/j.jhep.2018.09.006. PMID: 30297274.
17. Kim KW, Ramaiya NH, Krajewski KM, et al. Ipilimumab associated hepatitis: imaging and clinicopathologic findings. Investig New Drugs. 2013;31:1071–7.
18. Weber JS, Kahler KC, Hauschild A. Management of immune-related adverse events and kinetics of response with ipilimumab. J Clin Oncol. 2012;30:2691–7.
19. Kwak JJ, Tirumani SH, Van den Abbeele AD, Koo PJ, Jacene HA. Cancer immunotherapy: imaging assessment of novel treatment response patterns and immune-related adverse events. Radiographics. 2015;35:424–37.
20. Johncilla M, Misdraji J, Pratt DS, et al. Ipilimumab-associated hepatitis: clinicopathologic characterization in a series of 11 cases. Am J Surg Pathol. 2015;39:1075–84.
21. Chmiel KD, Suan D, Liddle C, et al. Resolution of severe ipilimumab-induced hepatitis after antithymocyte globulin therapy. J Clin Oncol. 2011;29:e237–40.
22. Cramer P, Bresalier RS. Gastrointestinal and hepatic complications of immune checkpoint inhibitors. Curr Gastroenterol Rep. 2017;19:3.
23. Michot JM, Bigenwald C, Champiat S, et al. Immune-related adverse events with immune checkpoint blockade: a comprehensive review. Eur J Cancer. 2016;54:139–48.
24. Friedman CF, Proverbs-Singh TA, Postow MA. Treatment of the immune-related adverse effects of immune checkpoint inhibitors: a review. JAMA Oncol. 2016;2:1346–53.
25. Tirumani SH, Ramaiya NH, Keraliya A, et al. Radiographic profiling of immune-related adverse events in advanced melanoma patients treated with ipilimumab. Cancer Immunol Res. 2015;3:1185–92.
26. Imafuku K, Yoshino K, Yamaguchi K, Tsuboi S, Ohara K, Hata H. Successful treatment of sudden hepatitis induced by long-term nivolumab administration. Case Rep Oncol. 2017;10:368–71.
27. Common Terminology Criteria for Adverse Events (CTCAE) version 4.0. US Department of Health and Human Services. 2009 .
28. Suzuki A, Brunt EM, Kleiner DE, et al. The use of liver biopsy evaluation in discrimination of idiopathic autoimmune hepatitis versus drug-induced liver injury. Hepatology. 2011;54:931–9.
29. Kleiner DE, Berman D. Pathologic changes in ipilimumab-related hepatitis in patients with metastatic melanoma. Dig Dis Sci. 2012;57:2233–40.
30. Mortele KJ, Segatto E, Ros PR. The infected liver: radiologic-pathologic correlation. Radiographics. 2004;24:937–55.
31. Widmann G, Nguyen VA, Plaickner J, Jaschke W. Imaging features of toxicities by immune checkpoint inhibitors in cancer therapy. Curr Radiol Rep. 2016;5:59.
32. Kumar V, Chaudhary N, Garg M, Floudas CS, Soni P, Chandra AB. Current diagnosis and management of immune related adverse events (irAEs) induced by immune checkpoint inhibitor therapy. Front Pharmacol. 2017;8:49.
33. Alessandrino F, Tirumani SH, Krajewski KM, et al. Imaging of hepatic toxicity of systemic therapy in a tertiary cancer centre: chemotherapy, haematopoietic stem cell transplantation, molecular targeted therapies, and immune checkpoint inhibitors. Clin Radiol. 2017;72:521–33.
34. Everett J, Srivastava A, Misdraji J. Fibrin ring granulomas in checkpoint inhibitor-induced

hepatitis. Am J Surg Pathol. 2017;41:134–7.
35. Zen Y, Yeh MM. Hepatotoxicity of immune checkpoint inhibitors: a histology study of seven cases in comparison with autoimmune hepatitis and idiosyncratic drug-induced liver injury. Mod Pathol. 2018;31:965–73.
36. Puzanov I, Diab A, Abdallah K, et al. Managing toxicities associated with immune checkpoint inhibitors: consensus recommendations from the Society for Immunotherapy of Cancer (SITC) Toxicity Management Working Group. J Immunother Cancer. 2017;5:95.
37. Postow MA, Chesney J, Pavlick AC, et al. Nivolumab and ipilimumab versus ipilimumab in untreated melanoma. N Engl J Med. 2015;372:2006–17.

第 9 章

患者报告的症状结局

Tito R. Mendoza

译者：程 超 李雪飞 苏春霞

摘要 抗肿瘤治疗具有毒性，新一代的抗肿瘤治疗，如免疫治疗产生的不良反应与传统治疗（如化疗）不同，被统称为免疫相关不良反应（immune-related adverse event，irAE）。这些 irAE 由医生评估，并通过美国国立卫生研究院（NIH）的 CTCAE 不良反应报告系统汇报。而实际上，这些治疗相关的症状及疾病的严重程度由患者自己来描述才是最准确的。虽然很多免疫治疗药物的重要研究都包含了健康相关的生活质量指标，但患者症状评估才更接近药物疗效和肿瘤负荷。本章阐述了如何更好地描述症状，合适的症状评估工具具备的特点，综述了目前可用的症状评估工具，并提供解读患者汇报结果（PRO）系统数据的方法，也会详细阐述将 PRO 整合进入肿瘤患者评估的可行性和获益，并描述目前免疫治疗中 PRO 的应用，指出哪些地方需要将来进一步的研究，以加强 PRO 在接受免疫治疗的肿瘤患者中的应用。

关键词 患者汇报结果 症状 免疫治疗 癌症

引言

癌症是一种可能伴有多种症状的疾病，这些症状显著影响患者的生活质量和活动能力。新的癌症治疗方法，如免疫治疗，通过重新激活原本被抑制的免疫系统而革新性地改变了癌症的治疗，但也会进一步加重癌症相关的症状。因为这种治疗重新打破了免疫平衡，从而引起了一系列独特的不良反应，称为免疫相关不良反应（immune-related adverse event，irAE）。这些 irAE 通常是由临床医生来评

T. R. Mendoza (✉)
Department of Symptom Research, The University of Texas MD Anderson Cancer Center, Houston, TX, USA
e-mail: tmendoza@mdanderson.org

© Springer Nature Switzerland AG 2018
A. Naing, J. Hajjar (eds.), *Immunotherapy*, Advances in Experimental Medicine and Biology 995, https://doi.org/10.1007/978-3-030-02505-2_9

估，可能与患者原本对自己症状的描述并不完全一致。为了更准确地量化这些症状，我们必须使用患者汇报结果系统（PRO）。

症状与健康相关生活质量（HRQOL）一样，属于 PRO，因为患者自己是最好的信息来源。然而与 HRQOL 不同的是，症状与治疗疗效和疾病本身关系更接近。"健康相关生活质量"这一概念的范围较"症状"更加宽泛。

本章阐述了如何使用 PRO 最好地量化症状，讨论心理躯体症状评估工具应具备的特点，综述目前的症状评估工具，为解读 PRO 数据提供方法，描述在几种不同癌症人群中使用 PRO 系统的可行性和获益，以及目前免疫治疗中 PRO 的应用，并指出哪些地方需要将来进一步的研究，以加强 PRO 在接受免疫治疗的肿瘤患者中的应用。

症状评估的重要性

如果患者不能耐受治疗相关的症状，通常也不能接受完整和有效的治疗疗程，而治疗相关的遗留症状也会影响缓解期患者的生活质量。大多数针对症状的干预手段都旨在减轻相关症状的严重程度和对患者的影响。因为在患者面临治疗选择的时候，多种治疗的抗肿瘤疗效类似，因此这些不同治疗引起的患者症状成了个体化治疗中治疗方法选择和新疗法开发的主要决定因素。因此，在评估各种不同的抗肿瘤疗法时，比较这些疗法所产生的治疗相关症状就显得尤为重要。患者的生活质量也与治疗相关症状的程度和强度相关，以上这些都需要准确的症状评估体系。

症状和患者报告结果

症状报告是患者对其受疾病或疾病相关治疗影响而产生的、干扰自身正常活动的描述。虽然症状的产生是源于复杂的生物学和行为学现象，但是作为主观经验，对症状的检测仍然仅限于患者自身报告。因为症状只能通过患者主观报告，自然而然的，症状就属于 PRO。相反的，体征或实验室检查结果，如疾病或治疗相关的白细胞计数升高或血红蛋白水平降低，则是客观证据。

近年来 PRO 的应用在逐步增加，原因如下：第一，NIH 在新的测量工具的研发中有很大投入，作为其"路标工程（roadmap program）"的一部分，该测量工具名为"患者报告结果测量信息系统"，目的是加强患者自报量表的测量准确性[1]；第二，FDA 给制药行业发布了患者报告的结果测量：用于医疗产品开发以支持标签声明用来指导如何在申请新药的过程中，使用患者报告评估方法陈述药物有效性[2]；第三，美国国家癌症研究所意识到，其常见不良事件评价标准（CTCAE）标准存在缺陷，所以批准开发包含患者报告结果版本的 CTCAE，名为 PRO-CTCAE[3]。

症状报告是首要的评估疾病和治疗的手段

患者报告结果可以采用多种形式，包括健康状况、患者满意度、症状严重程度及功能影响等。正如前文所提，症状通常被认为是 HRQOL 的子集。HRQOL 是多维度的体系，包含至少 4 个维度：生理功能（如日常活动、自理能力等），心理功能（如感情和精神状态、情绪等），社会角色功能（如社交、家庭关系等），以及疾病和治疗相关症状（如疼痛、恶心等）[4]。常用的 HRQOL 评估手段，包括[健康调查简表（SF-36）[5]、癌症治疗功能评估（FACT）[6]及欧洲癌症治疗研究组织生命质量测定量表（EORTC QLQ-C30）[7]等]检测主要的症状如疼痛、抑郁、疲乏和恶心。在 EORTC QLQ-C30 量表中，30 个项目中有 18 项是自报症状。HRQOL 量表也会问不同维度的患者感知问题，如社会角色功能和社会支持相关问题。在大多数对 HRQOL 的概念解释中，症状被认为是患者报告中对疾病过程和治疗反应与生理心理感知最贴近的指标[8]。

症状测量

症状仅能通过患者告知而获得，关于症状的陈述（如"我背痛得厉害"）是汇报者（患者）和接收者（临床医生或健康服务提供方）共有经验的描述。如果一个人从未经历过疼痛，那也可能很难准确描述疼痛。与身高和体重不同，疼痛、疲乏、悲伤等无法通过量尺或者体重计来直接测量。

症状测量依赖于经历这些症状的患者和需要了解这些症状的人关于症状的交流。因为自报症状都是主观性的，通常都是用"概念"，或者用不可测量的内心感受来描述。而且，我们是通过一系列相关的问题来推导出这些"概念"的，例如，为了了解"疼痛"这一概念，我们会问疼痛的严重程度和疼痛对日常生活的影响。这些概念作为症状的检测依赖于心理测量学，是源于教育领域的，旨在测量智力和教育效果的学科。我们可以问许多相关性更强的问题，而心理测量学的主要目标还是评估自报表的准确性。心理测量学主要的关注点是减少测量的误差，从而为我们想要理解的概念提供最多的信息[9]。两个常用的心理测量学指标是测量工具的可靠性和有效性。

症状测量应该具备的特点

可靠性测量

再次检测可靠性

如果患者在短期内被多次询问到关于他们症状的问题,则每次症状的评估应该类似。大体来看,不同次的同一症状打分如果相关性系数达到 0.7 或以上,则认为这样的评分是可靠的[10],这种可靠性称为"再次检测可靠性"。因为癌症患者症状可能快速变化,在检验这种"再次检测可靠性"的时候,应该选在患者症状和疾病状态相对稳定的时候。

内部一致可靠性

另外一个检测可靠性的指标是内部一致可靠性,或者说是某因素对整体的贡献与该因素测量值的一致性。内部一致可靠性最广泛使用的一个测量方法是 Cronbach alpha[11]。该方法可以被看作是使用两个半数检验得到的所有因素与其他因素相关性的平均值。

有效性检测

内容有效性

自报评估不仅需要稳定或可靠。"有效性"一词有时候被用来广义地描述一个自报评估工具所有的步骤。但是,用心理测量学更加专业的眼光来看,"有效性"指的是评估工具涵盖设计者希望其涵盖内容的比例。如果一种评估工具能够检测需要检测的概念,那么该工具就可以认为是具有实质有效性的。与实质有效性相对的是表面有效性,后者反映使用测量工具的人(健康服务提供者和患者)对该工具的评价,即该工具是否能检测到设计该工具时希望其能检测的内容。长期以来,专家和临床医生一直专注于(测量工具中)指标的选择,但是与教育系统检测标准不同的是,新的有效性标准中整合了患者反映的信息[12]。FDA 指南提出了"通俗标准",即一个 PRO 评估系统对使用它的患者来说需要"通俗易懂",且需要包含需要评估的疾病或治疗相关的症状[2,13]。因此在开发指标的过程中常包含患者采访和评论等过程,该方法称为"质量研究"或"认知采访"。如果一种新的测量工具被开发出来，那通常意味着其包含的指标和量表是有意义的，是可以被患者理解的[14]。如果某项研究使用已经存在的测量工具，认知报告会支持在该研究或试验中使用该工具的合理性。FDA 指南推荐，在药物档案——包括新的免疫治疗药物的档案中，需要包含认知报告研究，作为申请标签的支持材料[2]。

同证效度

同证效度是指使用相似但是独立的检测手段是否能得到与本检测手段类似的结果。通过使用新的检测手段与"金标准"检测方法所得的结果进行对比，从而来判定新方法对感兴趣的指标（症状）的检测效度。然而，在症状检测中，这样的"金标准"非常少。有一些同证效度的研究使用既往已经被验证过的检测手段，或者是 HRQOL 体系中的症状特异性子量表作为参照，如使用 SF-36 的疼痛量表或者是 Profile of Mood States 中的疲乏量表来检测同证效度。

已知组效度

已知组效度是指检测工具分辨可预测结果组别的能力。例如，在检测工具中，体力状态不佳、晚期的癌症患者中，其所检测到的症状负荷应该比良好体力状态、早期癌症患者更大。类似的，接受高强度治疗的患者，其接受治疗后的治疗相关症状（如疲乏），检测结果应该比治疗前更严重。

改变的敏感性

已知组效度为横断面指标，而一项检测手段的敏感性需要通过反复检测不断变化的症状来评估。敏感性通常包含一个时间维度，即在某段时间内检测手段所得到的具有某种趋势的改变。例如，疼痛严重程度评分，在服药前后的对比研究中，在患者接受适当的治疗后，其评分应该相应降低。类似的，接受强化疗的患者，随着治疗的进行，其治疗相关症状应该越来越严重，而症状评估工具需要能准确检测到这样意料之中的改变。

症状检测的实用性特点

理想的症状评估工具除了对变化敏感，并具备可接受的可靠性和有效性之外，还应简单易行，以减轻患者负担。如果该工具是用来多次评估一段时间内的症状改变的，则简洁性就显得尤为重要。症状评估工具同时也需要浅显易懂，最好是五年级的难度，这样即便受教育程度很低的患者也能尽量在没有协助的情况下完成。工具的多种语言版本也很重要，特别是在面向来自不同国家和语言背景患者的时候。最后，测量工具的结果（打分）要直观易懂，这样报告症状的患者和接收症状的医生都能很直观地理解所得结果。

常用的症状评估工具

疼痛评估工具

需要反映：①个体在经受疼痛时具体经历的内容；②在经过设计的治疗后疼痛应该会怎样变化。这些内容一直是 IMMPACT（临床试验中关于方法学、检测手段和疼痛评估的倡议，Initiative on Methods, Measurement and Pain Assessment in Clinical Trials，见 www.impact.org）的重要关注点。关于该工作组的出版物都在其官方网站上，这些资料也是症状相关临床试验工作者的重要资源。IMMPACT 细化了临床疼痛相关试验中的检测内容，如疼痛强度、牵涉痛，以及治疗对其他症状（包括情绪）的影响[15]。在这些工具中，有一个单症状、多因素的工具是简明疼痛评估（brief pain inventory，BPI），可检测上述各维度[16,17]。

其他癌症中常用的疼痛评估工具还有 McGill 疼痛问卷短表（近期有更新）[18]，SF-36 量表和 EORTC QLQ-C30 疼痛量表[7]等。

疲乏评估工具

疲乏是癌症患者最常描述的症状，在晚期癌症和癌症治疗过程中也很常见。关于疲乏，争论的焦点在于如何去准确测量，很多学者认为疲乏应该是多维度的，包含生理、心理甚至是情绪方面的因素。有学者提出，单因素疲乏评估和单症状、多因素疲乏评估均太简单，不能反映疲乏的复杂构成；相反的，想要准确反映疲乏复杂性的问卷常又有太多内容，所需要的时间太长，比短表对患者负担更大。

简易疲乏检测表（brief fatigue inventory，BFI）[19]为单症状、多指标评估手段，由 BPI 改变而来。BFI 可用于临床筛查和临床试验，对疲乏严重程度进行快速评估。根据 BPI 的条目开发出来该量表，并且比较了该量表在癌症住院或门诊患者与社区普通成年人中的心理躯体特点。与 BPI 一样，BFI 通过 3 个指标评估疲乏程度，6 个指标评估疲乏对日常行为能力的影响。开发 BFI 的目的是为了评估疲乏的程度和对日常生活的影响两方面，有几项研究显示，BFI 所包含的所有指标其实是指向同一个维度。该结果与 Lai 等的报道一致，他们在 555 例肿瘤患者中检测了 72 个疲乏指标，最后发现，癌症相关的疲乏其实是一个单维度的问题[20]。

其他单症状、多指标疲乏检测手段包括癌症疲乏量表[21]、疲乏症状检测表[22]、FACT 疲乏[23]、Lee 疲乏量表[24]、多维疲乏检测表[25]、改良 Piper 疲乏量表[26]和 Schwartz 癌症疲乏量表[27]等。

个体症状指标库

患者报告结果测量信息系统（patient-reported outcomes measurement information system，PROMIS）是 NIH 资助的项目，旨在开发更灵活、一致性好的 PRO 测量系统。PROMIS 已经开发出，并且在持续测验不同 PRO 相关指标，以期在临床研究中有效、准确地评估 PRO[1]。PROMIS 正在根据最初的线索，使用项目反应理论（IRT）原理来产生患者自报问题集。

PROMIS 的指标库和所用的 IRT 方法使其成为了 PRO 研发中的一项重大突破，但是仍然有大量的工作要做，来为 PRO 的实用性提供依据，从而使其被医生接受。

不良事件报告的指标库

为了补全 CTCAE（一般不良事件分级），美国 NCI 开发了患者报告结果版本的 CTCAE（PRO-CTCAE）。确认版 PRO-CTCAE 包含 124 个指标，能反映 78 个不良反应症状，每个不良反应都是用一个或者多个属性来描述，特别是有无该症状、频率、程度和（或）对日常生活能力的影响[28]。PRO-CTCAE 包含所有癌症治疗模块中全部的治疗相关症状。其频率、严重程度和对日常生活能力的影响打分均为 0~4 分（频率：0 分，意为从来没有；1 分，少见；2 分，偶尔；3 分，经常；4 分，几乎持续存在；严重程度：0 分，无；1 分，轻度；2 分，中度；3 分，严重；4 分，非常严重；对日常生活能力的影响：0 分，无；1 分，一点点；2 分，一些；3 分，不小；4 分，非常大）。对于症状是否存在的备选答案是：0 无，1 有。所有指标回顾的时间是过去 7 天。开发 PRO-CTCAE 是为了补全 CTCAE，其主要的目的是用来描述和阐明研究所用药物的毒性。PRO-CTCAE 已被一项大型多中心的研究证实是可行的[29]，但是由于这个系统是新开发的，还需要做很多工作来确认不同 PRO-CTCAE 打分的临床含义。

多症状评估工具

免疫疗法会产生一系列症状。一个理想的多症状评估工具应该包括最频繁发生和最令患者痛苦的症状。同时，评估应简短，易于理解。多症状评估工具量表可用于识别各种癌症和治疗中普遍存在和令人痛苦的各种症状。例如，医学博士安德森症量表（MDASI）是一个简单的衡量癌症相关症状严重程度和影响的工具，而不管癌症或治疗类型[30]。MDASI 是在我们之前评估单一症状的严重性和影响的基础上开发的，包括短期疼痛量表和短期疲劳量表[16,19]。MDASI 要求对癌症患者开始治疗后常见的 13 种症状的严重程度进行评分：疲劳、睡眠紊乱、疼痛、困倦、食欲缺乏、恶心、呕吐、呼吸急促、麻木、记忆困难、口干、痛苦和悲伤。患者用 11 点数字评分法（0~10 分），对过去 24 小时内出现的每种症状和最严重的程度进行评分，0 分代表"不存在"，10 分代表"你能想象到的最严重程度"。MDASI 还包含 6 个项目，用于评估在过去 24 小时内症状对患者生活各方面的影响程度：一般活动、情绪、行走能力、正常工作（包括户外工作和家务）、与他人的关系及享受生活。每一项也按 11 点数字评分法，0 分表示"没有影响"，10 分表示"完全影响"。

其他常用的多症状评估工具包括 EORTC QLQ C30[7]、鹿特丹症状量表[31]、症状困扰量表[32]、MSAS[33]、ESAS[34]和症状监测[35]。

患者报告的症状评分的解读，以及确定最小重要差异的方法

一种工具的广泛使用取决于临床医生和研究人员如何使用和解释该工具得出的分数。一旦确定了工具的有效性，下一步就是确定该工具在症状评分的最小临床重要差异（MCID），或最小重要差异（MID）。由于样本量足够大，症状评分的微小差异在统计学上可能是显著的，但对患者和做出治疗决定的医疗保健专业人员几乎没有价值。在与健康相关的生活质量领域确定 MCID 可以促进症状评分更容易理解。可使用两种方法确定 MCID：分布法和校标法[36]。其中一种方法并不优于另一种方法，专家共识[37]一致认为，每种方法并不完善，而是相互互补的，尤其是当它们各自的结果一致时。

分布法

将临床试验中出现的症状评分的变化与评分分布的变异性进行比较，如标准差、效应值或测量的标准误差（SEM）。对于疗效大小，通常使用所有试验患者基线时症状报告的可变性。然而，根据患者样本的异质性，不同的研究对差异的估计可能有所不同。

分步法是将症状评分的 1/2 标准差设置为 MCID 基线[38,39]。科恩效应值是把结果附加到效应的大小上,也有助于症状评分的理解[40]。通过计算 SEM,可以进一步缩小种群异质性的影响,计算方法为基线标准差乘以根号下(1 - 症状评分的可靠性)*;对于任何纵向研究,可以使用内部一致性或重测信度当中的一种方法。Wyrwich 等[41]研究表明,在确定慢性呼吸衰竭问卷和慢性心力衰竭问卷的 MCID 时,1 SEM 标准与效基法密切相关。

效基法

顾名思义,这种方法需要使用一个"锚",它通常是一个问题或一组问题,用于比较患者对与变化逻辑相关变量(如健康状况分级)的变化程度的判断。"锚"可以是针对个体的(单个"锚"),也可以是面向人群的(多个"锚")。这两种方法都要求"锚"本身是可解释的,并且"锚"与症状相关。举例说明单"锚"方法如下,"与您上次的治疗相比,您现在如何评估您的症状?"可能的回答选项是"更好""不变""更糟"。每个值对应的平均症状得分构成一个 MCID。该策略与用于慢性心力衰竭问卷[42]的 MCID 方法一致。对于多"锚"方法,可以通过使用候选变量(如疾病严重程度、疾病进展、治疗反应或治疗中断)来扩展此过程。

使用阈值点来确定治疗有效的患者

将症状分为轻度、中度或重度可能有助于理解临床症状水平的显著变化,并有助于确定临床试验中治疗反应的变化幅度。Serlin 等[43]展示了如何使用多变量方差分析确定的割点,将 0~10 分数学分级评分法(NRS)测量的癌症"最严重疼痛"分为轻度(1~4 分)、中度(5 分、6 分)或重度(7~10 分)。以往的研究表明,与轻度或无疼痛的患者相比,中度至重度疼痛的患者(如:0~10NRS 评分 5 分及以上),疼痛对机体功能的影响明显增加。利用 0~10NRS 疲劳量表将割点的推导方法应用于疲劳分析。一些研究人员在非肿瘤疾病(如糖尿病神经病[44]、下腰痛[45])中也使用这种方法,使用"平均疼痛"而不是"最剧烈疼痛"。割点把症状分为轻度、中度和重度,是临床医生在实践环境中评估患者症状的一种简单方法。

这种割点法也可用于临床试验中比较对治疗反应的患者[46,47]。例如,一个治疗有效者可以定义为"最剧烈疼痛"的患者从服药开始的中度或重度疼痛到干预

---

* 即基线标准差 $\times \sqrt{(1-症状评分的可靠性)}$。

治疗后的无或轻微疼痛。

在不同的肿瘤患者中 PRO 的可行性和实用性

本章讨论 PRO 尤其是本章前面介绍的 MDASI 在评估治疗毒性和治疗期间症状变化中的可行性和额外益处。这些包括接受治疗的肺癌、血液肿瘤和头颈部肿瘤患者。

症状的严重程度可以预测放射性肺炎的发生

在一项 152 例同时接受放化疗的非小细胞肺癌患者的研究中,MDASI 在化疗开始前进行,然后每周 1 次评估直至治疗结束后 6 个月。在控制性别、年龄和辐射剂量或体积的影响后,作者发现,在治疗完成后 6 个月,呼吸短促和咳嗽严重程度的上升与高级放射性肺炎有关[48]。总之,局部晚期非小细胞肺癌的同步放化疗与临床典型的放射性肺炎有关。

症状严重程度和症状对患者的影响可预测晚期肺癌的生存率

在一项研究中,我们跟踪了 94 例晚期非小细胞肺癌患者,我们收集了 MDASI 在第一个化疗周期前后的症状评分结果[49]。我们发现,基线是中度至重度咳嗽(0~10 分,等级≥5 分)的患者,预示着较差的总体生存率。此外,从基线开始到第一个化疗周期结束时,疲劳和呼吸急促的评分增加也预示着较差的总体生存率。在另一组晚期非小细胞肺癌患者中,我们发现,在总体生存率预测中,MDASI 测量的关于患者报告的症状对日常活动的影响,对东部合作肿瘤学组的肿瘤状态和癌症分级增加了预后信息[50]。

造血干细胞移植受者的症状负担

我们在 192 例患者接受造血干细胞移植患者中使用了 MDASI 的血液和骨髓移植模块(如 MDASI-骨髓移植),以评估症状的严重程度和症状对日常活动的干扰程度,收集造血干细胞移植后 20~100 天的 20 个时间点的数据,采用 MDASI-骨髓移植项目对症状严重程度或症状对日常活动的干扰程度的评分,再进行算术平均来计算症状严重程度和症状对日常活动的干扰程度。急性移植物抗宿主病（GVHD）患者的症状严重程度和症状对日常活动的干扰程度高于无 GVHD 患者[51]，最初预计症状会增加，但最终随着时间的推移会减少，这些症状的变化可以用 MDASI -骨髓移植可靠和有效地测量出来。值得注意的是 GVHD 和免疫治疗之间的共性，GVHD 是异基因造血干细胞移植的主要并发症之一[52]，无论是 GVHD 还是免疫治疗，症状都是由免疫反应引起的。

我们还发现，长期收集有关症状的评分是可行的。在一项对慢性髓系白血病患者的研究中，使用交互式语音反应系统，每 2 周评估 1 次 MDASI -慢性髓系白血病症状，为期 1 年，依从性良好：80%的患者至少完成了 50%的评估，51%的患者完成了 80%的评估[53]。

头颈部癌症患者的症状负担

在一项前瞻性研究中[54]，我们研究了头颈部癌症患者在放疗和同步化疗期间报告的症状模式，以便更有效地设计未来的症状干预和临床调查。一个由 149 例患者组成的队列在基于放射治疗的治疗过程中，每周完成 MDASI 的头颈模块。整体症状的严重程度（$P<0.001$）和症状对日常活动的干扰（$P<0.001$）在治疗过程中逐渐加重，同时接受化疗的患者症状更严重（$P<0.001$）。对于同时接受化疗的患者，其疲劳、嗜睡、食欲缺乏、口腔和咽喉黏液及味觉问题更为严重。在治疗结束前的 6~7 周，67%的患者出现了高症状负担。多变量分析显示，患者基线症状评分较低及接受同步化疗与症状增加有关。总之，本研究确定了局部和全身症状的模式，症状对日常活动的干扰程度在时间上是不同的，表现为个体症状等级的增加和变化，以及可识别的症状症候群。

症状 PRO 及免疫治疗

虽然有多个正在进行的单独治疗或与其他形式的治疗相结合的临床试验正在测试免疫治疗的安全性和有效性，但与肿瘤免疫治疗有关的患者报告的症状数据是缺乏的。虽然有少数研究[55,56]报道了 HRQOL 与免疫治疗的关系，但以症状为重点的 PRO 更具相关性，因为它接近于免疫治疗的效果。Bordoni 等最近的一项研究中[57]，确实使用了 EORTC-QLQ-C30，其中包括用 PRO 进行多症状评分。然而，评估的频率可能不利于精确的随访症状的变化。在 Bordoni 等的研究中，每个周期的第 1 天收集 PRO，直至治疗结束，每周的 PRO 评估可能提供有用的数据。如本章所述，PRO 评估不需要在临床访问时进行，但可以通过各种管理模式来完成。这种频繁的评估对临床医生来说是至关重要的，因为它能了解患者对预期肿瘤治疗的耐受能力，并改善以患者为中心的护理[58]。FDA 也关注癌症患者的症状及功能变化，其除了延长癌症患者的生存期外，症状 PRO 在药物开发中扮演的角色更为重要，尤其是对于新的免疫治疗药物。然而，随着时间的推移，对接受免疫治疗患者的症状数据收集的缺乏，阻碍了我们对这些症状变化及其对日常功能的干扰的理解。

在早期临床试验中的 PRO

在 52 个晚期癌症患者参加的真正人类单克隆抗体 MABp1 的 I 期临床试验中，在试验中的三个时间点，患者完成欧洲癌症治疗研究组织生命质量测定量表调查和 PRO 测量[59]，PRO 测量能够捕捉症状随时间的纵向变化，基线和第 8 周的 PRO 评估显示，第 3 周期第 1 天的社交（$P = 0.042$）、情感（$P = 0.032$）和角色功能评分（$P = 0.006$）有显著改善，疲劳（$P = 0.0084$）、疼痛（$P = 0.025$）和食欲下降（$P = 0.020$）也有所改善，患者报告总体生活质量评分显著提高，从 4.8 分提高到 5.4 分（$P = 0.021$）。这些结果表明，在接受单克隆抗体治疗的 I 期临床试验患者中可以观察到 PRO 的变化。

在最近的一项横断面研究中，George 等[60]探索了基于症状严重程度的症状模式和患者群体，并检查了相关因素。研究人员对 248 例患者进行了 I 期临床试验，只有 2 例患者拒绝参与，与未入组的患者相比，I 期临床试验的患者呼吸困难（$P<0.001$）和呕吐（$P<0.029$）更少，但患者组在其他症状方面没有差异。研究人员还评估了入组早期临床试验的晚期肿瘤患者的睡眠质量、症状负担和患者情绪之间的关系。结果显示，大多数患者的睡眠质量较差，而较差的睡眠质量与高的症状负担和症状相关的生活质量干扰极可能相关。

在 I 期临床试验中获得多个基线症状评估和频繁评估的可行性

在 MD Anderson 近期的一项针对癌症患者的研究中[61]，37 例接受免疫治疗的患者在开始治疗前约 2 周每天接受 1 次评估，在第 2 周期结束或疾病进展前 4~6 周每周 2 次评估。患者可以选择用纸、通过交互式语音响应系统或通过基于网络的电子平台进行反馈，大多数患者更喜欢电子回复。15 项潜在的最大基线评估的平均值为 10.2，标准差为 2.8，来自 8 例患者的评分显示，基线评估的中位数为 11，模式为 12，在 22 个潜在的最大治疗评估中，平均值为 11.8，标准偏差为 6.1，中位数为 13 和模式为 15。

PRO 管理模式

随着技术的进步，收集 PRO 数据出现了很多选择。患者的报告可以通过交互式语音响应系统或各种基于网络的数据收集版本来获得。这些选择的一个主要益处是能够收集更频繁和实时的评估，而不需要患者去诊所或医院。此外，缺失的数据最小化，这点在纵向研究中至关重要。

将 PRO 运用到免疫治疗研究中的潜在问题

在免疫治疗研究中使用 PRO 时，实用性、易于管理、患者（评估）负担水平和可解释性等问题是需要考虑的关键因素。免疫疗法在很多情况下都能延长患者的生存时间，但患者伴随生存益处的感受和机体功能尚不清楚。PRO 侧重症状负担的评估，可以提高对免疫治疗效果的理解。许多症状测量方法可以满足各种需求，但需要批判性地思考如何使用它们。我们可以向其他治疗模式的患者问类似的问题，治疗是否会减少目前的症状（如肺癌患者出现呼吸急促）或预防正常情况下预期会发生的症状（如某些癌症治疗引起的神经病变）？这种疗法是否对症状有快速的缓解效果？需要在短时间内反复评估，可能是每天或每周 3 次。或者说，这种疗法会对症状产生逐渐改善的效果，比如与姑息性放疗相关的疼痛减轻？如果对症状的影响是迅速的，重复使用简短和易于管理的症状测量方法可能是最好的选择，而如果症状变化缓慢，则应减少评估的频率，并可能包括额外的症状评估项目。

选择用于免疫治疗评估的症状项目是另一个挑战。包括 MDASI 在内的许多症状测量方法，包含针对疾病或治疗的特定项目，得到了进一步改善。例如，MDASI 的头颈部模块包括吞咽困难和口腔溃疡等项目，以强调影响头颈部的癌症的本质。然而，免疫治疗相关的综合全面的症状评估项目尚未确定，虽然与免疫相关的不良事件为这些症状评估提供了一些依据，但我们还需要通过实质性访谈询问患者本人，这也是一种被监管机构广泛接受的方法。

结论

与更普遍的和健康相关的生活质量相比，我们已经讨论了症状或集体症状负担如何更接近用于对疾病和治疗的效果的评估。在开发甚至使用症状测量方法时，我们需要认识到心理测量学上有效的可取性症状评估工具。我们回顾了现有的症状评估工具，首先只关注疼痛和疲劳，然后强调需要进行多症状评估是因为癌症及其治疗会产生多种症状。我们描述了推导最小重要性的两种主要方法的差异，效基法和分步法，以帮助解释 PRO 数据。

我们已经说明了症状评估的重要性，我们不能再争辩说，我们不能使用患者报告以相对较高的精确度来代表患者的症状，也不能满足标准临床评估和实验室测试所期望的"检测灵敏度"标准。根据患者报告测量的症状状态的变化对临床护理和实施症状控制的临床指南至关重要。质量保证和临床效果研究越来越需要对症状状态进行评估，以反映患者在临床试验或临床中遇到的情况。

最后，我们描述了将 PRO 用于不同癌症的实用性，讨论了 PRO 在免疫治疗中的应用现状，并确定了需要进一步研究的领域，以提高 PRO 在接受免疫治疗的癌症患者中的应用。随着免疫疗法的出现，FDA 等监管机构不仅对延长癌症患者的存活时间越来越感兴趣，而且对这些患者在接受癌症治疗时的感觉和功能也越来越感兴趣。了解患者的感觉，最好是使用 PRO 直接询问他们的症状。许多使用免疫治疗药物的研究已经开始将 PRO 纳入研究设计中。然而，许多研究仍处于起步阶段，许多涉及症状评估的问题尚未解决，如给药频率和所选症状列表是否足以涵盖免疫治疗的已知和未知效果，这些领域给未来的研究提供了一个潜在的丰富的研究空间。

声明

作者无相关利益。

参考文献

1. Patient-Reported Outcomes Measurement Information System. Welcome to PROMIS. Available from: http://www.nihpromis.org. Accessed 26 June 2018.
2. US Food and Drug Administration, Center for Drug Evaluation and Research, Center for Biologics Evaluation and Research, Center for Devices and Radiological Health. Guidance for industry. Patient-reported outcome measures: use in medical product development to support labeling claims. Available from: http://www.fda.gov/downloads/Drugs/GuidanceComplianceRegulatoryInformation/Guidances/UCM071975.pdf. Accessed 26 June 2018.
3. Basch E, Reeve BB, Mitchell SA, Clauser SB, Minasian LM, Dueck AC, et al. Development of the National Cancer Institute's Patient-Reported Outcomes Version of the Common

Terminology Criteria for Adverse Events (PRO-CTCAE). J Natl Cancer Inst. 2014;106(9). pii: dju244.
4. de Haes JC. Quality of life: conceptual and theoretical considerations. In: Watson M, Greer S, Thomas C, editors. Psychosocial oncology. Oxford: Pergamon Press; 1988. p. 61–70.
5. Ware JE Jr, Sherbourne CD. The MOS 36-item short-form health survey (SF-36). I Conceptual framework and item selection. Med Care. 1992;30(6):473–83.
6. Cella DF, Tulsky DS, Gray G, et al. The Functional Assessment of Cancer Therapy Scale: development and validation of the general measure. J Clin Oncol. 1993;11(3):570–9.
7. Aaronson NK, Ahmedzai S, Bergman B, et al. The European Organization for Research and Treatment of Cancer QLQ-C30: a quality-of-life instrument for use in international clinical trials in oncology. J Natl Cancer Inst. 1993;85(5):365–76.
8. Cleeland CS. Symptom burden: multiple symptoms and their impact as patient-reported outcomes. J Natl Cancer Inst Monogr. 2007;(37):16–21.
9. Crocker LM, Algina J. Introduction to classical and modern test theory. Pacific Grove: Wadsworth Publishing; 2006.
10. Litwin MS. How to measure survey reliability and validity, vol. 7: The survey kit. Thousand Oaks: Sage; 1995.
11. Nunnally JC, Bernstein IH. Psychometric theory, vol. 3. New York: McGraw-Hill; 1994. McGraw-Hill Series in Psychology
12. American Educational Research Association, American Psychological Association, National Council on Measurement in Education, Joint Committee on Standards for Educational and Psychological Testing. Standards for educational and psychological testing. 2nd ed. Washington, DC: American Educational Research Association; 1999.
13. Turner RR, Quittner AL, Parasuraman BM, Kallich JD, Cleeland CS. Patient-reported outcomes: instrument development and selection issues. Value Health. 2007;10(s2):S86–93.
14. Willis GB, Reeve BB, Barofsky I, Invited Paper C. The use of cognitive interviewing techniques in quality of life and patient-reported outcomes assessment. In: Lipscomb J, Gotay CC, Snyder C, editors. Outcomes assessment in cancer: measures, methods and applications. Cambridge: Cambridge University Press; 2004. p. 610–22.
15. Dworkin RH, Turk DC, Farrar JT, et al. Core outcome measures for chronic pain clinical trials: IMMPACT recommendations. Pain. 2005;113(1–2):9–19.
16. Cleeland CS, Ryan KM. Pain assessment: global use of the Brief Pain Inventory. Ann Acad Med Singap. 1994;23(2):129–38.
17. Cleeland CS. Measurement of pain by subjective report. In: Chapman CR, Loeser JD, editors. Issues in pain measurement, vol. 12: Advances in pain research and therapy. New York: Raven Press; 1989. p. 391–403.
18. Dworkin RH, Turk DC, Revicki DA, et al. Development and initial validation of an expanded and revised version of the Short-form McGill Pain Questionnaire (SF-MPQ-2). Pain. 2009;144(1–2):35–42.
19. Mendoza TR, Wang XS, Cleeland CS, et al. The rapid assessment of fatigue severity in cancer patients: use of the Brief Fatigue Inventory. Cancer. 1999;85(5):1186–96.
20. Lai JS, Crane PK, Cella D. Factor analysis techniques for assessing sufficient unidimensionality of cancer related fatigue. Qual Life Res. 2006;15(7):1179–90.
21. Okuyama T, Akechi T, Kugaya A, et al. Development and validation of the cancer fatigue scale: a brief, three-dimensional, self-rating scale for assessment of fatigue in cancer patients. J Pain Symptom Manage. 2000;19(1):5–14.
22. Hann DM, Jacobsen PB, Azzarello LM, et al. Measurement of fatigue in cancer patients: development and validation of the Fatigue Symptom Inventory. Qual Life Res. 1998;7(4):301–10.
23. Cella D. The Functional Assessment of Cancer Therapy-Anemia (FACT-An) Scale: a new tool for the assessment of outcomes in cancer anemia and fatigue. Semin Hematol. 1997;34(3 Suppl 2):13–9.
24. Lee KA, Hicks G, Nino-Murcia G. Validity and reliability of a scale to assess fatigue. Psychiatry Res. 1991;36(3):291–8.
25. Smets EM, Garssen B, Bonke B, de Haes JC. The Multidimensional Fatigue Inventory (MFI) psychometric qualities of an instrument to assess fatigue. J Psychosom Res. 1995;

39(3):315–25.
26. Piper BF, Dibble SL, Dodd MJ, Weiss MC, Slaughter RE, Paul SM. The revised Piper Fatigue Scale: psychometric evaluation in women with breast cancer. Oncol Nurs Forum. 1998;25(4):677–84.
27. Schwartz AL. The Schwartz Cancer Fatigue Scale: testing reliability and validity. Oncol Nurs Forum. 1998;25(4):711–7.
28. Dueck AC, Mendoza TR, Mitchell SA, Reeve BB, Castro KM, Rogak LJ, et al. Validity and reliability of the US National Cancer Institute's Patient-Reported Outcomes Version of the Common Terminology Criteria for Adverse Events (PRO-CTCAE). JAMA Oncol. 2015; 1(8):1051–9.
29. Basch E, Pugh SL, Dueck AC, Mitchell SA, Berk L, Fogh S, et al. Feasibility of patient reporting of symptomatic adverse events via the Patient-Reported Outcomes Version of the Common Terminology Criteria for Adverse Events (PRO-CTCAE) in a Chemoradiotherapy Cooperative Group Multicenter Clinical Trial. Int J Radiat Oncol Biol Phys. 2017;98(2):409–18.
30. Cleeland CS, Mendoza TR, Wang XS, et al. Assessing symptom distress in cancer patients: the M.D. Anderson Symptom Inventory. Cancer. 2000;89(7):1634–46.
31. de Haes JC, van Knippenberg FC, Neijt JP. Measuring psychological and physical distress in cancer patients: structure and application of the Rotterdam Symptom Checklist. Br J Cancer. 1990;62(6):1034–8.
32. McCorkle R, Young K. Development of a symptom distress scale. Cancer Nurs. 1978;1(5):373-378.
33. Portenoy RK, Thaler HT, Kornblith AB, et al. The Memorial Symptom Assessment Scale: an instrument for the evaluation of symptom prevalence, characteristics and distress. Eur J Cancer. 1994;30A(9):1326–36.
34. Bruera E, Kuehn N, Miller MJ, Selmser P, Macmillan K. The Edmonton Symptom Assessment System (ESAS): a simple method for the assessment of palliative care patients. J Palliat Care. 1991;7(2):6–9.
35. Hoekstra J, Bindels PJ, van Duijn NP, Schadé E. The symptom monitor. A diary for monitoring physical symptoms for cancer patients in palliative care: feasibility, reliability and compliance. J Pain Symptom Manage. 2004;27(1):24–35.
36. Revicki D, Hays RD, Cella D, Sloan J. Recommended methods for determining responsiveness and minimally important differences for patient-reported outcomes. J Clin Epidemiol. 2008;61(2):102–9.
37. Guyatt GH, Osoba D, Wu AW, Wyrwich KW, Norman GR. Methods to explain the clinical significance of health status measures. Mayo Clin Proc. 2002;77(4):371–83.
38. Norman GR, Sloan JA, Wyrwich KW. Interpretation of changes in health-related quality of life: the remarkable universality of half a standard deviation. Med Care. 2003;41(5):582–92.
39. Sloan JA, Dueck A. Issues for statisticians in conducting analyses and translating results for quality of life end points in clinical trials. J Biopharm Stat. 2004;14(1):73–96.
40. Cohen J. Statistical power analysis for the behavioral sciences. 2nd ed. Hillsdale: Lawrence Earlbaum; 1988.
41. Wyrwich KW, Tierney WM, Wolinsky FD. Further evidence supporting an SEM-based criterion for identifying meaningful intra-individual changes in health-related quality of life. J Clin Epidemiol. 1999;52(9):861–73.
42. Guyatt G, Walter S, Norman G. Measuring change over time: assessing the usefulness of evaluative instruments. J Chronic Dis. 1987;40(2):171–8.
43. Serlin RC, Mendoza TR, Nakamura Y, Edwards KR, Cleeland CS. When is cancer pain mild, moderate or severe? Grading pain severity by its interference with function. Pain. 1995;61(2):277–84.
44. Zelman DC, Gore M, Dukes E, Tai KS, Brandenburg N. Validation of a modified version of the brief pain inventory for painful diabetic peripheral neuropathy. J Pain Symptom Manag. 2005;29(4):401–10.
45. Keller S, Bann CM, Dodd SL, Schein J, Mendoza TR, Cleeland CS. Validity of the brief pain inventory for use in documenting the outcomes of patients with noncancer pain. Clin J Pain. 2004;20(5):309–18.

46. Cleeland CS, Portenoy RK, Rue M, et al. Does an oral analgesic protocol improve pain control for patients with cancer? An intergroup study coordinated by the Eastern Cooperative Oncology Group. Ann Oncol. 2005;16(6):972–80.
47. Wong GY, Schroeder DR, Carns PE, et al. Effect of neurolytic celiac plexus block on pain relief, quality of life, and survival in patients with unresectable pancreatic cancer: a randomized controlled trial. JAMA. 2004;291(9):1092–9.
48. Wang XS, Shi Q, Yue J, Chen TY, Xu T, Komaki R, et al. Predictive value of patient-reported outcomes on radiation pneumonitis related normal lung uptake of FDG on PET in patients with non-small cell lung cancer treated with concurrent chemoradiation [abstract 3015]. International Society for Quality of Life Research 23rd annual conference; Copenhagen, Denmark; Oct 19-22, 2016. Qual Life Res. 2016;25(Suppl 1):157–8.
49. Wang XS, Shi Q, Lu C, Basch EM, Johnson VE, Mendoza TR, et al. Prognostic value of symptom burden for overall survival in patients receiving chemotherapy for advanced nonsmall cell lung cancer. Cancer. 2010;116(1):137–45.
50. Barney BJ, Wang XS, Lu C, Liao Z, Johnson VE, Cleeland CS, et al. Prognostic value of patient-reported symptom interference in patients with late-stage lung cancer. Qual Life Res. 2013;22(8):2143–50. PMCID: PMC3724766.
51. Williams LA, Giralt SA, Wang XS, Mobley GM, Mendoza TR, Cohen MZ, et al., editors. Measuring the symptom burden of allogeneic hematopoietic stem cell transplantation in patients with and without acute graft-versus-host disease [abstract 49]. Biol Blood Marrow Transplant. 2009;15(Suppl 2):20–1.
52. Stewart BL, Storer B, Storek J, Deeg HJ, Storb R, Hansen JA, et al. Duration of immunosuppressive treatment for chronic graft-versus-host disease. Blood. 2004;104(12):3501–6.
53. Williams LA, Garcia Gonzalez AG, Ault P, Mendoza TR, Sailors ML, Williams JL, Huang F, Nazha A, Kantarjian HM, Cleeland CS, Cortes JE. Measuring the symptom burden associated with the treatment of chronic myeloid leukemia. Blood. 2013;122(5):641–7.
54. Rosenthal DI, Mendoza TR, Fuller CD, Hutcheson KA, Wang XS, Hanna EY, et al. Patterns of symptom burden during radiotherapy or concurrent chemoradiotherapy for head and neck cancer: a prospective analysis using The University of Texas MD Anderson Cancer Center Symptom Inventory-Head and Neck Module. Cancer. 2014;120(13):1975–84.
55. Long GV, Atkinson V, Ascierto PA, Robert C, Hassel JC, Rutkowski P, et al. Effect of nivolumab on health-related quality of life in patients with treatment-naive advanced melanoma: results from the phase III CheckMate 066 study. Ann Oncol. 2016;27:1940–6.
56. Schadendorf D, Dummer R, Hauschild A, Robert C, Hamid O, Daud A, et al. Health-related quality of life in the randomised KEYNOTE-002 study of pembrolizumab versus chemotherapy in patients with ipilimumab-refractory melanoma. Eur J Cancer. 2016;67:46–54.
57. Bordoni R, Ciardiello F, von Pawel J, Cortinovis D, Karagiannis T, Ballinger M, Sandler A, Yu W, He P, Matheny C, Felizzi F, Rittmeyer A. Patient-reported outcomes in OAK: a phase III study of Atezolizumab versus Docetaxel in advanced non-small-cell lung cancer. Clin Lung Cancer. 2018. pii: S1525-7304(18)30131-1. https://doi.org/10.1016/j.cllc.2018.05.011.
58. Basch E, Iasonos A, McDonough T, Barz A, Culkin A, Kris MG, et al. Patient versus clinician symptom reporting using the National Cancer Institute common terminology criteria for adverse events: results of a questionnaire-based study. Lancet Oncol. 2006;7:903–9.
59. Hong DS, Hui D, Bruera E, Janku F, Naing A, Falchook GS, Piha-Paul S, Wheler JJ, Fu SQ, Tsimberidou AM, Stecher M, Mohanty P, Simard J, Kurzrock R. MABp1, a first-in-class true human antibody targeting interleukin-1 alpha in refractory cancers: an open-label, phase 1 dose-escalation and expansion study. Lancet Oncol. 2014;15:656–66.
60. George GC, Iwuanyanwu EC, Anderson KO, Yusuf A, Zinner RG, Piha-Paul SA, et al. Sleep quality and its association with fatigue, symptom burden, and mood in patients with advanced cancer in a clinic for early-phase oncology clinical trials. Cancer. 2016;122:3401–9.
61. Mendoza TR, George G, Williams L, Shi Q, Naing A, Hong DS, et al, editors. Feasibility and added value of multiple baseline symptom assessments in early-phase clinical trials [abstract]. Presented at the International Society for Quality of Life Research (ISOQOL) 24th annual conference, Philadelphia; 2017.